Perspectives
in Neuropharmacology

A TRIBUTE TO JULIUS AXELROD

EDITED BY
SOLOMON H. SNYDER
Departments of Pharmacology and
Experimental Therapeutics and Psychiatry
The Johns Hopkins University School of Medicine

New York
OXFORD UNIVERSITY PRESS
London   1972   Toronto

Contributors

Jacques de Champlain
Centre de Recherches en Sciences
   Neurologiques
Faculté de Medecine
Université de Montréal

Arnold Joel Eisenfeld
Departments of Pharmacology
   and Internal Medicine
Yale University School of Medicine

John D. Fernstrom
Department of Nutrition and
   Food Sciences
Massachusetts Institute of Technology

Jacques Glowinski
Groupe Neuropharmacologie
   Biochimique
Collège de France

Georg Hertting
Institute of Pharmacology
University of Vienna

Leslie L. Iversen
Department of Pharmacology
University of Cambridge

Seymour S. Kety
Department of Psychiatry
Harvard Medical School

Irwin J. Kopin
Laboratory of Clinical Science
National Institute of Mental Health

Perry B. Molinoff
Department of Pharmacology
University of Colorado
   School of Medicine

Lincoln T. Potter
Department of Biophysics
University College London
After September 1972:
Department of Pharmacology
University of Miami School of Medicine

Sune Rosell
Department of Pharmacology
Karolinska Institutet

Solomon H. Snyder
Departments of Pharmacology and
   Experimental Therapeutics
   and Psychiatry
The Johns Hopkins University
   School of Medicine

Josef Suko
Institute of Pharmacology
University of Vienna

Kenneth M. Taylor
Department of Pharmacology
University of Otago
Dunedin, New Zealand

Hans Thoenen
Department of Pharmacology
Biocenter of the University of Basel

Richard J. Wurtman
Department of Nutrition and
   Food Science
Massachusetts Institute of Technology

Acknowledgments

A special note of gratitude is due to Hoffman-LaRoche, Inc. for a very generous contribution that helped bring the authors together in a conference that led to this book. For their assistance in this same effort we would also like to thank Eli Lilly and Company, Geigy Pharmaceuticals, McNeil Laboratories, Inc., the Merck Institute for Therapeutic Research, the New England Nuclear Corporation, E. R. Squibb and Sons, Inc., Sterling Drug Incorporated, Schering Corporation and the Bayer A. G. Company. We are particularly grateful to Dr. William Manger for enabling some of this work to be presented at the Catecholamine Club meeting in Chicago in 1971.

Chapter 2   The work reported in this chapter was supported by a grant from the British Medical Research Council.

Chapter 3   This research was supported by USPHS grants NS-07275, MH-18501, GM-16492, and NIMH Research Scientist Development Award K3-MH-33128 to SHS. The authors would like to thank Birgitta Brown for her inspired and devoted technical assistance. Some of these studies were conducted in collaboration with Michael J. Kuhar, Anne B. Young, Candace D. Pert, David G. Brown, and Eduard Gfeller.

Chapter 5   Original Research reported in this chapter was supported by Grants HD-02498 and CA 10748 and Contract NIH 70-2258.

Chapter 6   Studies performed in our laboratory were supported by grants from the United States Public Health Service (AM-11709 and AM-14228), the National Aeronautics and Space Administration (NGR-22-009-272), and the John A. Hartford Foundation.

Chapter 7   The work presented here has been supported by grants from the Swedish Medical Research Council (Grant No. B71-40X-731-06), Svenska Lakaresallskapet and Karolinska Institutet.

Chapter 8   This work was partly supported by grants to the Medical Research Council group in Neurological Sciences and by grants of the Quebec Heart Foundation.

The author wishes to acknowledge the stimulating collaboration with Dr. Julius Axelrod in the studies carried out on experimental hypertension. Without his advice, enthusiasm and encouragement these studies would not have been possible. The friendly and fruitful collaboration with Dr. Lawrence R. Krakoff and Dr. Robert A. Mueller has also been essential in pursuing these studies. The skillful technical help of Miss Marie-Reine Corbeil B.Sc. and Miss Solange Imbault, in more recent studies, is gratefully acknowledged. The author also wishes to express his gratitude to Miss Danielle Beauliey for her efficient secretarial assistance in the preparation of the manuscript.

Figures 2, 3, 4, 6, 7, 9, 12, 13, 14 have been reproduced from previously published work with kind permission of *Circulation Research*. Figures 10 and 15 have been reproduced from previously published studies in *L-DOPA and Parkinsonism*, 1970, with the kind permission of the F. A. Davis Co. (Philadelphia).

Chapter 11   This contribution was written in the author's private capacity. No official support nor endorsement by the U. S. Public Health Service is intended nor should be inferred.

Chapter 12   The author is very grateful to Mrs. M. H. Lévi and E. Monsonégo for their excellent assistance in the preparation of the manuscript.

The various investigations reported were supported in part by grants of the I.N.S.E.R.N., C.N.R.S., D.R.M.E., D.G.R.S.T., Fondation de la recherche médicale, Société des usines chimiques Rhône-Poulence, and N.I.M.H. (U.S.A.).

Contents

Perspectives in Neuropharmacology

1

Julius Axelrod: A Triumph for Creative Research

SEYMOUR S. KETY

Scientists, like journalists, are sometimes "scooped" by their colleagues, and it is not unusual, especially among those who work in the field of the catecholamines, to learn that one's very exciting finding has been anticipated by a group in Goteborg or Stockholm. We didn't realize, however, until quite recently, into what high circles in Sweden that tendency had penetrated.

More than a year ago, in January 1970, several former fellows of Julius Axelrod—Sol Snyder, Jacques Glowinski, Leslie Iversen, Hans Thoenen, and Linc Potter—met at a neurotransmitter conference in Paris, and decided to honor their mentor by arranging a grand reunion of all the fellows and associates with whom Axelrod had shared his genius, to be followed by the publication of a *Festschrift*. There was not the usual occasion for this since Julie was not about to reach some convenient chronological milestone and hadn't the remotest idea of retiring. It was simply a spontaneous expression of their affection and admiration for him and a recognition of his contributions to science. I was given the privilege of writing this introduction to the *Festschrift*—the only contribution which was to be personal.

It was decided to wait until the Federation meeting of 1971 and—the rest is history. On October 15, 1970, while he was sitting in a dentist's chair with his mouth full of cotton sponges, Julie learned that the Committee in Stockholm had awarded the Nobel Prize in Physiology and Medicine jointly to him, von Euler, and Katz. (It is rumored that there has been a sharp rise in the number of scientists coming for dental checkups since that time.)

Sol Snyder wrote me that day, exultant, but also concerned about how that affected the plans for the *Festschrift*. It was soon agreed, however, that the plans for this tribute were not to be altered, since the action of the Nobel Committee simply confirmed the conviction that we were on the right track!

It is clearly difficult to avoid the "halo" effect (that term has never seemed more appropriate) and to speak of Julie as we would have done last April. Yet the feelings we want to express are those which have been shared for a long time by all who were associated with him. His scientific contributions gained him international recognition but it is his human qualities which have so endeared him to his colleagues.

It is not necessary to do more than briefly summarize Axelrod's scientific contributions. A major segment of neuropharmacology and experimental psychiatry depends upon his elucidation of the biochemical and physiological processes involved in the storage, release, and inactivation of norepinephrine at the adrenergic synapse, which has made possible an understanding of the role of that amine in neurotransmission and a clarification of the mechanism of action of numerous drugs and hormones that affect adrenergic activity peripherally and centrally.

In 1957 he described the O-methylation pathway in the metabolism of catecholamines, and shortly thereafter demonstrated its importance in the inactivation of epinephrine in animals and man, characterizing the enzyme involved and its distribution in the mammalian organism. Within a few years and based largely upon his work, knowledge of the metabolism of catecholamines advanced from almost total ignorance to characterization of their major and minor pathways and metabolites. With Glowinski and Kopin he extended this knowledge to the metabolism of catecholamines in the brain.

His studies, with Whitby and Hertting, of the effects of psychotropic drugs on the uptake of ^{3}H-norepinephrine by sympathetically innervated tissues led to his recognition of the most important mechanism for the inactivation of norepinephrine at the adrenergic synapse and initiated a major area of current research activity on the anatomical, physiological, and pharmacological aspects of this process.

With Wurtman and Snyder he adduced evidence for the regulation of biogenic amine synthesis under environmental variations throughout the body but especially in the pineal gland, an organ resurrected by Wurtman and himself from historic neglect. Steroid hormones of the adrenal cortex were shown to regulate epinephrine formation in the adrenal gland. More recently, with Mueller and Thoenen, he has demonstrated what appears to be an induction of tyrosine hydroxylase following increased sympathetic activity. And currently, together with Weinshilbaum, Molinoff, and Coyle, he has explored the regulation of dopamine hydroxylase and its "exocytic" release by nerve impulses.

His scientific talents are so unusual that one senses them early in one's association with him. Ten years ago they impressed me in this way: "In all of his contributions success has been much less attributable to good fortune and much more to a unique ability to develop imaginative new concepts, to select and perform crucial experiments and to stimulate the activity and productivity of others in the field." These are some of the qualities which contribute to Axelrod's creativeness, but there are many more.

Sol Snyder describes the experience of many of the research associates who have come under his influence: "Perhaps the greatest lesson Julie taught was that science is fun and exciting . . . I was struck by his intense involvement in experiments he was doing. He would lean over the scintillation counter urging it on to higher and higher counts with impatient 'body English' (a trait I inherited, and a tradition that the new computerized machines sadly have laid to rest) . . . What was quite evident then . . . was his scientific vision. He saw (and still perceives) the farthest reaching implications of apparently trivial data. And he would put forth important ideas in such deceptively simple ways that, at first glance, they seemed incredibly naive."

The excitement which Julie derived from his experiments and his ability to read what apparently mundane results were saying are certainly two of his outstanding characteristics as a scientist, and they have played a crucial role in his most important discoveries. When he saw the abstract by Armstrong and McMillan in the Federation Proceedings reporting the presence of 3-methoxy-4-hydroxymandelic acid in the urine of patients with pheochromocytoma, he immediately recognized the importance of the possible direct O-methylation of catechols and carried out his first experiment that very afternoon. Incubating epinephrine with the soluble supernatant fraction of liver, ATP, and methionine, he saw the catecholamine disappear—"right before my eyes"—to be replaced by a new compound which appeared to be the methylated derivative. He communicated his excitement to Witkop, who with Senoh synthesized the authentic O-methyl-epinephrine in short order, providing Axelrod with a means of proving the identity of his new metabolite.

Another flash of insight led to the discovery of the reuptake mechanism as the major means by which the synaptic action of catecholamines is terminated. When he, Weil-Malherbe, and Tomchick examined the fate of tritiated epinephrine and, a little later, with Whitby, the disposition of norepinephrine, they found high concentrations of the labelled amines in certain tissues. I remember Julie excitedly telling me that the labelled catecholamines were concentrated in the tissues with the richest sympathetic innervation, convinced even then that they were taken up by the sympathetic nerve endings. Within a year Hertting and he had the evidence to permit their conclusion that reuptake of norepinephrine at sympathetic nerve endings occurred.

Perhaps the most remarkable thing about Julie is his ability to maintain an indomitable scientific conviction without losing his humility and warmth in human relationships. One of his associates wrote about him thus: "I would like to try to describe the personality of Julie from the point of view of a younger European scientist who has worked (and suffered) in the atmosphere of the 'Herr Professor and Geheimrat.' What a tremendous contrast to Julie's lab!" Hans Thoenen describes his human side in a way which needs no embellishing: "Besides his extraordinary scientific qualities Julie showed the ability to create a highly stimulating but at the same time pleasant atmosphere in his laboratory, determined by his kindness, tolerance, and great modesty. It certainly would be possible to find people with either the scientific or the human qualities of Julie, but the combination of both is unique in him."

There are some special meanings for many of us in Julie's achievements and the world-wide recognition they have so eminently deserved. He returned from Stockholm last December by way of Israel, where he received a hero's welcome. He gave strength and confidence to the Research Institutes in Bethesda and to the philosophy they have represented. He reinforced the viability of pharmacology as a challenging and intellectually satisfying discipline. But what he has done at an especially crucial time has been to exemplify the importance and the productivity of research which is undirected and untargetted, except by scientific insight.

Our society is now laboring under a well-meaning but nevertheless false assumption that the great needs we have belatedly recognized in the provision and distribution of physical and mental health care must necessarily compete with research and the acquisition of new knowledge. Arbitrary ceilings have thus been put on research funds and the training of new investigators. Moreover, like the goose that laid the golden eggs, even this commitment to research is being tampered with and operated on in the erroneous belief that by channeling them we can somehow accelerate the processes of creativity and scientific discovery. Axelrod is an emphatic refutation of that notion.

When I became chief of the Laboratory of Clinical Science in 1956, I felt that it would be worthwhile to test the hypothesis which was then current, that abnormal metabolites of epinephrine circulation in the blood were the cause of schizophrenia. If one could use a small dose of epinephrine with very high specific radioactivity, then, with the help of chromatography and the new liquid scintillation counters which were becoming available, one might hope to characterize some of the normal and abnormal metabolites. It wasn't a bad plan as targetted research goes, and I pursued it in the modest way it deserved so as not to disturb the ecology of the laboratory. Seymour Rothschild agreed to attempt the synthesis of tritium-labelled epinephrine of the required activity. In the year it took before the first successful batch arrived, Axelrod (who was not part of the plan) had discovered the O-methylation pathway and characterized the various metabolites of epinephrine. As a minor spin-off of his work, the search for abnormal metabolites of epinephrine in schizophrenia was greatly facilitated, but—much more important—his contributions have had implications for psychiatry which were simply undreamed of in 1956.

It is quite fortunate that there were no administrative or legislative directives to put the funds of the Laboratory into mission-oriented research at the expense of the individual creativity of its scientists, no cost-benefit analyses prematurely and inappropriately applied, no requirement to answer for duplication of effort.

Axelrod has courageously voiced his concerns regarding the dangers of constricting the funds, restricting the training of new investigators, and channeling research support into illusory hierarchies of relevance. We hope his advice is heeded, for no one knows better than he the ingredients of scientific discovery.

2

Isolation of Cholinergic Receptor Proteins

L. T. POTTER
P. B. MOLINOFF

Introduction

Scope and Definitions

Nerve cells have the ability to transmit information rapidly and precisely from one or a few cells to a limited number of other cells which are often far away. The mechanism developed for carrying impulses along nerve axons is electrical in nature and highly efficient for maintaining an unaltered message in hair-thin axons (Hodgkin, 1964). At almost all synapses in the central and peripheral nervous systems, each nerve terminal passes on a chemical messenger, or neurotransmitter, to special receptors on the next cell. Chemical transmission permits a marked amplification of the weak electrical signal in axons, and allows the nature of the message to be varied by changing the transmitter and/or the type of receptor. In addition, since the duration of action of neurotransmitters exceeds the duration of a nerve impulse, chemical transmission facilitates summation of the effects of many impulses.

Even before the first conclusive demonstration of a neurotransmitter (acetylcholine, ACh: Loewi, 1921), it was beginning to become apparent (Langley, 1906; cf. Dale, 1953) that chemical synaptic transmission requires a number of special adaptations: (a) synthesis of the transmitter; (b) a mechanism for coupling the arrival of impulses at a nerve terminal with rapid secretion of the transmitter (Katz, 1969); (c) a receptor for the transmitter on or in the postsynaptic cell; (d) a means of coupling an activated receptor to the required response; and (e) provision for removal of

9

the transmitter. This chapter is concerned with the chemical nature of receptors.

Receptors have always been defined operationally in terms of the cellular responses which they initiate. This fact has contributed to a widespread feeling that receptors may be part of macromolecular complexes in postsynaptic membranes which are too complicated, insoluble, and/or aggregated (as well as too scarce) to study biochemically (cf. discussions Ciba Symposium, 1970). For the purpose of discussing receptor isolation, receptors will be defined narrowly as the molecules in the above sequence which have the sites required for receiving the neurotransmitters involved; any associated molecules which are required for initiating cellular responses are considered to be part of the subsequent coupling mechanism. The isolated protein described in this chapter is one such receptor: it clearly reacts with ACh and several antagonists in solution, and it has been studied by the usual procedures for working with soluble proteins.

Given that receptors can be isolated, it becomes important to know how they are coupled to cell responses. In general, receptors are coupled to a mechanism for generating a change in the permeability or conductance of the postsynaptic membrane and this change serves to excite or inhibit action potentials in the remainder of the cell membrane. These action potentials become nerve impulses, or initiate muscle contraction or gland secretion, according to the cell involved. In a few tissues (e.g. the electric tissue of *Torpedo:* Bennett, 1961) the cells are heavily innervated and fully depolarized by synaptic potentials, and the action potential mechanism is absent. It is possible that receptors can in themselves cause the initial changes in ion fluxes. But the fact that there are electrically excitable "ionophores"* at a distance from receptors—those which subserve action potentials—suggests that there may also be distinct ionophores which are chemically excited via receptors. In some cases receptors may be coupled solely to a metabolic response, but even the responses mediated through adenyl cyclase (Robison, Butcher, and Sutherland, 1970) appear to be

---

* For convenience, the term "ionophore" will be used for any molecule or macromolecular complex which serves as an ion-selective carrier, channel, or pore. It is generally assumed that the conductance mechanism of synaptic potentials is metabolically independent, because the rate and direction of ion fluxes depend upon the electrochemical gradients present (Fatt and Katz, 1951; Takeuchi and Takeuchi, 1960), but even these fluxes may, or may sometimes, be metabolically dependent (Kehoe and Ascher, 1970).

coupled via an ionophore (Rasmussen, 1970). This subject is discussed further later.

Receptor Properties in situ

Our knowledge of receptors has been derived from a variety of sources. Their *specificity* for a particular transmitter has been established largely through bath applications of a wide range of transmitter analogues to isolated tissues (Paton, 1970). These pharmacological studies have established that a given receptor responds rapidly and efficiently only to one transmitter and its close structural analogues (agonists). A variety of receptor antagonists has been obtained from natural sources or has been synthesized. Their use has demonstrated that receptors exist which are able to distinguish not only between different excitatory and inhibitory transmitters but also between different isomeric forms of one transmitter.

The *location* of receptors has been established most clearly by the application of ACh focally through micropipettes onto different parts of striated muscle cells. Responsiveness in innervated muscles is very sharply localized at neuromuscular endplates (Thesleff, 1970), although some muscles are also sensitive near their tendons (Katz and Miledi, 1964). With denervation, sensitivity (Miledi, 1962) and the number of receptors (Miledi and Potter, 1971) increase over the whole cell. The distribution of receptors in innervated and denervated muscles has been confirmed by the use of radioactively labelled antagonists which bind to the receptors (Waser, 1970; Lee, Tseng, and Chiu, 1967; Miledi and Potter, 1971), and the results to date imply that receptors are not present (but uncoupled to cell responses) where ACh responsiveness is absent. A focal distribution of sensitivity has also been observed at nerve-nerve synapses (Harris, Kuffler, and Dennis, 1971) where the morphological appearance of a close synaptic junction is similar to that at endplates. Receptors are probably more widely distributed where ganglionic nerves diffusely innervate smooth and cardiac muscle, and glands. Muscle cells respond only to ACh applied externally (del Castillo and Katz, 1955), indicating that their receptors are associated with the cell membrane and face outwards. That ACh receptors are membrane-bound has been further demonstrated by showing ACh-linked permeability changes to sodium ions in isolated microsacs of postsynaptic membranes (Kasai and Changeux, 1970). At present it seems reasonable to assume that all neuroreceptors are membrane-bound, since all known and suspected neurotransmitters are ions which do not readily diffuse through lipid membranes, and since cell responses to them are very rapid. Even in those cases where transmitters are known to cause predominantly metabolic effects, the common metabolic pathway includes the membrane-bound enzyme, adenyl cyclase (Robison et al., 1970). The *number* as well as the location of receptor molecules on a cell membrane has long been assumed to parallel the sensitivity of a cell to its neurotransmitter, although it has also been clear that maximal responses of a cell can be produced even when most of its receptors are blocked by an irreversible antagonist (Paton, 1970). Direct evidence of the number and location of receptor molecules on several cells has been obtained by affinity labelling techniques. Not only are receptors on striated muscles localized at normal endplates where sensitivity is maximal (Waser, 1970; Lee et al., 1967; Miledi and Potter, 1971) but the number increases outside the endplate region in denervated muscles (Lee et al., 1967) with the same time course as the increase in sensitivity (Miledi and Potter, 1971). The number of receptor molecules per endplate (about 16, 47, and 1000 million for mouse, rat, and frog muscles, respectively: Miledi and Potter, 1971) is much larger than the number of molecules of ACh released by a nerve impulse (about 3 million in the rat diaphragm: Potter, 1970), and the muscle cells can be excited when 90 per cent of the receptors are irreversibly blocked. Both findings support the concept that there are many "spare receptors" at endplates. The fact that the number of receptors changes with alterations in muscle firing (Lømo and Rosenthal, 1971) suggests that long-term alterations in synaptic efficiency may derive in large part from changes in the number and/or density of receptors. At a higher level of organization such changes could subserve learning. The *chemical composition* of receptor molecules, which have a specificity comparable to that of enzymes, has long been believed to be protein (or lipoprotein) in nature. The fact that ACh receptors in electroplaques are blocked by reagents which reduce S-S bonds to SH groups, and that responsiveness is restored by the use of oxidizing agents which reverse this step, provided the first firm and direct evidence that these receptors are proteins (Karlin, Prives, Deal, and Winnik, 1970). The damaging effects of some proteases (Lu, 1957; Eldefrawi, Eldefrawi, and O'Brien, 1971) and the binding of ACh to lipoproteins (De Robertis, Lunt, and La Torre, 1971) and proteins (Changeux, Kasai, Huchet, and Meunier, 1970; Eldefrawi et al., 1971) extracted from electric tissue supported this conclusion.

The results described in this chapter confirm that ACh receptors are specific membrane proteins. Some evidence indicates that the *conformation* of receptors is altered by their reaction with a neurotransmitter. In particular, an alkylating derivative of decamethonium combines more rapidly with the receptors of muscles in the presence of ACh analogues than in their absence, suggesting that this blocking agent combines with and stabilizes an altered or reacted form of the molecule (Rang and Ritter, 1969, 1970a, 1970b). The reverse is true of α-bungarotoxin, which binds more slowly in muscles desensitized with ACh, indicating that it stabilizes a resting state of these ACh receptors (Miledi and Potter, 1971).

Recognition of Isolated Receptors

In intact tissues, receptors are defined operationally in terms of the cellular response which is initiated by the interaction between the appropriate neurotransmitter and the receptor. Once the tissue has been disrupted this response is no longer present, and other means of measuring the presence of receptors are required. Several means of recognizing receptors have been considered.

Reconstitution

The most direct means of receptor recognition would be to reincorporate the isolated substance back into a membrane under conditions where its original coupling with an ionophore or other molecule could be established. Reconstitution of an organized membrane macromolecule has been claimed to work with serotonin receptors (Wooley and Gommi, 1966) and with the sodium-potassium pump (Jaim, Strickholm, and Cordes, 1969). Since there are more convenient means for assaying receptors in solution, this method is unlikely to see use during attempts at receptor purification. The technique will probably be essential, however, for demonstrating that all the components of the receptor-ionophore mechanism are known, and it may prove useful for identifying the oligomeric form or forms which functional receptors may take in a membrane. We are attempting to reincorporate the protein units described in this chapter into lipid vesicles (Johnson and Bangham, 1969) made from other constituents of electric tissue membranes so as to study the receptor structure which reforms. The potential artifacts in such systems must, however, be considered; on one hand it is possible that the components of a complete receptor-ionophore system may be impossible to re-incorporate in their original functional state, and on the other, it is known that a protein which is not a receptor, acetylcholinesterase (AChE), can be introduced into black membranes in a form which causes depolarization of the membrane in the presence of ACh (del Castillo, Rodriguez, and Romero, 1967).

Conformational Studies

It is likely that receptors undergo conformational changes on interacting with appropriate agonists. It should be possible to observe these changes experimentally and to utilize them for an *in vitro* assay of receptor activity. There are several possible means for recognizing such changes, including measurements of optical absorbance (De Robertis, González-Rodríguez, and Teller, 1969), electron spin resonance, and nuclear magnetic resonance. The most promising technique would appear to be the use of "fluorescent probes," substances which bind to proteins and whose fluoresence changes when there is an alteration in the configuration of the protein (Stryer, 1970). Attempts have been made to use two such agents to demonstrate receptors in isolated membrane fragments of electric tissue: in one case agonists and antagonists had no effect on fluorescence intensity or polarization, and in the other, effects were observed but occurred also with noninnervated membranes (Changeux, Blumenthal, Kasai, and Podleski, 1970). More success is to be anticipated with preparations of soluble receptors, particularly purified preparations which do not contain other postsynaptic membrane proteins which are known to react with the transmitters involved, for example, AChE and choline carriers (cf. Potter, 1970), which both have specific sites for cholinomimetic compounds. There is reason to believe that considerable information concerning the active site of receptors may eventually be obtained by this approach.

Antibodies

In theory, a receptor antibody should have the ideal characteristics of specificity and irreversibility for labelling receptors. At least one attempt to make such antibodies, to membrane proteins from denervated rat muscles (Miledi and Potter, unpublished), was unsuccessful, possibly because any antibodies which formed reacted with receptors in the host rabbit. While one can foresee some interesting experiments in destroying a given kind of receptor in living animals by giving the receptor, further attempts to make antibodies to receptors should probably make use of receptors whose active sites have been chemically altered, or occluded with an alkylating agent. As an absolutely specific means for localizing receptors *in situ* (excepting those which react with α-bungarotoxin or similar compounds which have antibody-like specificity and tenacity already), it is difficult to imagine a better approach.

Reversible Agonists and Antagonists

Many attempts have been made to use the specificity of receptor interactions with reversible agonists and antagonists to count, localize, and/or isolate receptors. In almost every case the drug used has been made radioactive. The following conclusions may be drawn from these studies.

Because of the reversibility of specific interactions between receptors and drugs in aqueous solutions, it is generally necessary to measure either the clearance of the agent from the solution in contact with the receptors, or the amount of bound agent, without washing out unbound material. In order to reduce binding by ion exchange it is usually necessary, as well, to work with iso-ionic media. Where attempts have been made to study the amount of a drug which remains bound to washed tissues, membranes, or protein precipitates (Chagas, Penna-Franca, Nishie, and Garcia, 1958; Ehrenpreis, Fleisch, and Mittag, 1969; Namba and Grob, 1967) the results have generally been explicable on the basis of ion-exchange phenomena and the isolated substances have not had the characteristics of specific receptors (cf. Ehrenpreis et al., 1969). One possible exception to this rule concerns studies in nonaqueous media, in which it has been demonstrated that proteolipid extracts of synaptic membranes bind and retain considerable quantities of otherwise freely dissociable ions (De Robertis et al., 1971).

Only limited information can be gained with intact tissues. Despite the use of highly potent antagonists which are effective at concentrations as low as 10^{-9}M, and which might be expected to have considerable specificity, all attempts to label receptors *in situ* with reversible agents have shown that most of the agent used was bound elsewhere. Problems have included low specificity of the drug (methylene blue on heart tissue: Cook, 1926), far more nonspecific than specific binding (atropine on heart tissue: Clark, 1926; curare on electric tissue: Chagas et al., 1958; Ehrenpreis et al., 1969), solubility of the agent in lipids (propranolol on hearts: Potter, 1967), and diffusion of the agent into cells (hexamethonium on diaphragms: Taylor, Creese, and Scholes, 1964; Waser, 1970). The greatest success has been achieved with atropine on the abundant muscarinic receptors of gut smooth muscle; in this case despite more nonspecific than specific binding it was possible to correlate the kinetics of binding and receptor block (Paton and Rang, 1965). Apparent success has also been achieved with curarine on innervated diaphragmatic muscle, where the agent localizes well enough at endplates to permit wholemount radioautographs (Waser, 1970). The binding of curare does not increase significantly in denervated muscles, however, while the number of receptors increases markedly (Miledi and Potter, 1971). Although rough estimates, usually upper limits, of the receptor capacity for atropine, curarine, and propranolol have been made by these techniques, the results do not provide a firm basis for calculating the recovery of isolated receptors. The degree of specificity achieved in such experiments can be increased by "protection experiments," in which the desired receptors are first protected by a potent antagonist while nonspecific sites are irreversibly occluded with an alkylating agent; any excess of the latter is then removed, and the receptors are uncovered for study (Furchgott, 1966). This approach has been most successful when used in conjunction with irreversible tagging agents.

Greater success has been achieved by studying the binding of reversible agents to partially purified cell membranes and membrane proteins than to tissues. The "signal to noise ratio" is improved by removing nonspecific substances which have affinity for the tagging agent and by concentrating the receptors. It has been possible, for example, to demonstrate a saturable component of binding of propranolol to cardiac muscle membranes which was not observable with whole tissues (Potter, 1967). Binding sites for curare on microsomes from electric tissue were not found to saturate, however (Trams, 1964). Comprehensive experiments with membrane fragments and reversible agents have been carried out by O'Brien and his coworkers (Eldefrawi et al., 1971; O'Brien and Gilmour, 1969) and by Changeux and his coworkers (Kasai and Changeux, 1970;

Changeux, Kasai, Huchet, and Mennier, 1970; and Changeux, Kasai, and Lee, 1970b). The former group have used electric tissue membranes from *Torpedo*. These were exposed in ionic media to labelled muscarone, curarine, atropine, nicotine, and decamethonium, and the clearance of the drugs was measured after sedimentation of the fragments, or after equilibrium dialysis. Binding constants were of the order of 1 μM; cholinergic antagonists inhibited binding, whereas noncholinergic drugs had little or no effect; and the number of molecules reversibly bound was of the same order as the number of binding sites for α-bungarotoxin in the same tissue (Miledi, Molinoff, and Potter, 1971). Changeux's group have used "microsacs" of the electric tissue of *Electrophorus electricus,* and have studied their permeability to radiosodium in the presence of the agonists, carbachol and decamethonium, with or without the antagonists, d-tubocurarine, flaxedil, hexamethonium, and α-bungarotoxin. These studies demonstrate the presence of ACh-linked permeability changes which are inhibited to the degree expected from the effects of these agents on intact electroplaques. Many experiments have also been carried out with membrane material from mammalian brains, and the results suggest that synaptic membranes have high affinity for several transmitter analogues, including agonists and antagonists (De Robertis, Fiszer, and Soto, 1967). However, these experiments have been carried out under conditions in which binding by ion-exchange would be maximal, that is, in nonionic media and with assays of repeatedly washed membrane pellets; it is also curious that Triton X-100 did not solubilize binding sites for dimethyltubocurarine when it dissolved AChE, since both the enzyme and ACh receptors are readily dispersed from electric tissue membranes with this detergent (Miledi, Molinoff, and Potter, 1971).

Evidence that reversible agonists and antagonists are useful for the study of "soluble" receptors has been obtained by Changeux and his coworkers (1970c) and by the Eldefrawis and O'Brien (1971). The former group have dissolved membrane proteins from the electric tissue of *Electrophorus electricus* with the detergent desoxycholate, and the latter have studied soluble proteins from water homogenates of housefly brains, which are as rich in AChE as the electric tissue. By equilibrium dialysis against decamethonium, and the five antagonists noted above, respectively, these groups have shown the presence of saturable binding sites on heat-labile, nondialysable substances, and have demonstrated that binding is affected by several specific agonists and antagonists. Proteolytic enzymes reduced the binding to the fly brain protein. In the case of the electric tissue, affinity constants for several compounds are similar to those found with intact electroplax preparations; and high specificity is further indicated by the fact that α-bungarotoxin blocks a large fraction of the decamethonium-binding sites.

Affinity Chromatography

While it is becoming clear that readily reversible agents are useful for recognizing and assaying crude preparations of receptors, it is also obvious that equilibrium dialysis is an inconvenient means for following a receptor during the many stages in its purification. For the latter purpose a specific and nearly irreversible tagging agent like α-bungarotoxin is generally more useful. An exception to this generality concerns affinity chromatography, particularly since our knowledge of how to dissociate "irreversible" tagging agents from receptors (cf. Miledi, Molinoff, and Potter, 1971) is at present quite limited. In affinity chromatography a mixture of proteins to be purified is passed through a column containing an insoluble resin, to which a specific substrate, inhibitor, or other affinity ligand for one substance has been covalently attached. Substances without substantial affinity for the bound agent pass through the column, whereas those which are recognized by reversible or irreversible association with the attached molecule are retarded in proportion to the affinity constant between the two. Striking purifications of several enzymes (e.g. chymotrypsin: Cuatrecasas, Wilchek, and Anfinsen, 1968) and of a thyroxine-binding protein (Pemsky and Marshall, 1969) have been achieved by this technique. Several groups including ourselves are now attempting to apply the technique to the isolation of receptors, by using agonists, antagonists, and sulfhydryl-reactive compounds as the resin-bound agents (cf. Meunier, Huchet, Boquet, and Changeux, 1971).

Irreversible Tagging Agents

The ideal label for a receptor is a compound that reacts rapidly and irreversibly with the receptor and does not react with any other tissue component. Several attempts have been made to study cholinergic receptors with irreversible tagging agents, but in general the small molecules which have been used have lacked the required specificity.

One means of reducing nonspecific receptor labelling is to use a reversible agent having high specificity to protect the receptor sites, while nonspecific sites react with an unlabelled, irreversible reagent. The unlabelled reagent and the protecting compound are then washed out and the radioactively labelled reagent is added. An example of this approach was the use of tritiated dibenamine on the isolated smooth muscle strip of the dog small intestine (Takagi and Takahashi, 1968). Atropine was used to protect cholinergic receptors during a preliminary treatment with unlabelled dibenamine. However, the protecting agent in this type of experiment may not be entirely specific for the receptor, and Takagi and Takahashi found labelled dibenamine irreversibly bound to components in all seven protein fractions which they isolated.

To improve the specificity of labelling reactions, alkylating or arylating compounds which have a high degree of intrinsic affinity for the receptor have been used in addition to the use of protective agents. For example, p- (trimethylammonium) benzene-diazonium-fluoroborate (Tdf) is a structural analogue of phenyltrimethylammonium, which is a potent ACh receptor agonist. Tdf has a reactive diazonium group which forms a covalent bond with tyrosine, histidine, and lysine side-chains of proteins. When an isolated electroplax was exposed to Tdf, the cell became insensitive to receptor activators (Changeux, Podleski, and Wofsy, 1967). This effect was prevented by curare, so that curare could be used to protect the receptors. A high concentration of Tdf (10^{-4}M) was required for blockade, however, and much of the Tdf was presumably bound to nonspecific sites.

A modification of the affinity-labelling approach called photo-affinity labelling (Singer, 1970) uses an agent which is ordinarily unreactive, but which can be converted by photolysis to an exceedingly reactive intermediate. Aryl azides have been used to label the acetylcholine-binding site of the enzyme acetylcholinesterase on red blood cell membranes and the acetylcholine receptor at the neuromuscular junction of the frog sartorius muscle (Kiefer, Lindstrom, Lennox, and Singer, 1970). However, the specificity of these reactions remains to be established.

In experiments using dibenamine or Tdf, the specificity of the reaction is largely dependent on the specificity of the protecting agent. A cholinergic receptor antagonist resembling a choline ester (benzilylcholine mustard) has been synthesized by Gill and Rang (1967). This compound is itself highly potent (and therefore presumably quite specific) and is an essentially irreversible blocking agent of muscarinic receptors. The binding of benzilylcholine mustard is reduced by atropine but not by tubocurarine or physostigmine. This compound appears to be sufficiently specific to allow its use for the isolation of the muscarinic receptor.

The response of the electroplax to acetylcholine is also blocked by the disulphide reducing agent, dithiothreitol (Karlin and Bartels, 1966). This inhibition can be reversed by oxidizing agents like 5,5′-dithiobis (2-nitrobenzoate), or the reduced receptor can be alkylated by thiol alkylating agents like N-ethylmaleimide. A highly specific alkylation can be obtained using quaternary ammonium maleimide derivatives such as 4-maleimidobenzyltrimethylammonium iodide (MBTA), and this compound appears to act as an affinity label for the reduced receptor (Karlin and Winnik, 1969; Karlin, 1969; Karlin, Prives, Deal, and Winnik, 1970). Com-

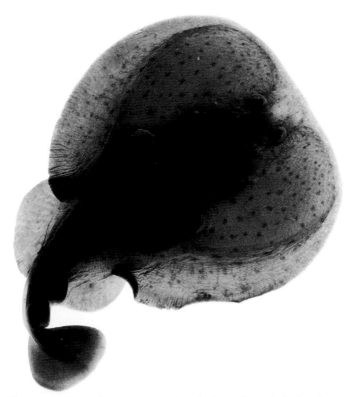

Figure 2-1   *Torpedo marmorata*—dorsal view. The paired electric organs, which are slightly less transparent than the edges of the fish, are seen to occupy a large percentage of the "wings" of the animal. This fish was only 10 cm across.

pounds like MBTA have an irreversible effect only after the receptor has been reduced. They act as completely reversible competitive inhibitors of the response to carbamylcholine in the absence of pretreatment with dithiothreitol. The binding of MBTA is prevented by prior treatment of the reduced receptor by the affinity oxidizing agent, cholinedisulphide, and is considerably decreased when it is added in the presence of hexamethonium. Using MBTA along with cholinedisulphide or hexamethonium, Karlin et al. (1970) have estimated that there are 26-75 $\times$ 10^{-14} moles of receptor per electroplax cell. This value is similar to the calculated amount of acetylcholinesterase in the cell.

Isolation of the Cholinergic Receptor of Torpedo Electric Tissue

Torpedo

Torpedo (Fig. 2-1) are bottom-feeding elasmobranchs (skates) which are common in the Atlantic ocean and Mediterranean sea. They vary in

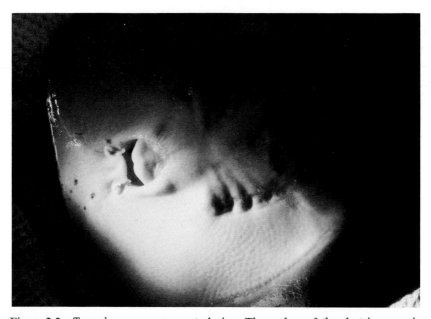

Figure 2-2 *Torpedo marmorata*—ventral view. The surface of the electric organ is puckered, and the bases of the stacks of cells are visible through the skin. These cells were about 2 mm across.

size from about 5 cm across, just after birth, to more than a meter, and their electric organs, which comprise about 25 per cent of the body weight, reach weights of many kilograms. The fish are readily caught in nets, especially when they come into shallow bays to breed, and they survive well in cold sea water for many weeks without feeding. They apparently use their electric organs to stun shrimp and other food, but they are easy to handle (in sizes under 30 cm) in the laboratory, and do not commonly produce large shocks unless treated unkindly.

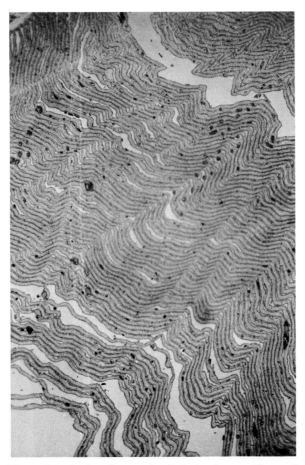

Figure 2-3   Light micrograph of electroplaques. The section was stained in 1 per cent toluidine blue, and shows an edge-on view of the cells. The thickness of these cells was about 5 μm.

Each electric organ is composed of about 500 stacks or columns of cells; the columns run from dorsal skin to ventral skin, and through the latter, the hexagonally shaped flat faces of the cells are readily seen (Fig. 2-2). Each column has several hundred to several thousand electroplaques (Fig. 2-3), which vary in thickness from 5 to 10 μm, and in breadth from 1 to 10 or more mm, depending upon the size of the fish. The number of cells in a stack determines the voltage output of the organ, which is usually only 20 to 60 volts, but the surface area of organ is so large that the current output of a large fish can reach 50 amperes. Each cell is innervated over most of its ventral surface (Sheridan, 1965; Nickel and Potter, 1970) by cholinergic nerve terminals (Feldberg and Fessard, 1942; Israel, 1970), and the ventral cell membrane needs to be and is only excitable chemically (Bennett, 1961). We have estimated that the infolded postsynaptic membrane has a total area of about 70 m^2 per kg of tissue (Miledi, Molinoff, and Potter, 1971).

Torpedo electric tissue was chosen as a source of cholinergic receptors because of its dense innervation and relatively immense area of postsynaptic membrane. The plaques of *Torpedo* are thinner and more densely innervated then the cells from *Electrophorus electricus*. This suggests that there are more receptors in the electric organs of the fish than the eel, which appears to be the case (O'Brien, Eldefrawi, Eldefrawi, and Farrow, 1971). The fish are also easier to obtain and to keep. Their AChE and receptors are more resistant to solubilization with salts (probably because the fish live in salt water) and by sonication than are those of *Electrophorus,* which makes handling the membranes, and washing other proteins off them before dissolving the receptors, quite convenient.

Alpha-bungarotoxin

Bungarus multicinctus is a banded krait (a snake several feet long with white rings; Fig. 2-4) which is common in Taiwan; it prefers to live in wet places like rice paddies, and is known for its nonaggressive behavior to man, if not to frogs. The curare-like action of its venom was first analyzed in detail by Chang in 1960, and components of the venom which produce pre- and postsynaptic effects were further studied by Chang and Lee (1963), Lee and Chang (1966), Lee and Tseng (1966), and Lee, Tseng, and Chiu (1967). One of four crude toxin fractions obtained by starch-block electrophoresis, and called α-bungarotoxin (61 per cent of

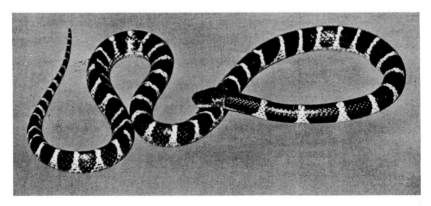

Figure 2-4   *Bungarus multicinctus.*

the venom protein), was found to block synaptic potentials produced by acetylcholine at vertebrate neuromuscular junctions, without affecting resting or action potentials, or the release of ACh from motor nerve terminals. Pretreatment of muscles with curare prevented the blocking action of the toxin, while neostigmine, if anything, increased the rate of blockade. After the exposure of mouse diaphragms to ^{131}I-labelled toxin, and washout of unbound material for four hours, whole-mount radioautographs showed sharp localization of the radioactivity at normal endplates, and diffuse localization in denervated muscles. From these experiments it was concluded that α-bungarotoxin specifically and irreversibly blocks the acetylcholine receptors of striated muscles. By electron microscopic radioautography, the toxin has been found only at endplates in muscles (Barnard, Wieckowski, and Chiu, 1971) and associated with the innervated membranes of eel electric tissue (Bourgeois et al., 1971).

In 1969 a sample of the dried venom of *B. multicinctus* was provided by Lee, and several grams of the dry venom, obtained from hundreds of snakes, were purchased from a source in Taiwan. (The venom is also obtainable from Sigma Corp.) Twelve pure proteins were isolated from the venom by chromatography on Sephadex G-50 fine and subsequent cation-exchange chromatography at pH 7.5 on CM-Sephadex (Miledi and Potter, unpublished). The major component of the venom, comprising 20 to 25 per cent of its protein had the properties described for α-bungarotoxin (Miledi, Molinoff, and Potter, 1971; Miledi and Potter, 1971), and will be so designated. It gave a single band when subjected to electrophoresis on 7.5 per cent cross-linked acrylamide at pH 8.5, and a single peak by chromatography on Sephadex G-50. By the latter method its molecular weight, determined by co-chromatography with glucagon, ribonuclease, and soybean trypsin inhibitor, was 8000. Lee and his coworkers (personal communication) have isolated the same protein by cation-exchange chromatography, and are in the course of determining its sequence.

The isolated toxin was found to block neuromuscular transmission in frog sartorius muscles, at concentrations as low as 10^{-8}M, without affecting resting or action potentials, or spindle discharges (Miledi and Potter, 1971). Synaptic potentials could be blocked in less than a minute in surface fibers. Because the block persisted undiminished despite washout of the drug for as long as 8 days at 4°C, for practical purposes it may be considered that the toxin binds irreversibly with acetylcholine receptors. The toxin similarly blocks the action of ACh on electroplaques in *Torpedo* electric tissue, but its action in this tissue, like that of curare, is very slow, probably because access of the toxin to the very narrow synaptic clefts is limited (Miledi, Molinoff, and Potter, 1971).

Alpha-bungarotoxin is an exceptionally stable protein: we have kept a stock solution of 7 mg/ml as long as 6 months at 4°C in sodium phosphate buffer, pH 7.5, and 0.02 per cent sodium azide, without significant protein denaturation, or observable loss in biological potency.

In order to measure trace amounts of the toxin bound to receptors, the toxin was labelled (Pressmen and Eisen, 1950) with carrier-free ^{131}iodine of the highest available specific activity. Routinely, we have used 10 mCi of ^{131}I with 700 μg of the toxin, and, after isolation of the labelled protein on a 1 × 50 cm column of Sephadex G-25, have obtained initial specific activities of about 23,000 curies/mole. The molecular weight of the toxin is increased by only a few grams at this level of iodination. Even maximal iodination has no observable effect on the potency of the toxin.

Preparation and Labelling of Membranes, and
"Solubilization" of the Receptor

(A summary of the steps used for the following experiments is given in Table 2-1.)
When homogenates of fresh or frozen electric tissue were made in isotonic or hypotonic media, and were treated with subsaturating amounts of labelled α-toxin, more than 80 per cent of the toxin and of the total AChE of

Table 2-1   Preparation of soluble membrane proteins, including labelled receptors, from *Torpedo* electric tissue. All operations are carried out at 1 to 4°C in 20 mM sodium phosphate, pH 7.5.

Electric Tissue

Tissue ± skin is homogenized in a Waring blender at top speed for 2 min in buffered 0.4 M NaCl, 4 g/g tissue, and the homogenate is poured through a sieve.

Centrifuged at 23,000 $\times$ g_{max} for 30 min in plastic bottles.

First Pellet

Resuspended with Polytron blender (20,000 rpm $\times$ 1 min) in buffer, 1 to 2 ml/g original tissue.

^{131}I-α-bungarotoxin is added, 1 to 5 μg/g original tissue.

Centrifuged as before after 30 min.

Unbound toxin is discarded.

Membranes resuspended by swirling in buffer and centrifuged as before.

Toxin-Labelled Membranes

Resuspended by swirling in buffer containing 1.5 per cent Triton X-100, w/w, 0.5 ml/g original tissue.

Centrifuged at 100,000 $\times$ g_{avg} for 60 min after 30 min.

Dispersed Membrane Proteins

---

the tissue (0.78 mmol acetylthiocholine hydrolized per min per g of tissue) could be sedimented with membrane fragments by low speed centrifugation. Attempts to isolate the toxin-labelled membranes (presumably the postsynaptic membranes) from such homogenates (Fig. 2-5) showed that they could be separated from several other particulate fractions. For the initial experiments, however, we chose to recover most of the receptors by collecting most of the cell membranes, and used conditions designed to remove as much soluble protein as possible. The tissue was first blended in isotonic NaCl, and the membranes from this homogenate were then further disintegrated and osmotically shocked in dilute buffer, to remove any protein trapped in artifactually formed membrane vesicles. The final membrane pellet retained about 24 per cent of the tissue protein (total = 23 mg/g tissue), 82 per cent of its AChE, and 85 per cent of the toxin-binding sites. Binding of the toxin to the isolated membranes was dependent upon concentration and time (Fig. 2-6); saturation was achieved with 7.43 μg of toxin for the membranes from 1 g of tissue. On the basis of the recovery figures it was estimated that a gram of tissue has 6.6 $\times$ 10^{14} binding sites; assuming that AChE is a protein of molecular weight (MW) 240,000, with 4 active sites/molecule and an activity of 12.5 moles ACh hydrolyzed per min per g of en-

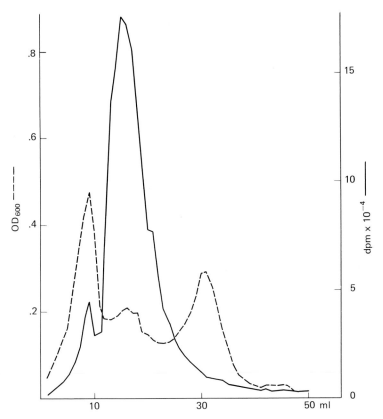

Figure 2-5 Localization of α-toxin in subcellular fractions of electric tissue. La-belled membranes from 2 grams of tissue (Table 2-1) were spun into a sucrose density gradient, 0 to 47 per cent (w/w), for 2.5 hours at 63,500 × g_{avg}. The peak of ^{131}I was at 33 per cent sucrose (S.G. = 1.144). A small amount of toxin was apparently trapped in association with membranes of the first light-scattering peak, which have been identified by electron microscopy and their content of Na^+-K^+-activated ATPase as dorsal electroplaque membranes. The third and fourth light-scattering peaks have been identified as myelin (peak at 20 per cent sucrose) and microsomes, respectively, by electron microscopy. In other experiments, the toxin was found not to bind to intact mitochondria from electric tissue (peak at 41 per cent sucrose), or to vesicles containing ACh (13 per cent sucrose).

zyme (Kremzner and Wilson, 1964; cf. Millar and Grafius, 1970), the number of active sites of the enzyme was 6.3×10^{14} per g of tissue (Miledi, Molinoff, and Potter, 1971).

Binding of the toxin to isolated membranes was inhibited by curare, a

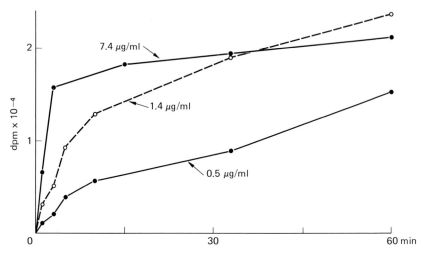

Figure 2-6 Time course of binding of [131] I-α-toxin. Membranes (first pellet, Table 2-1) from about 200 mg of electric tissue were incubated at 20°C in 1 ml of 20 mM phosphate buffer, pH 7.4, with bovine serum albumin, 10 μg/ml, and ^{131}I-α-toxin at the indicated concentrations. At the times shown the membranes were sedimented by centrifugation at 20,000 × g for 1 min. The pellet was washed twice and was then dissolved in an alkaline solvent for liquid scintillation spectrometry.

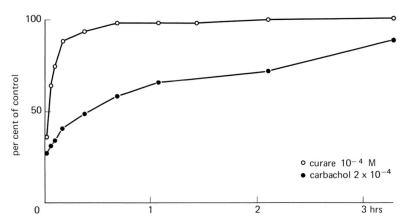

Figure 2-7 Effect of d-tubocurarine and carbamylcholine on the binding of ^{131}I-α-toxin. Membranes from approximately 200 mg of electric tissue were incubated at 20°C in 1 ml of buffer with or without curare or carbachol. The reactions were stopped at the indicated times as described in Fig. 2-6. Results are expressed as per cent of toxin-binding without these drugs.

competitive antagonist at the receptors, and by carbachol (Fig. 2-7), an ACh analogue which is effective in blocking the toxin apparently because the toxin does not bind efficiently to desensitized receptors (Miledi and Potter, 1971).

Several possible means of dissolving toxin-tagged receptors from the membranes were investigated (Table 2-2). Sonication in dilute or strongly ionic solutions did not remove the labelled material, indicating that it is tightly bound to the membrane. Moderately vigorous agitation of two-phase suspensions in butanol or chloroform-methanol did not yield the material in solution in either the aqueous or organic solvent phases. Treatment with chloroform-methanol (in the manner used by De Robertis

Table 2-2 Solubilization of membrane proteins. Aliquots of toxin-labelled membranes (about 15 mg protein, usually in 20 mM sodium phosphate, pH 7.5) were subjected to the procedures indicated at 4°C in a final volume of 10 ml, and particulate material was then sedimented by ultracentrifugation. Samples of the supernatant fluids were assayed for ^{131}I before and after centrifugation. Samples of the fluid after treatment with Triton, urea, and NaBr were analyzed for protein-bound toxin vs. free toxin (Fig. 2-8).

Treatment	Method	Per Cent Unsedimented ^{131}I
Sonication	30 sec $\times$ 6 in buffer or buffered 0.4 M NaCl	0-2
n-Butanol	5 ml aqueous suspension + 5 ml butanol shaken 1 min	0 (most at interface)
Chloroform: methanol 2:1 by vol	Freeze-dried membranes blended by Polytron 1 min at top speed	0
	5 ml aqueous suspension + 5 ml organic phase shaken 1 min	0 (most at interface)
NaI	2 M with 5 mM EDTA 1 hour	76
Urea	7.2 M, 1 hour	85
Na decyl SO$_4$ or Na dodecyl SO$_4$	1 per cent in buffer, 30 min	100
Triton X-100	1.5 per cent by weight in buffer for 1 hour	75 to 95
	1.5 per cent + 1M NaCl	100

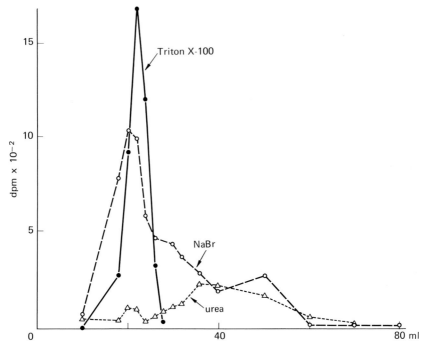

Figure 2-8   Dissociation of α-toxin from receptor protein. Labelled membranes from approximately 500 mg of electric tissue were sedimented by centrifugation at 34,000 × g_{max} for 10 min. The pellet was then suspended in 8 M urea, 6 per cent Triton X-100 or 25 per cent NaBr (w/w). After 1 hour a 1 ml aliquot of the fluid was chromatographed on a 1.5 × 25 cm column of Sephadex G-50 fine which had been prewashed with urea, Triton, or NaBr. In each case forty-2 ml fractions were collected. Radioactivity is in dpm/100 μl.

and coworkers, 1971, followed by freeze-drying) also prevented subsequent binding of the toxin to previously unlabelled membrane material, presumably because the organic solvents denatured the toxin-binding sites. Sodium bromide, urea, and sodium dodecyl sulfate (SDS) alone, partially or fully dissociated the toxin from its binding sites (Fig. 2-8 and subsequent sections), and both NaI and urea prevented subsequent binding of the toxin to treated proteins after their dialysis against dilute buffer. Of the procedures studied, the use of low concentrations of Triton X-100 (at least 2 mg/kg protein), a nonionic detergent, was most satisfactory, because it gave high recovery of the toxin-labelled material and AChE in a dispersed state which was not sedimented at 100,000 × g for 1 hour, and

Table 2-3   Binding of ^{131}I-α-bungarotoxin to soluble receptor protein. Fifty μl of soluble membrane protein, 50 μl of 20 mM NaPO$_4$ buffer pH 7.5, 0.5 μg ^{131}I-α-bungarotoxin, and the drugs indicated were mixed at 20°C and allowed to incubate for 10 minutes. Labelled receptor protein was then separated from free toxin on a 1.2 ml column of Sephadex G-50 fine in the presence of the drugs used.

Treatment	Per Cent Control
Carbachol 10^{-3}M	32
Carbachol 2×10^{-4}M	50
Physostigmine 10^{-5}M	100

permitted the same degree of binding of the toxin to dispersed protein as was achieved with the membranes. About 7 per cent of the tissue protein was recovered at this stage (Miledi et al., 1971). Addition of salt or anionic detergents to Triton-solubilized material changed its state as indicated in later sections.

Binding of the toxin to Triton-dispersed material was unaffected by physostigmine (Table 2-3), which inhibits AChE. Toxin-binding was inhibited by carbachol, however, indicating that the toxin-receptive site and the cholino-receptive site are on the same molecule or macromolecule

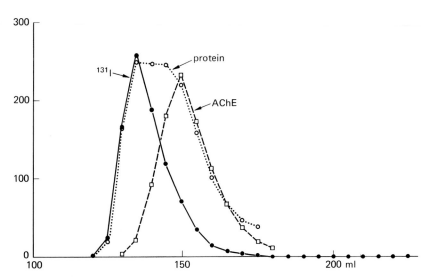

Figure 2-9   Molecular sieving on Sephadex G-200. Soluble membrane proteins were layered onto a 2.5 × 90 cm column of Sephadex G-200 in 20 mM phosphate buffer, pH 7.4, containing 1.5 per cent Triton X-100. Protein is in μg/ml, AChE, in μmol acetylthiocholine hydrolyzed per min per 10 ml, and ^{131}I as dpm/0.05 μl.

(Table 2-3). This result also suggests that the conformational changes produced in the receptor by agonists occur in dispersed forms of the protein as well as in the intact membrane.

Molecular Sieving

Samples of Triton-dispersed, partially labelled material were chromatographed on Sephadex G-200 (Fig. 2-9) and Sepharose 6B. In each case the labelled protein was eluted before AChE, indicating that the active enzyme is a protein distinct from the receptor. On Sephadex, all, and on Sepharose, about half of the labelled protein was excluded from the resin. The disruption of hydrophobic bonds between the receptor and other membrane constitutents, by Triton, was thus insufficient to obtain the receptor in a monodispersed form.

Addition of 1 or 2 M NaCl to Triton-treated proteins caused all of the toxin-labelled material to appear in a single symmetrical peak after the void volume on Sephadex G-200 (Fig. 2-10), just before AChE, which has a molecular weight of 260,000 (cf. Millar and Grafius, 1970). The

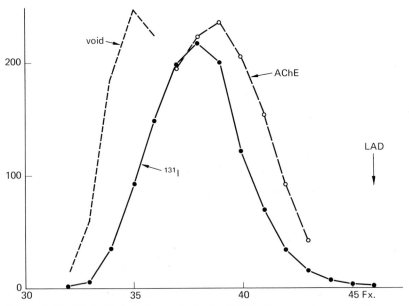

Figure 2-10   Molecular sieving on Sephadex G-200. The experiment was the same as described in Fig. 2-9, except that 1 M NaCl was present throughout. LAD shows the peak position of liver alcohol dehydrogenase.

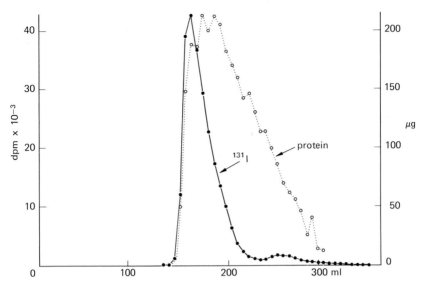

Figure 2-11   Molecular sieving on Sephadex G-200 in the presence of 0.5 per cent sodium dodecylsulfate (SDS). The same column was used as in Fig. 2-10. Before the sample was loaded, the column was equilibrated with 0.5 per cent SDS. The radioactivity peak begins just after the void volume, as determined in separate experiments with Blue Dextran. Protein is expressed as $\mu g/0.5$ ml and radioactivity as dpm/50 μl.

toxin-labelled material thus moved as would a globular protein having a molecular weight of about 300,000. Other studies, however, indicate that NaCl causes toxin-receptor complexes to move more slowly than expected during molecular sieving, and more rapidly during ultracentrifugation; the most likely explanation for these results is that salt causes the complexes to become, or to become more, rod-shaped (Molinoff and Potter, 1972).

Addition of cold 0.5 per cent SDS to Triton-dispersed material similarly caused the toxin-labelled protein to appear just after the void volume on Sephadex G-200 (Fig. 2-11). In addition a small amount of radioactivity was found in a position that would correspond to a globular protein of molecular weight about 90,000. We previously suggested that this smaller peak might represent a subcomponent of the material eluted in the main peak. However, further experiments have shown that α-toxin behaves anomalously on Sephadex in the presence of SDS, and it is probable that this small peak represents α-toxin which has been dissociated from the receptor by SDS. After treatment of toxin-labelled membranes with 1 per cent SDS at 37°C for 15 or more minutes, with or without 1 per cent Triton or 1 per cent β-mercaptoethanol, most of the radio-activity eluted from Sephadex G-200 was found in this anomalous position for α-toxin.

Ultracentrifugation

Freshly prepared membrane proteins and several fractions from Sephadex G-200 were subjected to ultracentrifugation in density gradients of sucrose or glycerol. The fresh toxin-receptor complex moved in Triton X-100 as one of the largest or most dense of the dispersed membrane proteins (Fig. 2-12), in keeping with the results obtained by molecular sieving. But

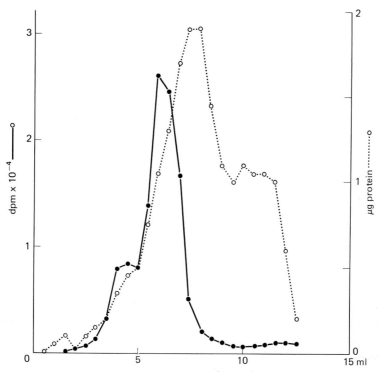

Figure 2-12   Sedimentation of ^{131}I-labelled proteins. Soluble membrane proteins were layered onto a density gradient formed from sucrose and 20 mM phosphate buffer, and containing 1 per cent Triton X-100. The gradient ran from 5 to 25 per cent sucrose (w/w). Centrifugation was for 22 hours at 39,000 rpm in Spinco SW 40 Ti tubes. Radioactivity is expressed as dpm per fraction, and protein as μg per fraction.

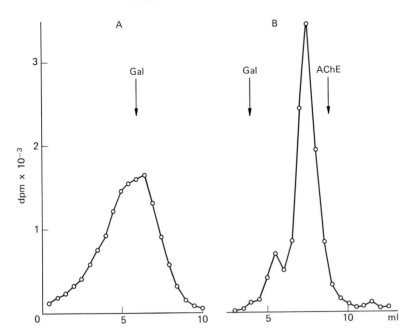

Figure 2-13   Ultracentrifugation of toxin-labelled protein. Soluble membrane proteins were subjected to molecular sieving on Sephadex G-200. Samples from the peak of Fig. 2-9 were diluted to 0.5 ml with 50 mM Tris HCl, pH 8, in 50 mM KCl-0.1 mM EDTA, and a small amount of β-galactosidase was added. The samples were spun into linear density gradients of glycerol prepared in the same solution (12 ml, 10 to 30 per cent glycerol (w/w) in Spinco SW 40 Ti tubes) at 3°C for 15 hours at 37,000 rpm (A) or for 22 hours at 39,000 rpm (B). The peaks of β-galactosidase (Gal) and of acetylcholinesterase (AChE) are indicated by arrows. The glycerol solutions used in B contained 1.0 per cent Triton X-100.

whereas much of the labelled material in Triton had been excluded from beads of Sephrose 6B, indicating a molecular weight in excess of 2 million, similarly treated material moved during centrifugation primarily in one peak between the markers β-galactosidase (molecular weight about 540,000) and AChE (Fig. 2-13B). A small amount of a slightly larger or denser material was also present. The apparent difference in size of the toxin-labelled material as shown by sieving and ultra-centrifugation may be the consequence of some lipid constituent of the receptor: a lipoprotein would be less dense than a pure protein, and would move, therefore, more slowly during centrifugation. After removing Triton, the labelled material moved further into the gradients, as would soluble proteins of 0.5 to 2 million molecular weight (Fig. 2-13A).

Samples of the toxin-receptor complex obtained by chromatography on Sephadex G-200 in Triton and SDS (main peak of Fig. 2-11) were found to move in gradients in multiple peaks, depending upon the presence or type(s) of detergent used (Fig. 2-11). At present it is not clear whether these results depend upon reversible aggregation and disaggregation of

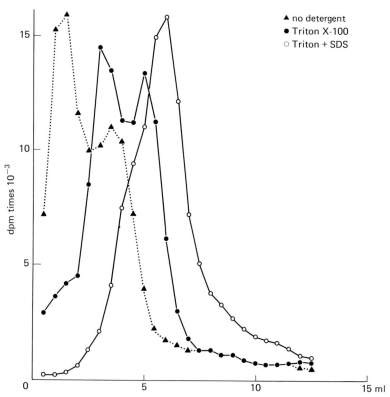

Figure 2-14 Ultracentrifugation of SDS-treated, toxin-labelled protein. Toxin-labeled proteins were subjected to molecular sieving on Sephadex G-200 in the presence of 0.5 per cent SDS. Samples (0.5 ml) from the first peak in Fig. 2-11 were layered onto sucrose density gradients running from 5 to 24 per cent sucrose (w/w). The sucrose solution used contained 20 mM PO_4 buffer. Two of the gradients contained 1 per cent Triton X-100 and one of these also contained 0.5 per cent SDS. The gradients were spun for 22 hours at 39,000 rpm in Spinco SW 40 Ti tubes. Radioactivity is expressed as dpm per 50 μl of each 0.5 ml fraction.

toxin-receptor complexes, upon changes in the density and size of a complex with addition or subtraction of the detergents, or both.

Ion-Exchange Chromatography

In 20 mM sodium phosphate buffer containing Triton X-100, most of the dispersed protein and all of the labelled protein bound to DEAE-Sephadex by anion exchange at pH values at and above pH 6.4, and to CM-Sephadex by cation exchange at pH values below 5. Gradient elution of the toxin-receptor complex from a column of DEAE-Sephadex at pH 6.4 (Fig. 2-15) demonstrated that the material behaved predominantly as a single ionic species.

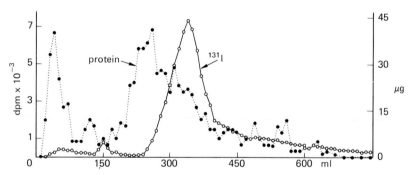

Figure 2-15   Ion exchange chromatography. Toxin-labelled proteins (15 ml) were layered onto a 30 ml column of DEAE-Sephadex (A-50) in 20 mM phosphate buffer, pH 6.4, containing 1:5 per cent Triton X-100. The column was washed with 50 ml of the same buffer and the sample was eluted with a linear gradient of NaCl, formed from 500 ml of buffer and 500 ml of 1 M NaCl. Radioactivity is dpm per 50 μl of each 10 ml fraction, and protein is μg/0.3 ml.

Discussion

We believe that α-bungarotoxin is a specific labelling agent for nicotinic receptors for the following reasons.

(a) The toxin blocks physiological and pharmacological responses to ACh in electric tissues and skeletal muscles without affecting resting or action potentials, the release of ACh, or acetylcholinesterase.

(b) Binding of the toxin is restricted to those regions of electroplaques, and of innervated and denervated muscle cells, which are sensitive to ACh.

(c) Binding of the toxin to intact muscles is inhibited by desensitization of receptors with ACh.

(d) After density gradient centrifugation of homogenates of *Torpedo* electric tissue, almost all of the toxin is found in a single peak, distinct from the majority of the tissue proteins.

(e) Binding of the toxin to membrane fragments and to detergent-dispersed membrane materials is inhibited by nicotinic agonists and antagonists which are believed to act on the receptor molecule.

(f) The toxin-binding material appears to be a single ionic species by ion-exchange chromatography.

From the number of binding sites for the toxin per kilogram of electric tissue (6.6×10^{17}), and our estimate of the area of postsynaptic membrane ($70 \, m^2/kg$), it is possible to roughly estimate the average number of receptors in the membrane as $10,000/\mu^2$ (Miledi et al., 1971). This number of sites corresponds to about 1 μmole/kg. If one assumes that one binding site is carried by a spherical unit of molecular weight 40,000, and that the protein occupies approximately 1 A^3 for each 0.7 g of molecular weight, the combined frontal area of 10,000 units would be about 0.1 μ^2. Despite the crudity of these estimates, and our lack of knowledge as to the arrangement of the receptors in or on the postsynaptic membrane, there is reason to anticipate that a large fraction of the area of postsynaptic membranes is taken up by receptors.

The reason for the similarity in the numbers of active sites of receptors and AChE is not clear, since the active enzyme is clearly separable from toxin-labelled protein and since, with denervation, the number of receptors increases (Miledi and Potter, 1971) while the activity of AChE decreases (Guth, Brown, and Watson, 1967). Three possibilities for the similarity in numbers are that the receptors and AChE share a common subunit; that the two molecules are normally part of one polymer in the membrane; or that there is one operon for the two (and perhaps for an ionophore) which is read off by molecules of messenger RNA.

The partial isolation of one receptor protein suggests that others can be obtained by similar means. At present it would appear better to obtain well-washed postsynaptic membranes from a good source for the receptor concerned, and to solubilize membrane protein from them, *before* attempting to assay the receptors with an agent which may not have absolute specificity, rather than to work with cells or homogenates.

References

Barnard, E. A., Wieckowski, J., and Chiu, T. H. 1971. *Nature* 234:207.
Bennett, M. W. V. 1961. *Ann. N. Y. Acad. Sci.* 94:458.
Bourgeois, J.-P., Tsuji, S., Boquet, P., Pillot, J., Ryter, A., and Changeux, J.-P. 1971. *FEBS Letters* 16:92.
Chagas, C., Penna-Franca, E., Nishie, K., and Garcia, E. J. 1958. *Arch. Biochem. Biophys.* 75:251.
Chang, C. C., and Lee, C. Y. 1963. *Arch. Int. Pharmacodyn.* 144:241.
Changeux, J.-P., Podleski, T. R., and Wofsy, L. 1967. *Proc. Nat. Acad. Sci. U.S.* 58:2067.
Changeux, J.-P., Kasai, M., and Lee, C. Y. 1970b. *Proc. Nat. Acad. Sci. U.S.* 67:1241.
Changeux, J.-P., Kasai, M., Huchet, M., and Meunier, J.-C. 1970c. *C.R. Acad. Sci. Paris* 270:2864.
Changeux, J.-P., Blumenthal, R., Kasai, M., and Podleski, T. 1970a. In Ciba Symposium *Molecular Properties of Drug Receptors,* A. Porter and M. O'Connor (Eds.), J. & A. Churchill, London, p. 197.
Ciba Symposium, *Molecular Properties of Drug Receptors,* A. Porter and M. O'Connor (Eds.), J. & A. Churchill, London, 1970.
Clark, A. J. 1926. *J. Physiol. (Lond.)* 61:547.
Cook, R. P. 1926. *J. Physiol. (Lond.)* 62:160.
Cuatrecasas, P., Wilchek, M., and Anfinsen, C. B. 1968. *Proc. Nat. Acad. Sci. U.S.* 61:636.
Dale, H. H. 1963. *Adventures in Physiology,* Pergamon Press, London.
Del Castillo, J., and Katz, B. 1955. *J. Physiol.* 128:157.
Del Castillo, J., Rodriguez, A., and Romero, C. A. 1967. *Ann. N.Y. Acad. Sci.* 144:803.
De Robertis, E., Fiszer, S., and Soto, E. F. 1967. *Nature* 158:928.
De Robertis, E., González-Rodríguez, J., and Teller, D. 1967. *FEBS Letters* 4:4.
De Robertis, E., Lunt, G. S., and La Torre, José L. 1971. *Mol. Pharmacol.* 7:97.
Eldefrawi, M. E., Eldefrawi, A. T., and O'Brien, R. D. 1971. *Mol. Pharmacol.* 7:104.
Ehrenpreis, S., Fleisch, J. H., and Mittag, T. W. 1969. *Pharmacol. Rev.* 21:131.
Fatt, P., and Katz, B. 1951. *J. Physiol.* 115:320.
Feldberg, W., and Fessard, A. 1942. *J. Physiol.* 101:200.
Furchgott, R. F. 1966. *Adv. Drug. Res.* 3:21.
Gill, E. W., and Rang, H. P. 1966. *Mol. Pharmacol.* 2:284.
Guth, L., Brown, W. C., and Watson, P. K. 1967. *Exper. Neurol.* 18:443.
Harris, A. J., Kuffler, S., and Dennis, M. 1971. *Proc. Roy. Soc. B.* 177:541.
Hodgkin, A. L. 1964. The Sherrington Lectures VII, Liverpool University Press.
Israël, M. 1970. *Arch. d'Anat. Microscop.* 59:5.
Jaim, M. K., Strickholm, A., and Cordes, E. H. 1969. *Nature* 222:871.
Johnson, S. M., and Bangham, A. D. 1969. *Biochim. Biophys. Acta* 193:82.
Karlin, A., and Bartels, E. 1966. *Biochim. Biophys. Acta* 126:525.
Karlin, A., and Winnik, M. 1968. *Proc. Nat. Acad. Sci. U.S.* 60:668.
Karlin, A. 1969. *J. Gen. Physiol.* 54:245.
Karlin, A., Prives, J., Deal, W., and Winnik, M. 1970. In Ciba Symposium *Molecular Properties of Drug Receptors,* A. Porter and M. O'Connor (Eds.), J. & A. Churchill, London, p. 247.

Kasai, M., and Changeux, J.-P. 1970. *C.R. Acad. Sci. Paris* 276:1400.

Katz, B., and Miledi, R. 1964. *J. Physiol. (Lond.)* 170:379.

Katz, B. 1969. The Sherrington Lectures X, Liverpool University Press.

Kehoe, J., and Ascher, P., quoted in T. W. Rall and A. G. Gilman, "The Role of Cyclic AMP in the Nervous System," *Neurosciences Res. Prog. Bull.* 8:273, 1970.

Kiefer, H., Lindstrom, J., Lennox, E. S., and Singer, S. J. 1970. *Proc. Nat. Acad. Sci. U.S.* 67:1688.

Kremzner, L. T., and Wilson, I. B. 1964. *Biochemistry* 3: 1902.

Langley, J. N. 1906. *J. Physiol.* 36:347.

Lee, C. Y., and Chang, C. C. 1966. *Mem. Inst. Butantan Simp. Internac.* 33:555.

Lee, C. Y., and Tseng, L. F. 1966. *Toxicon* 3:281.

Lee, C. Y., Tseng, L. F., and Chiu, T. H. 1967. *Nature* 215:1177.

Loewi, O. 1921. *Pflugers Arch. Physiol.* 189:239.

Lømo, T., and Rosenthal, J. 1971. *J. Physiol.* 216:52D.

Lu, F. C. 1957. *Rev. Can. Biol.* 16:108.

Meunier, J.-C., Huchet, M., Boquet, P., and Changeux, J.-P. 1971. *C.R. Acad. Sci. Paris* 272:117.

Miledi, R. in Ciba Symposium *Enzymes and Drug Action,* J. L. Morgan and A. U. S. de Rueck (Eds.), Little, Brown, Boston, 1962, p. 220.

Miledi, R., and Potter, L. T. 1971. *Nature* 233:599.

Miledi, R., Molinoff, P., and Potter, L. T. 1971. *Nature* 229:554.

Millar, D. B., and Grafius, M. A. 1970. *FEBS Letters* 12:61.

Molinoff, P. B., and Potter, L. T. 1972. In *Studies of Neurotransmitters at the Synaptic Level,* E. Costa and L. L. Iversen (Eds.), Raven Press (in press).

Namba, T., and Grob, D. 1967. *Ann. N.Y. Acad. Sci.* 144:772.

Nickel, E., and Potter, L. T. 1970. *Brain Research* 23:95.

O'Brien, R. D., Eldefrawi, M. E., Eldefrawi, A. T., and Farrow, J. T. 1971. In *Cholinergic Ligend Interactions,* D. J. Triggle, E. A. Barnard, and J. F. Moran (Eds.), Academic Press, New York, p. 49.

O'Brien, R. D., and Gilmour, L. P. 1969. *Proc. Nat. Acad. Sci. U.S.* 63:496.

Paton, W. D. M., and Rang, H. P. 1965. *Proc. Roy. Soc. B* 163:1.

Paton, W. D. M., in Ciba Symposium *Molecular Properties of Drug Receptors,* R. Porter and M. O'Connor (Eds.), J. & A. Churchill, London, 1970, p. 3.

Pensky, J., and Marshall, J. S. 1969. *Arch. Biochem. Biophys.* 135:304.

Potter, L. T. 1967. *J. Pharmacol.* 155:91.

Potter, L. T. 1970. *J. Physiol.* 206:145.

Pressman, D., and Eisen, H. N. 1950. *J. Immunol.* 64:273.

Rasmussen, H. 1970. *Science* 170:404.

Rang, H. P. 1967. *Ann. N.Y. Acad. Sci.* 144:765.

Rang, H. P., and Ritter, J. M. 1969. *Mol. Pharmac.* 5:394.

Rang, H. P., and Ritter, J. M. 1970a. *Mol. Pharmac.* 6:357.

Rang, H. P., and Ritter, J. M. 1970b. *Mol. Pharmac.* 6:383.

Robison, G. A., Butcher, R. W., and Sutherland, E. W. in *Fundamental Concepts in Drug Receptor Interactions,* J. P. Danielli, D. J. Triggle, J. F. Moran (Eds.), Academic Press, New York, 1970, p. 59.

Sheridan, M. N. 1965. *J. Cell. Biol.* 24:129.

Singer, S. J., in Ciba Symposium *Molecular Properties of Drug Receptors,* R. Porter and M. O'Connor (Eds.), J. & A. Churchill, London, 1970, p. 229.

Stryer, L., in Ciba Symposium *Molecular Properties of Drug Receptors,* R. Porter
    and M. O'Connor (Eds.), J. & A. Churchill, London, 1970, 133.

Takagi, K., and Takahashi, A. 1968. *Biochem. Pharmac.* 17:1609.

Takeuchi, A., and Takeuchi, N. 1960. *J. Physiol.* 154:52.

Taylor, D. B., Creese, R., and Scholes, N. W. 1964. *J. Pharmac. Exp. Ther.* 144:293.

Thesleff, S. in Ciba Symposium *Molecular Properties of Drug Receptors,* R. Porter
    and M. O'Connor (Eds.), J. & A. Churchill, London, 1970, p. 33.

Trams, E. G. 1964. BBA 79:521.

Waser, P. G. in Ciba Symposium *Molecular Properties of Drug Receptors,* R. Porter
    and M. O'Connor (Eds.), J. & A. Churchill, London, 1970, p. 59.

Wooley, B. W., and Gommi, B. W. 1966. *Arch. Int. Pharmacodyn.* 159:8.

3

Histamine in the Brain: A Neurotransmitter?

SOLOMON H. SNYDER
KENNETH M. TAYLOR

Julius Axelrod always urges his students to develop their own new methods to solve new research problems, admonishing that "Major breakthroughs always seem to depend on developing ways of measuring body constituents that are sensitive, specific and perhaps most importantly, simple and reproducible." This is certainly true in the case of early research on histamine. Sir Henry Dale was able to open up the field of histamine research largely because histamine could be shown to contract smooth muscle in minute doses, providing a relatively simple and somewhat specific bioassay. In more recent years, histamine research, especially in the brain, has faltered largely because of difficulties in measuring histamine in the brain with adequate sensitivity, specificity, and *ease*. Accordingly, the first section of this review will focus on methodology for the assay of histamine in nervous tissue. Initially, however, let us consider the criteria for establishing whether or not histamine might be a probable neurotransmitter in the brain.

It is almost impossible to establish with rigor that any chemical is a neurotransmitter in the brain. Ideally, one would want to show release of the putative transmitter from a particular synapse and demonstrate at that synapse that application of the chemical in question mimics the actions of the natural transmitter. Presupposed in the statement that one should identify release of the transmitter is the assumption that the transmitter occurs in the appropriate nerve terminals along with metabolic machinery to synthesize it and that some means of inactivating its synaptic effects is available. In the brain one can rarely if ever confine one's attention to particular synapses in evaluating all of these parameters. More and more, neuropharmacologists are satisfying themselves with either neurochemical or neurophysiological evidence, rarely with both. Thus serotonin is an impressive candidate on neurochemical grounds, but neurophysiological evidence is almost wholly lacking for its transmitter role. Serotonin is localized to specific neuronal tracts in the brain (Fuxe, 1965), and subcellular localization studies indicate that it is present predominantly in nerve terminals (Michaelson and Whittaker, 1963; De Robertis, 1967; Kuhar et al., 1971). Moreover, it can be accumulated into nerve terminals by specific transport systems which could serve to inactivate its synaptic effects (Blackburn et al., 1967; Shaskan and Snyder, 1970). There is even strong evidence that the serotonin neuronal systems, the raphe nuclei and their projections, have a specific physiologic role in the regulation of sleep and in mediating the behavioral effects of psychedelic drugs. Despite all these neurochemical niceties, there is negligible direct evidence that the application of serotonin to particular neurons in the brain mimics the effects of the release of the natural transmitter.

With amino acids such as glycine, an inverse situation exists. There is strong neurophysiological evidence that glycine mimics the actions of the natural inhibitory transmitter in spinal cord (Werman et al., 1968), while supporting neurochemical evidence is much sparser. For histamine there is essentially no neurophysiological data to support a neurotransmitter role at any place in the body. However, several biochemical findings in recent years have strongly suggested an analogous role of brain histamine to that of the other biogenic amines, the catecholamines and serotonin. It is to these neurochemical observations that the remainder of this review will be devoted.

Histamine Estimation in Brain Tissue

Using chemical techniques, as long ago as 1919, John Jacob Abel and S. Kubota identified histamine in the pituitary gland (Abel and Kubota, 1919). With a bioassay procedure, Kwiatkowski found histamine in the brain, more in gray than in white matter (Kwiatkowski, 1943). The key fact that in the brain histamine is most highly localized to the hypothalamus was established by Geoffrey Harris and his collaborators in 1952 with a bioassay procedure (Harris et al., 1952), a finding which was confirmed and amplified by Adam (1961).

The introduction of a fluorometric assay for histamine in animal tissues (Shore et al., 1959) promised a sensitive, specific, and fairly simple technique for measuring histamine in brain tissue. Unfortunately, interference in brain tissue of spermidine with the histamine assay (Green, 1970; Kremzner and Pfieffer, 1965) required that the technique be modified by the introduction of fairly laborious purification in order to measure brain histamine reliably (Kremzner, 1966; Michaelson and Coffman, 1967; Medina and Shore, 1966). Recently we have been able to measure brain histamine with sensitivity, selectivity, and simplicity by a few modifications of an enzymatic-isotopic procedure (Snyder et al., 1966a).

The original enzymatic-isotopic technique for histamine assay (Snyder et al., 1966a) was developed when one of us (S.H.S.) was a student in the laboratory of Julius Axelrod. The idea came out of an experiment Dr. Axelrod was performing with frog brain. He was incubating extracts of frog brain with ^{14}C-S-adenosylmethionine, extracting into an organic solvent and examining for the presence of new methylated metabolites in a quest for new methylating enzymes. Although the frog's brain methylated a great deal of endogenous material, all the methylated radioactivity turned out to be methylhistamine, reflecting the activity of histamine methyltransferase, a well-known enzyme which Axelrod had described together with Brown six years earlier (Brown et al., 1959). Instead of being discouraged that no "new" enzyme emerged from the experiment, Julie suggested, "Sol, since the enzyme is methylating the endogenous histamine in the frog's brain, perhaps this might be a way to develop an assay for histamine."

The enzymatic-isotopic technique that eventuated depends on the methylation of endogenous histamine in tissues by added histamine methyltransferase using ^{14}C-S-adenosylmethionine as the methyl donor. A tracer amount of ^{3}H-histamine is added to correct for the varying degree of histamine methylation in different samples. ^{14}C-^{3}H-methylhistamine is separated from ^{3}H-histamine and ^{14}C-S-adenosylmethionine by extracting into chloroform from a salt-saturated alkaline solution (Fig. 3-1). Endogenous S-adenosylmethionine is destroyed by boiling the tissue, a procedure which also serves to precipitate protein. Unfortunately, there were difficulties in the application of the assay, as first developed, to the estima-

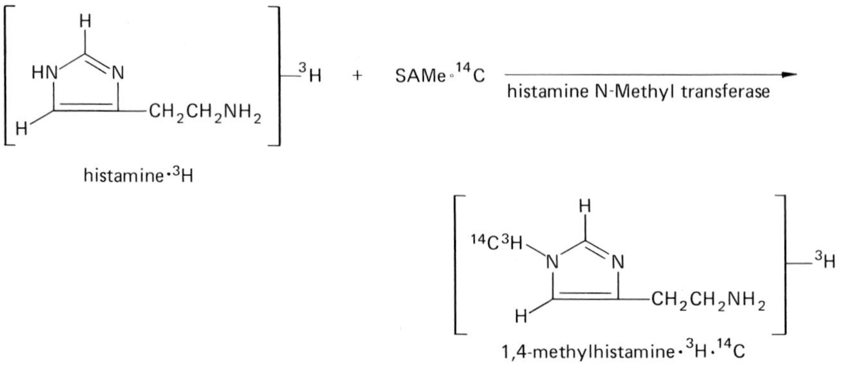

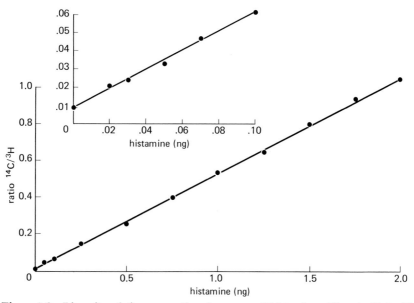

Figure 3-1   Enzymatic formation of ^{14}C-^{3}H-methylhistamine.

Figure 3-2   Linearity of the enzymatic microassay of histamine. Aliquots (1 to 20 μl) of standard solutions of histamine in 0.05 M sodium phosphate buffer, pH 7.9, containing 0.1 per cent Triton X-100 were placed in microfuge tubes (400 μl capacity; A. Thomas Co.) and were made up to 20 μl with the phosphate buffer. This was followed by the addition of 10 μl of the histamine methyltransferase reactant solution. This solution was prepared at 4°C immediately before addition and consisted of 1 part S-adenosyl-L-methionine-methyl-^{14}C (47.2 mCi/mmole, 0.64 μCi/ml),

tion of histamine in brain tissue, apparently related to its very low levels in brain and the presence of substances that interfered with the activity of histamine methyltransferase.

Recently by modifying the volume of the reaction mixture and the concentration of reactants, we have been able to enhance the sensitivity of the method so that in a macrosystem as little as 0.2 nanograms of tissue histamine can be detected in brain tissue, and employing a micro version of the assay, 0.02 ng can be detected reliably (Fig. 3-2) (Taylor and Snyder, 1971a, 1972a; Snyder and Taylor, 1971). Moreover, since in the microsystem virtually 100 per cent of added histamine is always methylated, we now use only a single isotope, ^{3}H-S-adenosylmethionine whose specific activity is 20 times that of the ^{14}C-isotope. Accordingly, presently we can reliably assay 0.004 ng of tissue histamine.

---

one part ^{3}H-histamine (7.26 Ci/mmole, 5 μCi/ml) and two parts of the guinea pig histamine methyltransferase preparation (3.8 mg protein/ml). Ten μl of this solution contained 1.6 nC (0.22 pmol) ^{3}H-histamine and 12.5 nC (0.28 nmol) AMe-^{14}C.

The mixture was incubated for 1 hour at 37°C. The reaction was stopped by the addition of 5 μl 1 M NaOH, the solution was saturated with NaCl and the methylhistamine formed in the reaction was extracted into 250 μl chloroform by applying a vortex to the capped microfuge tubes for 30 seconds, using a Lab-line Supermixer (A. Thomas Co.).

The aqueous phase was removed by aspiration and the organic phase was washed with 100 μl 1 M NaOH by applying a vortex for 10 seconds. The aqueous phase was carefully removed by aspiration and the organic phase was transferred to a glass vial and evaporated to dryness in a stream of air. Then 1 ml ethanol and 10 ml of toluene phosphor (0.4 per cent 2,4-diphenyloxazole benzene in toluene) were added and the radioactivity of ^{14}C and ^{3}H was measured in a Packard tri-carb liquid scintillation spectrometer for a counting period of 10 to 30 minutes. The efficiency of counting both ^{3}H and ^{14}C was found to be constant. Each assay was performed on triplicate samples.

^{3}H and ^{14}C were counted at an efficiency of 24 per cent and 61 per cent respectively. There was a 9 per cent overlap of ^{14}C into the tritium chanel but no overlap of ^{3}H into the ^{14}C channel. This overlap was allowed for in the calculation of the ratio of ^{14}C/^{3}H.

To demonstrate the presence of a single radioactive product the chloroform extracts were evaporated to a small volume and chromatographed on Whatman #1 paper with ethyl acetate-butanol-glacial acetic acid-water (1:1:1:1) or with ethanol-0.1 N HCl (9:1). A single peak of radioactivity was found in both solvent systems which corresponded in R_f to authentic methylhistamine. The amount of ^{14}C-methylhistamine, ^{3}H-histamine, and S-adenosyl-L-methionine-methyl-^{14}C extracted into chloroform in the above assay was 84 per cent, 4 per cent, and 0 per cent respectively. More than 85 per cent of the histamine in the samples was methylated by the above procedure.

Table 3-1   The Regional Localization of Histamine in the Monkey Brain (*Macaca mulatta*)

Cerebral Hemispheres	Histamine (mµg/mg protein)	Thalamus (cont.)	Histamine (mµg/mg protein)
Precentral gyrus cortex	0.81 ± 0.11	7 Ventral posterior nucleus	
Postcentral gyrus cortex	0.75 ± 0.08	thalamus	1.46 ± 0.10
Visual cortex Area 17	0.58 ± 0.07	Periventricular gray of	
Auditory cortex Area 41	0.48 ± 0.06	thalamus	3.84 ± 0.28
Insular cortex	1.09 ± 0.12	Habenula	1.74 ± 0.14
White matter	0.54 ± 0.05	Lateral geniculate body	1.82 ± 0.11
Corpus callosum	0.52 ± 0.04	Caudate nucleus	0.77 ± 0.03
Limbic Cortex		*Extrapyramidal Nuclei*	
Olfactory trigone	0.74 ± 0.09	Putamen	0.63 ± 0.02
Hippocampus	0.46 ± 0.04	Internal pallidum	1.76 ± 0.15
Amygdaloid nucleus	0.69 ± 0.07	External pallidum	0.63 ± 0.02
Septal nuclei	1.27 ± 0.12	Caudal medial nigra	1.16 ± 0.07
Pituitary and Pineal		Caudal lateral nigra	1.43 ± 0.14
		Rostral lateral nigra	1.92 ± 0.15
Pineal body	14.65 ± 1.56	*Midbrain*	
Posterior pituitary	4.49 ± 0.87		
Anterior pituitary	0.84 ± 0.12	Superior colliculus	0.71 ± 0.08
Hypothalamus		Interior colliculus	1.17 ± 0.08
		Interpeduncular nucleus	0.22 ± 0.03
Supraoptic nucleus	20.59 ± 6.79	Red nucleus	1.61 ± 0.11
Paraventricular nucleus	7.09 ± 0.66	Nucleus raphe	3.01 ± 0.23
Median eminence	11.42 ± 0.89	Central gray	3.61 ± 0.29
Infundibulum	5.21 ± 0.72	*Cerebellum and Lower Brain Stem*	
Preoptic nucleus	6.16 ± 0.31		
Ventromedial nucleus	17.01 ± 1.08	Pons	0.86 ± 0.04
Ventrolateral nucleus	15.78 ± 1.47	Cerebellar cortex	0.15 ± 0.01
Mammillary bodies	26.19 ± 0.98	Dentate nucleus	0.68 ± 0.05
Thalamus		Inferior olive	0.83 ± 0.05
		Dorsal motor nucleus	
Anterior nucleus		vagus	1.41 ± 0.08
thalamus	2.64 ± 0.16	Nucleus gracilis	0.95 ± 0.08
Dorsomedial nucleus			
thalamus	1.51 ± 0.09		

Three female monkeys (mid-cycle) and two male monkeys (1800 to 2200 g) were sedated with sodium pentobarbital (50 mg/kg i.p.) and bled to death. Their brains were rapidly removed, placed on crushed ice, and dissected by Dr. E. Gfeller, Department of Anatomy, on a cold glass slab in a cold room at 4°C.

Brain samples (5 to 20 mg) were homogenized in 10 volumes of 0.01 M sodium phosphate buffer, pH 7.9, containing 0.1 per cent Triton X-100 in microfuge tubes (400 µl capacity, A. Thomas Co.), using a moulded epon pestle. Samples of the homogenate were analyzed for histamine (Taylor and Snyder, 1972a) and protein (Lowry, Rosebrough, Farr, and Randall, 1951). Each value is the mean ± S.E.M. of five to ten determinations.

Regional Localization of Histamine in Mammalian Brain

Knowledge of the regional localization of neurochemicals has aided considerably in understanding their function in the brain. For the biogenic amines norepinephrine and serotonin, their localization to the hypothalamus and limbic forebrain enabled investigators to link them to the regulation of emotional behavior, long before there was strong evidence that they might be neurotransmitters. In 1952, careful bioassay revealed a localization of histamine to the hypothalamus (Harris et al., 1952). Subsequent investigations using a variety of assay procedures have reconfirmed the localization of histamine to the hypothalamus (Green, 1970). Adam (1959) examined the concentration of histamine in a few subdivisions of the hypothalamus. Employing the micro version of the enzymatic-isotopic assay for histamine, we have recently been able to explore the regional localization of histamine in monkey brain in considerable detail, focusing on individual nuclei of the hypothalamus and other brain regions (Table 3-1) (Taylor, Gfeller, and Snyder, 1972). In confirmation of earlier studies, the highest concentrations of histamine were found in the hypothalamus. However, there was as much as a 25-fold variation in histamine levels among the various nuclei of the hypothalamus (Table 3-1). The mammillary bodies had the highest levels of histamine, 250 times greater than the lowest found in the brain, i.e. in the cerebellum, and 5 times higher than concentrations in the infundibulum. The ventromedial and supraoptic nuclei had levels of histamine almost as high as those of the mammillary bodies. Histamine concentration in the paraventricular and preoptic nuclei was about 35 per cent that in the mammillary bodies but still 3 times higher than that in the infundibulum. While there was excellent consistency in values for most hypothalamic nuclei among the five monkeys, histamine concentration in the supraoptic nucleus varied as much as 10-fold in different animals.

Such findings may provide hints about the function of histamine in the brain. For instance, the supraoptic nucleus is thought to be predominantly concerned with the elaboration of neurosecretory granules containing the antidiuretic hormone (ADH). Conceivably, histamine neurons in this part of the brain may play a role in regulating the activity of these neurosecretory neurons. Perhaps the varying supraoptic histamine levels in different monkeys are related to episodic "stress-induced" discharge of ADH. Experiments are under way to examine the effects of water restriction or hypertonic saline on histamine synthesis in this area of the hypothalamus. The ventromedial region of the hypothalamus, among other functions, is involved in the regulation of eating behavior and, perhaps, histamine neurons may play a relevant role.

The catecholamines and serotonin have been shown by histochemical techniques (Fuxe, 1965; Dahlstrom and Fuxe, 1964) to have cell bodies localized to discrete areas of the brain stem. Although concentrations of these biogenic amines are highest in the nerve terminals, substantial levels also occur in areas of the brain rich in their cell bodies. If postulated histamine neurons were also to have cell bodies located in the brain stem, the existence of relatively high levels of histamine in discrete regions of the brain stem might indicate areas rich in the cell bodies of histamine neurons. Accordingly, it is of interest that there were marked differences in the levels of histamine throughout the brain stem. For instance, some of the highest levels occurred in the raphe nucleus and central gray, which contained six times the levels of histamine found in the superior colliculus. Within the substantia nigra, elevated histamine levels were restricted to an area rostro-medial within the zona compacta.

High concentrations of histamine also were observed in the median eminence and the pineal body. Since in most of the body outside of the brain histamine is largely confined to mast cells (Riley, 1959), it is probable that in the median eminence and pineal body, both of which contain mast cells, histamine is localized to mast cells. In mammalian brain, however, there is strong evidence that no mast cells are present (Riley, 1959; Kelsall and Lewis, 1964; Adam, 1959). Accordingly, it is unlikely that histamine in most regions of the brain is in mast cells. Indeed, subcellular fractionation studies to be discussed subsequently definitively established that mammalian brain histamine is localized to nerve terminals and not to mast cell granules.

The Subcellular Localization of Histamine and
Histamine Methyltransferase in Rat Brain

Subcellular fractionation is a valuable tool for determining the intracellular localization and possible function of numerous chemicals in the brain. When brain tissue is homogenized in isotonic sucrose, nerve terminals pinch-off to form membrane-bound sacs containing synaptic vesicles and cytoplasm which are referred to as "synaptosomes" (Whittaker, 1965; De Robertis, 1967). A high degree of synaptosomal localization for a compound has been considered an important criterion for neurotransmitter candidates. A number of putative neurotransmitters such as acetylcholine, norepinephrine, γ-aminobutyric acid, and serotonin are localized in brain synaptosomes.

Brain histamine in several mammalian species has been reported to be present predominantly in particulate subcellular fractions (Green, 1970). Some workers have reported the majority of brain histamine to be confined to the crude mitochondrial pellet (Michaelson and Coffman, 1967), while others have reported a greater proportion of brain histamine in microsomal fractions (Carlini and Green, 1963; Kataoka and De Robertis, 1966). The difference between these results may be related to the conditions of centrifugation used for preparing the crude mitochondrial fractions. Thus, studies showing histamine to be localized in the mitochondrial fraction involved centrifuging the supernatant fluid of nuclear pellets for longer times at higher centrifugal forces than did those experiments which reported histamine in the microsomal fraction. Kataoka and De Robertis (1966) and Carlini and Green (1963) compared the subcellular localization of histamine with that of other putative neurotransmitters such as serotonin and acetylcholine. In these studies histamine-containing particles sedimented more slowly than did those containing acetylcholine or serotonin, indicating that the histamine-storing particles do differ in sedimentation properties from particles containing other biogenic amines. In the microsomal fractions that were enriched in histamine in rat cerebral cortex, Kataoka and De Robertis (1966) observed numerous small nerve terminals in which they suggested histamine may be stored.

Recently by centrifuging linear continuous sucrose density gradients for brief periods of time, a procedure referred to as "incomplete equilibrium sedimentation," we were able to resolve populations of synaptosomes con-

Table 3-2   Subcellular Distribution of Histamine and Histamine Methyltransferase (HMT) in Five Rat Brain Regions

Region	Histamine				HMT			
	P_1	P_2	S	$\dfrac{P_1 + P_2}{S}$	P_1	P_2	S	$\dfrac{P_1 + P_2}{S}$
Hypothalamus	277	406	395	1.7	561	930	885	1.7
Striatum	52	111	150	1.1	255	405	612	1.1
Cerebral cortex	111	175	133	1.8	186	385	368	1.6
Cerebellum	20	26	90	0.5	904	126	183	5.7
Medulla oblongata-pons	31	60	92	1.0	272	492	645	1.2

Five rats were decapitated, their brains rapidly removed, and five regions were dissected and pooled. After homogenization in 0.32 M sucrose (0.005 M sodium phosphate buffer, pH 7.4), "nuclear" (designated P_1) and "crude mitochondrial" (designated P_2) pellets and supernatant fluids (S) were analyzed for histamine content and for histamine methyltransferase (HMT) activity. Histamine is expressed as ng/g protein, and HMT activity is expressed as mμmoles of methylhistamine/90 min/g protein. The results presented are the averages of two experiments whose results varied by less than 25 per cent.

taining different putative neurotransmitters (Kuhar et al., 1970). Synaptosomes storing serotonin as well as those storing catecholamines localized in denser portions of the gradients than did those containing γ-aminobutyric acid. With the sensitive enzymatic-isotopic method for histamine assay, we examined its subcellular localization as well as that of histamine methyltransferase (HMT), using the technique of incomplete equilibrium sedimentation (Kuhar et al., 1971a).

Initially, we evaluated the relative localization of histamine and HMT in different particulate fractions prepared from various regions of rat brain (Table 3-2). In all brain regions histamine tended to be localized predominantly to the crude mitochondrial fraction which is enriched in synaptosomes as well as free mitochondria. In most brain regions the relative localization of histamine and HMT in particulate fractions paralleled each other. In the cerebellum, however, HMT was highly localized to the "nuclear" fraction which contained more than five times as much enzyme activity as the crude mitochondrial or supernatant fractions. Mossy fiber endings in the cerebellum are known to form synaptosomes which sediment with the nuclear fraction (Israel and Whittaker, 1965) and which might constitute the major repository of HMT in the cerebellum.

In order to ascertain whether the histamine in the crude mitochondrial pellet occurred in synaptosomes or in free mitochondria, this pellet was layered on continuous sucrose gradients (1.5 to 0.32 M) and centrifuged for 90 minutes to apparent density equilibrium, a procedure which resolves free mitochondria from synaptosomes. Under these conditions, histamine (assayed in 15 discrete fractions after centrifuging each to form a pellet for histamine assay) was localized to an area of the gradient corresponding to the maximal potassium and lactic acid dehydrogenase activity. The highest levels of histamine occurred in a portion of the gradient less dense than the peak activity for monoamine oxidase, a marker for mitochondria. Hypotonic shock released histamine into the supernatant fluid. Since potassium and lactic acid dehydrogenase are markers for cytoplasm occluded within synaptosomes, and since synaptosomes but not mitochondria can be lysed by hypotonic shock, these data indicate that the histamine was localized to synaptosomes.

To determine how the sedimentation characteristics of the histamine-

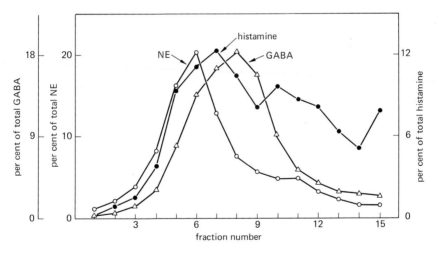

Figure 3-3   The subcellular distribution of hypothalamic ^{3}H-norepinephrine, histamine, and histamine methyltransferase in linear continuous sucrose gradients. The hypothalamic areas from 9 rats were excised, incubated with ^{3}H-NE, homogenized in 0.32 M sucrose in 0.005 M sodium phosphate buffer, pH 7.4, and a crude mitochondrial pellet was isolated by differential centrifugation. The pellet was resuspended and layered on a continuous gradient (0.32 to 1.5 M sucrose) and centrifuged at 100,000 × g for 20 minutes. Tritium, histamine, and histamine methyltransferase activities were determined in each gradient fraction. The experiment was replicated three times.

storing synaptosomes compared with those of sypnaptosomes storing other putative neurotransmitters, crude mitochondrial pellets were centrifuged in sucrose gradients by incomplete equilibrium sedimentation techniques (Fig. 3-3). Prior to homogenization hypothalamic slices were incubated with ^{3}H-norepinephrine (^{3}H-NE) to label the norepinephrine synaptosomes. Histamine showed a different pattern of localization from ^{3}H-NE. HMT and ^{3}H-NE displayed single discrete peaks in the same region of the gradient. Endogenous histamine content was distributed in two areas, one similar to that for HMT and ^{3}H-NE while a smaller peak of endogenous histamine was in a less dense region of the gradient. To compare the localization of histamine with that of γ-aminobutyric acid (GABA) as well as NE, in parallel experiments hypothalamic slices were incubated with ^{3}H-NE or ^{3}H-GABA and centrifuged by incomplete equilibrium sedimentation with subsequent assay of histamine as well as ^{3}H-NE and ^{3}H-GABA in individual fractions (Fig. 3-4). As had been observed previously (Kuhar et al., 1970), this centrifugal procedure separated the

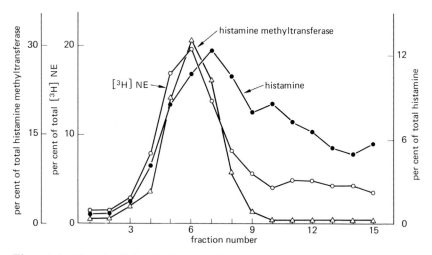

Figure 3-4   The subcellular distribution of hypothalamic norepinephrine (NE), histamine, and γ-aminobutyric acid (GABA) in linear continuous sucrose gradients. The hypothalamic areas from 9 rats were excised, incubated with either ^{3}H-NE or ^{3}H-GABA, homogenized in 0.32 M sucrose in 0.005 M sodium phosphate, buffer pH 7.4, and subjected to differential centrifugation. The pellet was resuspended and layered on a continuous gradient (0.32 to 1.5 M sucrose) and centrifuged at 100,000 × g for 20 minutes. Histamine and radioactivity were measured in each of 15 fractions. The experiment was replicated five times.

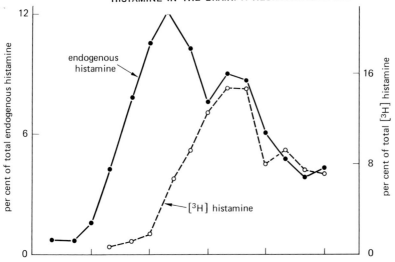

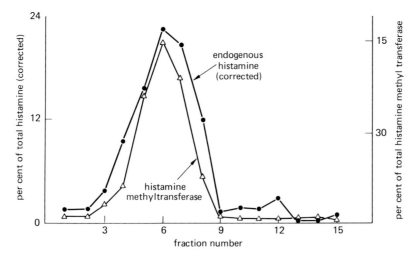

Figure 3-5 The subcellular distribution of histamine, histamine methyltransferase activity, and ³H-histamine added to hypothalamic tissue at 4°C in linear continuous sucrose gradients. Gradients were prepared in the same way as for Fig. 4 except that 1 μCi of ³H-histamine was added to the tissue at 4°C prior to homogenization to examine binding to subcellular particles. The profiles of endogenous histamine and ³H-histamine are compared (upper), and the profiles of "corrected" histamine and histamine methyltransferase are compared (lower). The "correct" histamine profile was produced by adjusting the height of the ³H-histamine peak to coincide with the second, lighter, endogenous histamine peak and subtracting the ³H-histamine values from those for endogenous histamine in each fraction. The experiment was replicated twice.

NE and GABA peaks with a minor peak of endogenous histamine again in a less dense region of the gradient.

Earlier we had found that exogenous histamine bound to a minor extent to particular fractions (Snyder et al., 1966b). To examine the distribution of exogenous histamine, brain slices were homogenized in ice-cold 0.32 M sucrose to which was added a tracer amount of ³H-histamine. When the crude mitochondrial pellet prepared from those slices was centrifuged by incomplete density equilibrium sedimentation, the ³H-histamine profile was exactly superimposable upon the minor peak of endogenous histamine (Fig. 3-5). This strongly suggests that this minor peak was produced by redistribution of endogenous histamine during homogenization and subsequent rebinding to particulate matter less dense than the majority of hypothalamic synaptosomes. If this is the case, subtracting this "redistributional component" from the profile of "apparent" endogenous histamine should provide an indication of the true distribution of endogenous histamine. When the profile of exogenous ³H-histamine was subtracted from that of apparent endogenous histamine, the resultant curve (Fig. 3-5) showed a single peak of distribution in a denser portion of the gradient, resembling the distribution of HMT activity.

Does exogenous histamine bind only to synaptosomes? How much more does it bind to particulate fractions than do other amines? To answer these questions, hypothalamic slices were homogenized together with ³H-histamine, ³H-NE, or ³H-inulin; and nuclear, crude mitochondrial and microsomal pellets as well as the supernatant fluid were assayed for tritium (Table 3-3). ³H-inulin and ³H-NE showed similar patterns of subcellular distribution with more than 70 per cent of the radioactivity confined to the supernatant fluid. In each particulate fraction there was about twice as much ³H-histamine as ³H-NE or ³H-inulin. This suggests that at low temperatures exogenous histamine can bind to a significant extent to a variety of subcellular fractions of brain tissues.

Thus, although redistribution of histamine during homogenization interferes with studies of its intracellular localization, it is evident that a major portion of brain histamine is localized to nerve terminals. This is an important piece of evidence in support of the case for histamine as a possible neurotransmitter in the brain. Moreover, it certainly rules out the possibility that histamine in the brain is localized to mast cell granules. Mast cell granules would sediment with the nuclear fraction which contained only a small portion of brain histamine.

Table 3-3 Subcellular Distribution of [³H]Histamine, [¹⁴C]Norepinephrine, and [³H]Inulin Added at 4°C to Rat Hypothalamus

Subcellular Fraction	[³H]Histamine	[¹⁴C]NE	[³H]Inulin
1000 × g, 10 min. pellet	21.0	11.0	13.0
17,000 × g, 20 min. pellet	22.5	12.0	12.0
100,000 × g, 60 min. pellet	5.0	2.5	2.7
Supernatant Fluid	51.5	74.5	72.3

Individual rat brain hypothalami were homogenized at 4°C in 2 ml of 0.32 M sucrose (O.OO5 M sodium phosphate buffer, pH 7.4) containing 0.1 μC of tritiated histamine, norepinephrine, or inulin. Three pellets and a supernatant fluid were obtained by differential centrifugation; radioactivity was determined in each. Results are the average of two experiments whose results differed by less than 15 per cent and are expressed as per cent of the total content of the homogenate (= 100 per cent).

Nuclear Localization of Histamine in Neonatal Rat Brain

In neonatal animals neurons actively proliferate and most neurotransmitters increase in concentration with age. Thus the observation that histamine levels in the brains of neonatal rats were five times higher than in adults was somewhat perplexing (Pearce and Schanberg, 1969; Ronnberg and Schwartz, 1969). It certainly suggested that most of the histamine in the brains of neonatal rats was not behaving like a neurotransmitter. Since the high levels of histamine occurred at times of rapid neuronal growth, one might suspect a role for histamine in the growth processes of the neonatal brain. This would be consistent with the suggestion that histamine is involved in certain cases of rapid tissue growth in which its synthesis is greatly enhanced (Kahlson and Rosengren, 1968). To clarify some of these questions we studied the subcellular localization of histamine in neonatal rat brain (Young et al., 1971).

We confirmed the observations that histamine levels are markedly elevated in neonatal rat brain. In the telencephalon and diencephalon, the time course of changes in histamine content showed a peak of 5 to 10 days with a gradual decline by 17 days to adult levels (Fig. 3-6). In the rhombencephalon, fluctuations in histamine levels were not as marked. The differences among these regions may relate to well-known patterns of growth in different parts of the brain. Brain maturation proceeds in a caudocephalic direction so that the rhombencephalon may have already undergone in fetal life rapid growth processes which, in the telencephalon and diencephalon, take place during the neonatal period.

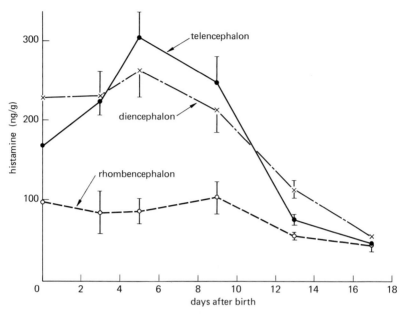

Figure 3-6 Developmental changes in concentrations of histamine in the rat brain. Rats were decapitated at various ages. Brains were dissected into telencephalon, diencephalon, and rhombencephalon and assayed for histamine content.

In subcellular fractionation studies employing differential centrifugation, about 90 per cent of brain histamine in the diencephalon at ages 3 to 13 days was confined to the crude nuclear fraction (Table 3-4). In other experiments the neonatal telencephalon and rhombencephalon showed the same subcellular distribution as the diencephalon. At 21 days the distribution pattern resembled that of adult rat brain with almost half of the histamine in the supernatant fluid and the remainder distributed between the crude nuclear and crude mitochondrial fraction. Unlike the situation of the minor peaks of histamine in sucrose gradients of adult rat brain, we could find no evidence of redistribution of neonatal brain histamine during homogenization. When a tracer quantity of ^{3}H-histamine was added to neonatal brains prior to homogenization, resultant centrifugation indicated that 90 per cent of the ^{3}H-histamine was confined to the supernatant fluid.

Crude nuclear fractions prepared by differential centrifugation may be contaminated by non-nuclear tissue constituents. To determine if hista-

Table 3-4   Change in the Subcellular Localization of Histamine During Development of the Rat Diencephalon

Age (days)	Histamine (ng/g of tissue)					Per Cent Total Histamine Content of Tissue			
	P_1	P_2	P_3	S	Total	P_1	P_2	P_3	S
3	129	12	0	0	141	91	9	0	0
5	188	7	2	3	200	94	4	1	1
7	210	23	2	2	237	88	10	1	1
13	139	16	0	7	162	87	10	0	3
21	14	18	2	26	60	23	30	3	44

Rats were decapitated at various ages, and brains were dissected into telencephalon, diencephalon, and rhombencephalon. The diencephalon regions from rats at various ages were homogenized with a Teflon pestle in 15 volumes of ice-cold 0.32 M sucrose. Differential centrifugation was employed according to the following scheme. The P_1 pellet was obtained by centrifuging the homogenate for 10 minutes at 1000 $\times$ g. The resulting supernatant fluid was centrifuged for 35 minutes at 18,000 $\times$ g to obtain the P_2 pellet. The supernatant fluid from the P_2 fraction was centrifuged for 1 hour at 100,000 $\times$ g to obtain the P_3 pellet and a soluble supernatant fraction (S). Recovery values obtained when exogenous histamine was added to subcellular fractions ranged from 90 to 100 per cent. The sum of the histamine content of the four subcellular fractions was 90 to 99 per cent of the total histamine content of the appropriate homogenate. Data presented are the mean values obtained from four different experiments whose results varied less than 20 per cent.

mine was indeed within nuclei in the neonatal rat brain, it would be desirable to prepare purified nuclear preparations. With the sucrose gradient technique of Blobel and Potter (1966) we obtained nuclear fractions which by light microscopic examination contained only nuclei and were free of contamination with unbroken cells or mast cell granules. In these purified nuclei 90 per cent of the histamine content of crude nuclear pellets was retained as was all of the DNA (Table 3-5).

To determine if histamine and DNA were stored in a similar fashion, we studied the retention of histamine and DNA within purified nuclei after washing with an isotonic medium with or without heparin (Table 3-5). Washing with the heparin-free buffer solution released 80 per cent of the nuclear histamine into the supernatant fluid, while all of the DNA remained in the nuclear fraction. Heparin causes swelling of nuclei from a variety of tissues and a partial release of DNA (Coffey and Kramer, 1970). Washing with the heparin-containing buffer medium did not release from the nuclei any more histamine than did washing with the buffer solution alone. However, heparin treatment resulted in a leakage of about

Table 3-5 The Differential Retention of Histamine and DNA Within Purified Nuclei from Neonatal Rat Brain

| | *Per Cent Histamine* | | *Per Cent DNA* | |
| | | *Supernatant* | | *Supernatant* |
Treatment	*Nucleus*	*Fluid*	*Nucleus*	*Fluid*
Blobel-Potter (1966)				
purification of P_1	91	9	100	0
Resuspension of nuclei				
Wash (TKM)	18	82	100	0
Heparin	21	79	51	49

Whole brains of 10 to 12 six-day-old littermate rats were homogenized at 0 to 4°C in 5 volumes of 0.32 M sucrose in TKM (50 mM Tris-HCl, pH 7.5 at 25°; 5 mM $MgCl_2$; 25 mM KCl) buffer with a Teflon pestle and centrifuged for 10 minutes at $1000 \times g$ to obtain the P_1 pellet. The pellets were resuspended with a Dounce homogenizer in 1.5 M sucrose in TKM buffer in the same volume as the original homogenate, and 5 ml portions were transferred into Corex tubes. A 10 ml syringe was used to underlay this suspension with about 7 ml of 1.8 M sucrose in TKM. The tubes were centrifuged for 1 hour at $40,000 \times g$; the supernatant fluid was decanted and the sides of the tubes were wiped with gauze. The pellets were resuspended by rapid vibration for 10 seconds in 2 ml of isotonic TKM buffer or the same buffer to which 0.2 mg/ml heparin had been added. The suspension was maintained at 4°C for 15 minutes and then was centrifuged at $1000 \times g$ for 10 minutes. The pellet and supernatant fluid were assayed for DNA and histamine. When ^{3}H-histamine was added before homogenization in these experiments, 99 per cent of the cpm was recovered in the $40,000 \times g$ supernatant. In these experiments, the total amount of DNA and of histamine recovered from the purified nuclei represented about half of the homogenate values. Data presented are the means of five different experiments in which values varied less than 15 per cent.

50 per cent of the nuclear DNA content into the supernatant fluid. The differential response of nuclear histamine and DNA to these treatments suggests that histamine and DNA are not stored in the same way. It is not clear why the storage of histamine in the nucleus survives differential and sucrose gradient centrifugation, yet can be washed out of the purified nuclei.

What might be the function of histamine in the nuclei of neonatal rat brains? Presumably it plays some role in the rapid growth processes of the brain and is probably involved with functions of the nucleus in regulating rapid growth. Histamine is a very basic compound. The polyamines, also highly basic, have been proposed as regulators of nucleic acid function in rapidly growing tissues, conceivably displacing histones from their binding sites on DNA or serving to stabilize ribosomal RNA (Tabor and Tabor, 1964; Cohen, 1970; Raina and Janne, 1970; Snyder, Kreuz, Medina, and Russell, 1970). It is possible that in the neonatal rat brain histamine plays a role analogous to that proposed for the polyamines.

Histamine Turnover in Rat Brain

Measuring the activity of particular classes of neurons in the brain with neurophysiologic techniques is quite difficult. The ability to measure the turnover rate of the catecholamines and serotonin has proved a valuable biochemical tool reflecting the activity of neurons which store these amines. We attempted to detect the synthesis of histamine *in vivo* in rat

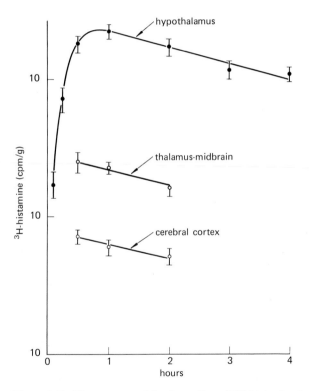

Figure 3-7   Time course of the formation of ^{3}H-histamine in regions of the rat brain after the intraventricular injection of 20 μCi of ^{3}H-histidine (20 μl). Each value is the mean $\pm$ S.E.M. of eight determinations. At early time intervals the radioactivity present in the thalamus-midbrain was less than double background values and is not depicted.

brain by administering tracer doses of ^{3}H-histidine intraventricularly and developing techniques to separate ^{3}H-histidine from the ^{3}H-histamine synthesized as well as from other metabolites (Taylor and Snyder, 1971a,b). Substantial synthesis of histamine was detected in the hypothalamus, with maximal formation about 1 hour after administration of ^{3}H-histidine and a gradual decline thereafter (Fig. 3-7). This corresponded to about 4 per cent of the ^{3}H-histidine concentration in the brain. In the thalamus-midbrain only about one-tenth as much ^{3}H-histamine was formed as in the hypothalamus, and in the cerebral cortex only about one-fortieth as much histamine was synthesized as in the hypothalamus. In the cerebellum, corpus striatum, and medulla-pons ^{3}H-histamine formation was considerably lower than in the cerebral cortex, and levels were less than double the blank values. White (1960) also observed the greatest formation of histamine from intraventricularly injected histidine in the hypothalamus of the cat brain.

Histidine can be decarboxylated to histamine in mammalian tissues by a "specific" histidine decarboxylating enzyme which can be inhibited by α-hydrazino-histidine or NSD-1055 (Schayer, 1957; Hakanson, 1963; Levine et al., 1965), or by the aromatic amino acid decarboxylase which also decarboxylates dihydroxyphenylalanine and 5-hydroxytryptophan and is inhibited by α-methyl-DOPA (Lovenberg et al., 1962). In order to determine whether histamine synthesized *in vivo* in rat brain was formed by the action of the specific histidine decarboxylase or by aromatic amino acid decarboxylase, we examined the effects of pretreatment with α-hydrazino-histidine, NSD-1055, α-methyl-DOPA, or saline 30 minutes prior to intraventricular administration of ^{3}H-histidine. Presumably, if histamine formation is attributable to aromatic amino acid decarboxylase, α-methyl-DOPA might be expected to inhibit its synthesis. Alpha-hydrazino-histidine and NSD-1055 both markedly lowered levels of ^{3}H-histamine in the hypothalamus and thalamus-midbrain, while in the cerebral cortex only α-hydrazino-histidine was effective. Alpha-methyl-DOPA failed to alter ^{3}H-histamine levels in any brain region. Although the lowering of ^{3}H-histamine would appear to reflect inhibition of histamine synthesis, such an effect could also be produced by alterations in the pools of endogenous histidine or ^{3}H-histidine. Accordingly, ^{3}H-histidine and endogenous histidine levels were assayed after treatment with these drugs (Table 3-6). None of the drugs produced any changes in the concentration of endogenous or tritiated histidine. These results suggest that the

Table 3-6   The Effect of α-Hydrazino-Histidine, NSD-1055, and α-Methyl-DOPA on Endogenous Histamine Levels and on the Formation of ^{3}H-Histamine from ^{3}H-Histidine

	Histidine μg/g	Histamine μg/g	^{3}H-Histidine cpm $\times$ 10^{-2}/g	^{3}H-Histamine cpm/g
Hypothalamus				
0.9 per cent NaCl	6.30 ± .54	0.192 ± .010	7654 ± 842	32570 ± 2100
α-hydrazino-histidine	6.14 ± .66	0.134 ± .009***	7746 ± 706	13390 ± 940***
NSD-1055	6.58 ± .55	0.117 ± .015***	8064 ± 632	19515 ± 1432***
α-methyl-DOPA	5.99 ± .60	0.186 ± .010	7448 ± 864	39620 ± 2433
Thalamus-Midbrain				
0.9 per cent NaCl	1.54 ± .26	0.068 ± .004	4686 ± 334	4395 ± 445
α-hydrazino-histidine	1.68 ± .35	0.035 ± .002***	4933 ± 286	2266 ± 291**
NSD-1055	1.43 ± .29	0.040 ± .005***	4328 ± 390	2426 ± 310**
α-methyl-DOPA	1.40 ± .28	0.062 ± .006	5064 ± 482	3825 ± 517
Cerebral Cortex				
0.9 per cent NaCl	0.92 ± .15	0.058 ± .004	1096 ± 107	896 ± 61
α-hydrazino-histidine	0.86 ± .17	0.043 ± .003**	1174 ± 94	499 ± 64**
NSD-1055	0.98 ± .26	0.049 ± .004	1004 ± 83	866 ± 85
α-methyl-DOPA	0.97 ± .19	0.051 ± .006	1234 ± 119	1035 ± 84

Drugs (200 mg/kg) were injected i.p. 30 minutes before rats received an intraventricular injection of 20 μl ^{3}H-histidine (20 μC). One hour later rats were sacrificed by immersion in liquid nitrogen, decapitated, their brains removed and dissected. Each value is the mean ± S.E.M. of eight determinations. Significance of difference between means of treated and control values: ***p < .001, **p < .01.

synthesis of histamine in rat brain *in vivo* is mediated by a specific histidine decarboxylase, a finding which is supported by recent *in vitro* studies of this enzyme in the rat brain (Schwartz et al., 1970).

Levine et al. (1965) found that α-hydrazino-histidine and NSD-1055 lowered histamine levels in several peripheral tissues, presumably by inhibiting the formation of histamine from histidine. If these drugs were to lower histamine levels in the brain similarly, they might provide a means of assessing the turnover rate of histamine. Accordingly, these drugs as well as α-methyl-DOPA were injected into rats at various doses and their hypothalami assayed for histamine (Table 3-7). At 100 mg/kg, α-hydrazino-histidine and NSD-1055 failed to alter histamine levels. However, at 200 mg/kg and at all higher doses, both drugs lowered histamine levels by about 40 per cent. Interestingly, doses as high as 500 mg/kg did not lower histamine levels by more than 40 per cent, suggesting that there was a drug-resistant pool of histamine. In all doses examined, α-methyl-DOPA failed to alter hypothalamic histamine levels. Similar effects were

Table 3-7   The Effect of Increasing Doses of α-Hydrazino-Histidine, NSD-1055, and α-Methyl-DOPA on the Concentration of Histamine in the Rat Hypothalamus

	Histamine Concentration (Per Cent of Control)		
Dose mg/kg	*α-Hydrazino-Histidine*	*NSD-1055*	*α-Methyl-DOPA*
100	89 ± 7	91 ± 8	84 ± 9
200	58 ± 5*	58 ± 3*	89 ± 8
300	50 ± 6**	57 ± 5*	113 ± 11
400	53 ± 6**	57 ± 6*	104 ± 8
500	58 ± 4*	60 ± 5*	84 ± 8

Rats received i.p. injections of drugs three hours before sacrifice. Each value is the mean ± S.E.M. of six determinations. Results are expressed as percentages of the mean control value in each experiment. Significance of difference from control concentration: ** $p < .01$, * $p < .05$.

obtained in the cerebral cortex, corpus striatum, and thalamus-midbrain. However, no depletion of histamine by these drugs was observed in the medulla-pons and cerebellum. In the hypothalamus, thalamus-midbrain, and cerebral cortex, after a single injection of 200 mg/kg of α-hydrazino-histidine or NSD-1055, the partial depletion was maintained for 24 hours. At 48 hours histamine levels in these brain regions had recovered to normal values.

When the early phases for the decline of hypothalamic histamine after α-hydrazino-histidine or NSD-1055 were plotted on a semilogarithmic

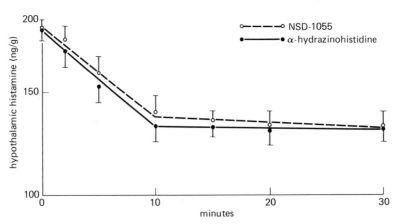

Figure 3-8   Time course of the depletion of histamine in the rat hypothalamus by α-hydrazino-histidine (200 mg/kg i.p.) and NSD-1055 (200 mg/kg i.p.). Each value is the mean ± S.E.M. of six determinations.

scale, the half-life for the decline for the "depletable" pool of hypothalamic histamine could be estimated (Fig. 3-8). With both drugs this portion of hypothalamic histamine fell with a half-life of about 5 minutes. It is not clear why these drugs failed to deplete brain histamine by more than 40 per cent. Perhaps this is related to the observation that they did not completely suppress the formation of histamine from intraventricularly administered histidine. Nonetheless, assuming that the partial depletion of brain histamine by these drugs is related to inhibition of histamine synthesis, the rate of decline may reflect the turnover rate of at least a portion of brain histamine. If so, our findings suggest that a pool of brain histamine, perhaps comprising about 40 per cent of brain levels, turns over much more rapidly than brain norepinephrine and serotonin, whose half-lives are several hours (Tozer et al., 1966; Iversen and Glowinski, 1966; Lin et al., 1969). The rapid turnover rate we have observed more closely resembles that reported for acetylcholine (Schuberth et al., 1969).

It is still conceivable that the lowering of brain histamine by NSD-1055 and α-hydrazino-histidine could have represented displacement or some other effect rather than inhibition of synthesis. If so, other drugs might be expected to alter histamine levels. Accordingly, we examined the effects of a large number of drugs. Reserpine in doses from 2.5 to 10 mg/kg at intervals from 1 hour to 24 hours failed to alter hypothalamic histamine levels in rat brain although we have observed a 50 per cent depletion of hypothalamic histamine with this drug in the mouse (Taylor and Snyder, 1972b), and Adam and Hye (1966) have observed a lowering of cat brain histamine. Chlorpromazine (10 mg/kg) and quinacrine (10 to 100 mg/kg), drugs which inhibit histamine methyltransferase, also failed to alter hypothalamic histamine levels 1 to 4 hours after administration. Moreover, pargyline (50 mg/kg), iproniazid (150 mg/kg), and tranylcypromine (25 mg/kg), inhibitors of monoamine oxidase, also did not change hypothalamic histamine concentration 2 or 24 hours after drug administration. In the cat, chlorpromazine and inhibitors of monoamine oxidase have been reported to produce modest elevations of brain histamine (Adam and Hye, 1966). Menon et al. (1970) reported that parachlorophenylalanine and 4-thiazolylmethoxyamine, markedly lowered rat brain histamine. We found that 4-thiazolylmethoxyamine, a potent inhibitor of histidine decarboxylase, depleted rat brain histamine to the same extent as NSD-1055 and α-hydrazino-histidine, whereas p-chlorophenylalanine was without effect (Taylor and Snyder, 1971a,b,c).

Acceleration of Brain Histamine Turnover
and Partial Depletion by Stress

In the case of serotonin and the catecholamines, valuable information regarding their physiological role has been obtained by examining the influence of varying environmental factors on their turnover rates. Thus far we have studied the influence of only a few procedures on rat brain histamine turnover. Initially, we used the stresses of cold exposure or restraint (Taylor and Snyder, 1971a,b). Rats were immobilized in plastic restraint boxes, placed in individual cages in a cold room (4°C), or maintained in the restraint boxes at 4°C, thus being subjected to both cold exposure and restraint. Thirty minutes of treatment by these procedures failed to alter histamine concentration in any brain regions examined. However, after 1 or 2 hours of cold exposure, restraint, or a combination of the two, histamine concentrations in the hypothalamus, thalamus-midbrain, and cerebral cortex were lowered (Table 3-8), while levels in the medulla-pons

Table 3-8   The Effect of Cold Exposure and Restraint on the Concentration of Histamine in Different Regions of the Rat Brain

| | Histamine (ng/g) | | | |
	Hypothalamus	Thalamus-midbrain	Cerebral cortex	Medulla-oblongata-pons
Control	182 ± 15	61 ± 7	59 ± 6	22 ± 5
Restraint				
0.5 hour	160 ± 16	63 ± 9	58 ± 9	19 ± 6
1 hour	$137 \pm 12^*$	58 ± 8	48 ± 7	20 ± 5
2 hour	$120 \pm 11^{**}$	48 ± 8	$37 \pm 6^*$	19 ± 4
Cold				
0.5 hour	149 ± 16	60 ± 9	55 ± 8	22 ± 4
1 hour	$129 \pm 16^*$	51 ± 8	$39 \pm 5^*$	24 ± 6
2 hour	$114 \pm 14^{**}$	42 ± 8	$35 \pm 5^*$	19 ± 4
Restraint & Cold				
0.5 hour	$141 \pm 11^*$	55 ± 8	49 ± 8	22 ± 5
1 hour	$119 \pm 10^{**}$	44 ± 6	$38 \pm 4^*$	24 ± 5
2 hour	$117 \pm 12^{**}$	$42 \pm 6^*$	$36 \pm 5^*$	20 ± 4

Rats were restrained in plastic restraint boxes or were placed in individual cages in a cold room maintained at 4°C or were maintained at 4°C in restraint boxes. Significance of difference between control and stressed groups, $** \ p < .01$, $* \ p < .05$. Each value is the mean $\pm$ S.E.M. of six determinations.

were unaffected. In preliminary experiments we found that histamine concentration in the cerebellum and corpus striatum were also unaltered by restraint or exposure to cold. In the hypothalamus, thalamus-midbrain and cerebral cortex, the maximal depletion of histamine was about 35 to 40 per cent, similar to the maximum lowering of histamine in these areas by histamine synthesis inhibitors. Interestingly, the brain regions whose histamine concentration was unchanged by cold or restraint were the same areas in which histamine levels were not lowered by NSD-1055 or α-hydrazino-histidine.

The role that histamine turnover might play in the partial depletion of brain histamine by restraint and cold exposure was studied by measuring the formation *in vivo* of hypothalamic histamine. Rats were subjected to restraint and cold exposure for 30 minutes, removed from the cold room for 5 minutes to receive an intraventricular injection of ^{3}H-histidine, and then returned to the cold room for periods varying from 15 minutes to 2 hours. The animals were then killed and their hypothalami assayed for ^{3}H-histidine, ^{3}H-histamine, and endogenous histidine. In control animals, allowed to move about freely in individual cages at room temperature, there was a rapid increase in ^{3}H-histamine levels with peak values at 1 hour, which fell about 30 per cent in the second hour (Fig. 3-9). Restraint and cold exposure markedly increased the initial formation of ^{3}H-histamine. At the earliest time interval examined, 15 minutes after ^{3}H-histidine administration and 45 minutes after the beginning of restraint and cold exposure, hypothalamic ^{3}H-histamine concentration was double control values, and by 30 minutes after ^{3}H-histidine adminstration it was almost triple control levels. One and 2 hours after injection of ^{3}H-histidine, ^{3}H-histamine levels in restrained and cold-exposed animals were slightly lower than those of control animals. ^{3}H-histidine and endogenous histidine in hypothalamus, thalamus-midbrain, cerebral cortex, and medulla-oblongata-pons of rats subjected to restraint and cold exposure for 15, 30, 60, or 120 minutes did not differ from those of control animals, indicating that changes in the formation of ^{3}H-histamine were not related to alterations in the size of the pool of histidine available for histamine formation.

Thus, in animals subjected to restraint and cold exposure, the depletion of hypothalamic histamine was associated with a marked enhancement of its synthesis. This suggests that these stresses lowered brain histamine levels by releasing the amine at a rapid rate, and an apparent compensa-

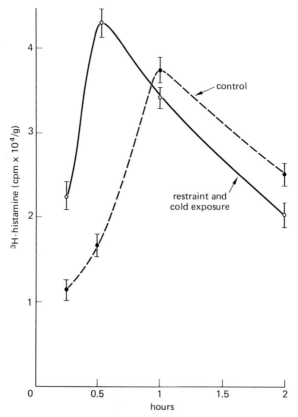

Figure 3-9   Time course of the effect of cold and restraint stress on the formation of ³H-histamine from ³H-histidine in the rat hypothalamus. Rats were placed in plastic restraint boxes in a cold room (4°C) for 30 minutes before receiving an intraventricular injection of 20 μCi (1 mμmole) of ³H-histidine. They were then returned to the restraint boxes in the cold room and sacrificed 15 to 120 minutes later. ³H-histamine, ³H-histidine, endogenous histamine, and endogenous histidine were determined in the hypothalamus (Taylor and Snyder, 1971c). In control and stressed groups at all time intervals there was no difference in the concentration of endogenous histidine and ³H-histidine in the hypothalamus. Each group consisted of 8 rats.

tory enhancement of histamine synthesis could not keep pace with the rate of amine release so that endogenous histamine levels were partially depleted.

Histamine Release by Depolarization of Brain Tissue

One of the classical criteria for a neurotransmitter is that it be released from neurons upon depolarization. With the catecholamines and serotonin, release from brain tissue by electrically or potassium-induced depolarization has been readily demonstrable by making use of the uptake systems for these amines (Baldessarini and Kopin, 1967; Chase et al., 1969). Brain slices are incubated with radioactive catecholamines or serotonin which are actively taken up and appear to mix with endogenous stores. Chemical or electrical depolarization enhances the base line efflux of radioactivity. Thus relatively small amounts of release are easily detected,

Table 3-9　The Release of Histamine from Slices of Rat Brain Hypothalamus

Experimental Condition	Histamine Per Cent Released	Histidine Per Cent Released
No additions　0°C	9.1 ± 0.5*	4.7 ± 0.4
No additions　37°C	19.7 ± 0.8	5.0 ± 0.5
Ca^{++} deleted	17.8 ± 0.9	5.1 ± 0.6
+ K$^+$ 60 mM	29.7 ± 1.1*	5.4 ± 0.4
+ EDTA 6 mM	13.6 ± 0.9	6.5 ± 0.7
+ Tetrodotoxin 10^{-5} M	21.1 ± 1.5	6.6 ± 0.6
+ K$^+$ 60 mM + EDTA 6 mM	19.2 ± 1.8	7.4 ± 0.8

Male Sprague-Dawley rats (200 to 240 g) were sacrificed by cervical dislocation. The brain was quickly removed and the hypothalamus was dissected into 1 mm wide strips which were placed on a McIlwain tissue chopper and sliced so that uniform slices of $1.0 \times 0.1 \times 0.1$ mm were prepared. The slices were washed twice by resuspension in 10 volumes of Krebs-Ringer solution at 4°C, and centrifuged at 10,000 $\times$ g for 10 minutes. They were then resuspended in 10 volumes of cold Krebs-Ringer solution and 50 μl samples were transferred to microfuge tubes (400 μl capacity, A. Thomas Co.). Aliquots (5 to 10 μl) of K$^+$, EDTA, or tetrodotoxin in Krebs-Ringer solution were added and the microfuge tubes were incubated at 37°C for 10 minutes in a flow of 95 per cent O$_2$ and 5 per cent CO$_2$. The tubes were cooled in an ice bath and centrifuged (10,000 $\times$ g for 10 min). Aliquots of the supernatant fluid were assayed for histamine and histidine (Taylor and Snyder, 1971d). The remainder of the supernatant fluid was removed and the pellet was resuspended in 50 μl of Krebs-Ringer solution. The tubes were placed in a boiling water bath for 10 minutes, cooled, and centrifuged at 15,000 $\times$ g for 10 minutes. Aliquots of the supernatant fluid were assayed for histamine and histidine (Taylor and Snyder, 1971d). Results are expressed as the percentage of total histamine or histidine released in each microfuge tube during the 10-minute incubation period. Each value is the mean ± S.E.M. of four determinations. The concentrations of additives are expressed as the final concentration in the incubation mixture.

* Significantly different from "no additions 37°" condition p < .001.

a critical factor, because less than 10 per cent of the tissue content of radioactive amine is generally released in these experiments. Since it is not possible to label the endogenous stores of histamine with radioactive amine, we have attempted to measure the efflux of endogenous histamine in small slices of rat hypothalamus depolarized with potassium (Table 3-9) (Taylor and Snyder, in preparation). The spontaneous efflux of histamine into the medium was greater at 37°C than at 4°C. Potassium depolarization of the hypothalamic slices elicited a further release of histamine.

In most neuronal systems, transmitter release requires calcium ions. When hypothalamic slices were incubated in a calcium-free medium, potassium released less histamine. EDTA, which chelates calcium ions, blocked completely the ability of potassium to release histamine. Interestingly, although the potassium-induced release of ^{3}H-norepinephrine from brain slices is reduced in calcium-free medium (Baldessarini and Kopin, 1967), ^{3}H-serotonin release in similar systems occurs normally in the absence of added calcium (Chase et al., 1969).

Under some experimental conditions, numerous investigators have found a variety of non-neurotransmitter compounds to be released by depolarization. Accordingly, we measure the efflux of histidine from hypothalamic slices, which was not altered by potassium depolarization (Table 3-9).

Thus depolarization of brain tissue can elicit a release of histamine in much the same way as norepinephrine and serotonin release has been demonstrated previously. For the latter two amines, it has been possible only to show release of exogenous ^{3}H-amine thought to label endogenous stores. In the case of histamine, we were able to detect the release of the endogenous amine. We assume that the histamine released originated in nerve terminals, because subcellular fractionation studies showed endogenous histamine to be localized in synaptosomes. Thus, histamine satisfies the important transmitter criterion of "release upon neuronal depolarization."

Unanswered Questions

Histamine in the brain shows many characteristics resembling the other biogenic amines. It is distributed unevenly throughout the brain. Its high concentration in selected hypothalamic nuclei may suggest specific functions for presumed histaminergic tracts which terminate in these areas.

Subcellular fractionation reveals that a major proportion of the histamine content in adult rat brain is localized to nerve terminals. Further subcellular fractionation in our laboratory now suggests that the histamine within these nerve terminals is concentrated in synaptic vesicles. Unlike other presumed neurotransmitters, histamine concentration is higher in the neonatal rat brain than in the adult. This appears to be related to its nuclear localization so that brain histamine in the neonatal rat plays some role other than that of a neurotransmitter, apparently connected with nuclear function. The exact significance of nuclear histamine in the neonatal rat brain remains perplexing.

Histamine is synthesized *in vivo* maximally in the hypothalamus, which contains the highest levels of endogenous histamine. At least a portion of brain histamine is stored in a dynamic state and turns over extremely rapidly. Stressful procedures such as cold exposure and restraint also accelerate histamine turnover and partially deplete its levels. Such stresses are nonspecific. Further experimentation will be needed to pinpoint the physiological role of brain histamine.

For most neurotransmitters there exists some mechanism whereby their synaptic activities may be terminated. Acetylcholine has its acetylcholinesterase. For the catecholamines (Iversen, 1967), serotonin (Blackburn et al., 1967; Shaskan and Snyder, 1970), γ-aminobutyric acid (Iversen and Neal, 1969), and conceivably glutamic acid and glycine (Neal and Pickles, 1968; Logan and Snyder, 1971; Johnston and Iversen, 1971), there exist selective high affinity uptake systems at nerve terminals. Using brain slices and synaptosomal preparations from a variety of brain regions and employing a wide range of ^{3}H-histamine concentrations, we have attempted to discern if brain tissue can accumulate histamine. Thus far, we have failed to demonstrate any temperature sensitive "uptake" of histamine by brain tissue to levels above those in the medium. It is still conceivable that there are uptake systems for histamine in nerve terminals of the histaminergic neurons which escape detection. Brain histamine levels are only about one-tenth the concentrations of serotonin and the catecholamines. Accordingly, the presumably small number of histaminergic nerve terminals may not suffice to produce a marked degree of histamine accumulation. We are currently examining brain areas rich in histamine, such as the mammillary bodies of the hypothalamus, for possible histamine uptake.

Ideally, one would prefer a histochemical technique to map with precision the neuronal tracts storing a putative neurotransmitter. Initial attempts at developing histamine-associated histochemical fluorescence in the hypothalamus with o-phthaladehyde have not been successful (Kuhar and Aghajanian, personal communication). Currently experiments are under way in our laboratory examining the effects of selective brain lesions on the histamine content of various areas of the rat brain (Logan and Snyder, in preparation). Detailed studies of the regional localization of histamine in the monkey brain have provided some hints as to areas that may be rich in histamine cell bodies or nerve terminals.

References

Abel, J. J., and Kubota, S. 1919. *J. Pharmacol. Exptl. Ther.* 13:243.
Adam, H. M. 1961. In *Regional Neurochemistry,* S. S. Kety and J. Elkes (Eds.), Pergamon Press, London, p. 293.
Adam, H. M., and Hye, H. K. A. 1966. *Brit. J. Pharmacol. Chemother.* 28:137.
Baldessarini, R. J., and Kopin, I .J. 1967. *J. Pharmacol. Exptl. Ther.* 156:31.
Blackburn, K. J., French, P. C., and Merrills, R. J. 1967. *Life Sci.* 6:1653.
Blobel, G., and Potter, V. R. 1966. *Science* 154:1662.
Brown, D. D., Tomchick, R., and Axelrod, J. 1959. *J. Biol. Chem.* 234:2948.
Carlini, E. A., and Green, J. P. 1963. *Brit. J. Pharmacol. Chemother.* 20:264.
Chase, T. N., Katz, R. I., and Kopin, I. J. 1969. *J. Neurochem.* 16:607.
Coffey, D., and Kramer, R. J. 1970. *Biochim. Biophys. Acta* 224:568.
Cohen, S. S. 1970. *Ann. N.Y. Acad. Sci.* 171:869.
Dahlstrom, A., and Fuxe, K. 1964. *Acta Physiol. Scand.* 67:481.
De Robertis, E. 1967. *Science* 156:907.
Fuxe, K. 1965. *Acta Physiol. Scand.* 64:37.
Green, J. P. 1970. *Handbook of Neurochemistry* 4:221.
Håkanson, R. 1963. *Biochem. Pharmacol.* 21:1289.
Harris, G. W., Jacobson, D., and Kahlson, G. 1952. In *Ciba Foundation Colloquia on Endocrinology,* G. E. W. Wolstenholme (Ed.), vol. 4, Churchill Press, London, p. 186.
Israel, M., and Whittaker, V. P. 1965. *Experientia* 21:325.
Iversen, L. L. 1967. *The Uptake and Storage of Noradrenaline in Sympathetic Nerves,* Cambridge University Press, London and New York.
Iversen, L. L., and Glowinski, J. 1966. *J. Neurochem.* 13:671.
Iversen, L. L., and Neal, M. J. 1968. *J. Neurochem.* 15:1144.
Johnston, G. A. R., and Iversen, L. L. 1971. *J. Neurochem.* (in press).
Kahlson, G., and Rosengren, E. 1968. *Physiol. Res.* 48, 155.
Kataoka, K., and De Robertis, E. 1966. *J. Pharmacol. Exptl. Ther.* 156, 114.
Kelsall, M. A., and Lewis, P. 1964. *Fed. Proc.* 23:1107.
Kremzner, L. T. 1966. *Analyt. Biochem.* 15:270.
Kremzner, L. T., and Pfieffer, C. C. 1965. *Biochem. Pharmacol.* 14:1189.
Kuhar, M. J., Green, A. I., Snyder, S. H., and Gfeller, E. 1970. *Brain Res.* 21:405.

Kuhar, M. J., Shaskan, E. G., and Snyder, S. H. 1971. *J. Neurochem.* 18:33.

Kuhar, M. J., Taylor, K. M., and Snyder, S. H. 1971a. *J. Neurochem.* 18:1515.

Kwiatkowski, H. 1943. *J. Physiol.* 102:32.

Levine, R. J., Sato, T. L., and Sjoerdsma, A. 1965. *Biochem. Pharmacol.* 14:139.

Lin, R. C., Costa, E., Neff, N. H., Wang, C. T., and Ngai, S. H. 1969. *J. Pharmacol. Exptl. Ther.* 170:232.

Logan, W. J., and Snyder, S. H. 1971. *Nature* (in press).

Lovenberg, W., Weissbach, H., and Udenfriend, S. 1962. *J. Biol. Chem.* 237:89.

Lowry, O. H., Rosebrough, N. J., Farr, A. L., and Randall, R. T. 1951. *J. Biol. Chem.* 193:263.

Medina, M., and Shore, P. A. 1966. *Biochem. Pharmacol.* 15:1627.

Menon, M. K., Aures, D., and Clark, W. G. 1970. *Pharmacologist* 12:205.

Michaelson, I. A., and Coffman, P. Z. 1967. *Biochem. Pharmacol.* 16:2085.

Michaelson, I. A., and Whittaker, V. P. 1963. *Biochem. Pharmacol.* 12:203.

Neal, M. J., and Pickles, H. G. 1969. *Nature* 222:679.

Pearce, L. A., and Schanberg, S. M. 1969. *Science* 166:1301.

Raina, A., and Janne, J. 1970. *Fed. Proc.* 29:1568.

Riley, J. F. 1959. *The Mast Cells,* E. and S. Livingstone, Edinburgh and London.

Ronnberg, A. L., and Schwartz, J. C. 1969. *C.R. Acad. Sci. Paris* 268:2376.

Schayer, R. W. 1957. *Am. J. Physiol.* 189:533.

Schwartz, J. C., Lampart, C., and Rose, C. 1970. *J. Neurochem.* 17:1527.

Shaskan, E. G., and Snyder, S. H. 1970. *J. Pharmacol. Exptl. Ther.* 175:404.

Shore, P. A., Burkhalter, A., and Cohn, V. P. 1959. *J. Pharmacol. Exptl. Ther.* 127:182.

Snyder, S. H., Baldessarini, R. J., and Axelrod, J. 1966a. *J. Pharmacol. Exptl. Ther.* 153:544.

Snyder, S. H., Glowinski, J., and Axelrod, J. 1966b. *J. Pharmacol. Exptl. Ther.* 153:8.

Snyder, S. H., Kreuz, D. S., Medina, V. J., and Russell, D. H. 1970. *Ann. N.Y. Acad. Sci.* 171:749.

Snyder, S. H., and Taylor, K. M. 1971. In *Methods in Neurochemistry,* R. Rodnight and N. Marks (Eds.), Plenum Press, New York (in press).

Tabor, H., and Tabor, C. W. 1964. *Pharmacol. Rev.* 16:245.

Taylor, K. M., and Snyder, S. H. 1971a. *Science* 172:1037.

Taylor, K. M., and Snyder, S. H. 1971b. *Fed. Proc.* 30:501.

Taylor, K. M., and Snyder, S. H. 1971c. *J. Pharmacol. Exptl. Ther.* (in press).

Taylor, K. M., and Snyder, S. H. 1972a. *J. Neurochem.* (in press).

Taylor, K. M., and Snyder, S. H. 1972b. *J. Neurochem.* (in press).

Taylor, K. M., Gfeller, E., and Snyder, S. H., 1972. (in preparation).

Tozer, T. N., Neff, N. H., and Brodie, B. B. 1966. *J. Pharmacol. Exptl. Ther.* 153:177.

Werman, R., Davidoff, R. A., and Aprison, M. H. 1968. *J. Neurophysiol.* 31:81.

White, T. 1960. *J. Physiol.* 152:299.

Whittaker, V. P. 1965. *Progr. Biophys. Molec. Biol.* 15:39.

Young, A. B., Pert, C. D., Brown, D. G., Taylor, K. M., and Snyder, S. H. 1971. *Science* 173:247.

4

The Uptake, Storage, Release, and Metabolism of GABA in Inhibitory Nerves

LESLIE L. IVERSEN

Those readers familiar with the literature on adrenergic neurotransmission may have noticed that I have substituted GABA for noradrenaline in one of Julie Axelrod's favorite titles. In other chapters of this volume are summarized some of the remarkable advances in our understanding of adrenergic neurotransmission which have been made by the application of biochemical methods; studies pioneered and catalyzed in very large part by his work and guidance. From this explosion of knowledge in the catecholamine field has come real progress in understanding the basic mechanisms of drug actions on adrenergic neurons. The pharmacology of neurotransmission had traditionally been devoted to the study of drug actions on *postsynaptic* receptors, at which drugs may mimic or antagonize the actions of the naturally occurring neurotransmitter substance. It is now clear, however, that drugs can also modify many aspects of the biochemical functions of the *presynaptic* nerve terminal. Thus, drugs may inhibit the biosynthesis of the neurotransmitter, the catabolic breakdown, or the storage of the transmitter in intraneuronal vesicle sites. The inactivation of the transmitter by uptake into the synaptic terminal or by metabolism can also be inhibited, with a consequent enhancement of its normal postsynaptic effects. Other drugs may take the place of the natural transmitter and act as "false transmitters." Although the details of these processes are most clearly understood for adrenergic synapses, such pharmacological mechanisms could in principle also operate at synapses in which other transmitters are involved. At cholinergic synapses certain drug actions can already be explained in this way. Thus, in addition to cholinergic agonist and antagonist drugs, compounds are known which modify cholinergic transmission by inhibiting the inactivation of acetylcholine by acetylcholinesterase, and we know of at least one drug with a presynaptic site of action—namely, hemicholinium.

In this chapter I will attempt to explore how a similar approach can be applied to synaptic transmission involving the neurotransmitter gamma-aminobutyric acid (GABA). This will often prove a difficult task, since by comparison with the adrenergic systems so little is known about the pharmacology of GABA-inhibitory mechanisms. However, the time may now be ripe for this subject to be examined more thoroughly. We may hope that our understanding of the biochemistry and pharmacology of adrenergic synapses will prompt us to ask the right questions about GABA synapses, so that progress in this area may be quite rapid.

Since it is only recently that GABA has attained respectability as a neurotransmitter substance, I will first review briefly the evidence in favor of the view that it does indeed serve such a function. I will then give a highly personal account of the biochemical and pharmacological properties of GABA synapses, and indicate some of the large gaps that exist in our understanding and knowledge of such systems.

GABA as an Inhibitory Neurotransmitter Substance

In Crustaceans

The crustacean nervous system offers an attractive model for the study of inhibitory synapses, since these occur peripherally in such organisms. For example, crustacean muscles receive a dual innervation by both excitatory and inhibitory motor nerves, and the inhibitory neuromuscular junctions are readily accessible for experiment. In contrast, the inhibitory synaptic processes involved in vertebrate motor pathways take place entirely within the brain and spinal cord, and are consequently extremely inaccessible for experimental study. The studies of inhibitory neuromuscular transmission in crustaceans by Fatt and Katz (1953) and later by Dudel and Kuffler (1961) established two fundamental principles in our understanding of the neurophysiology of inhibitory synaptic transmission. First that the inhibitory transmitter may stabilize the resting membrane potential of the postsynaptic cell by producing selective changes in the ionic permeability of this membrane; and second that inhibitory transmitters can also be released and act as synapses on presynaptic excitatory nerve terminals to reduce the number of quanta of excitatory transmitter released. The two principal types of inhibitory synaptic transmission, postsynaptic and presynaptic, both occur in crustacean neuromuscular transmission. Neither adrenergic nor cholinergic drugs were active either in exciting or inhibiting crustacean muscles (for review see Furshpan, 1959), so it was clear that other transmitters were involved. The possible role of GABA in inhibitory transmission was suggested by the finding of Bazemore, Elliott, and Florey (1957), that GABA was the most important inhibitory substance in an extract of mammalian brain that inhibited discharges in the crustacean stretch receptor (another invertebrate preparation in which peripheral inhibitory synapses occur). GABA was soon found also to have potent inhibitory effects on crustacean muscles (for review, see Kuffler, 1960). Detailed studies of the effects of inhibitory nerve stimulation and those of applied GABA on the membrane potential of crayfish muscle cells showed that the actions of GABA very closely mimicked those of the naturally occurring inhibitory neuromuscular transmitter. Both compounds acted by causing a selective increase in the permeability of the muscle membrane to chloride ions, thus tending to stabilize the membrane potential at or near to the chloride equilibrium potential (Boistel and Fatt, 1958; Grundfest et al., 1959; Kuffler, 1960; Takeuchi and Takeuchi, 1965). Takeuchi and Takeuchi (1965) also showed that the surface of the muscle membrane in the immediate vicinity of motor nerve terminals was very much more sensitive to GABA than other areas, suggesting that GABA receptors were concentrated at the motor endplate regions. Furthermore, GABA was not effective when injected inside the muscle fibers, indicating that the GABA receptors occurred only on the outside surface of the muscle membrane.

Pharmacological identity between the naturally occurring inhibitory transmitter and GABA was also suggested by the finding that postsynaptic inhibition was blocked by picrotoxin, which also blocked the postsynaptic actions of GABA (Florey, 1957). The actions of GABA and the natural inhibitory transmitter were also similar at presynaptic inhibitory synapses in the crustacean neuromuscular innervation, and again both actions were blocked by picrotoxin (Dudel and Kuffler, 1961; Dudel, 1965a, b).

Considerable weight was added to the hypothesis that GABA was the naturally occurring inhibitory transmitter at crustacean neuromuscular junctions by the finding that GABA was the most potent inhibitory sub-

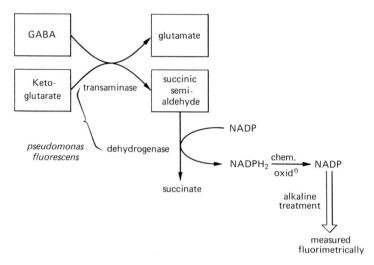

Figure 4-1   Enzyme fluorimetric assay for GABA. GABA-T and SSA-dehydrogenase partially purified from a bacterial source are used as reagents for a sensitive and specific assay of GABA, which is converted to succinate in the presence of an excess of α-ketoglutarate and NADP. NADPH₂ formed during this conversion is assayed by sensitive fluorimetric procedures. For details see Kravitz and Potter (1965) and Otsuka et al. (1966).

stance in extracts of lobster motor nerves, lobster CNS, and crab muscles (Dudel et al., 1963; Kravitz et al., 1963). These studies established unequivocally that GABA was present in considerable amounts in the lobster nervous system. Later the concentrations of GABA were determined by an enzymic microassay procedure (Fig. 4-1) in extracts of physiologically identified inhibitory and excitatory motor axons of the lobster (Kravitz et al., 1963; Kravitz and Potter, 1965). It was found (Table 4-1) that GABA was present in very much higher concentrations in the inhibitory (I) fibers than in excitatory (E). The enzyme responsible for the biosynthesis of GABA, glutamate decarboxylase, was later found to be detectable only in I axons and not in E axons (Kravitz et al., 1965; Hall et al., 1970). In a further elegant extension of these studies it was possible to show that not only the axons of I neurons but also the cell bodies of I neurons in lobster abdominal ganglia contained much higher concentrations of GABA than did those of E neurons (Table 4-1) (Otsuka et al., 1967).

If GABA is the inhibitory transmitter released by I motor neurons it

Table 4-1   GABA and related enzymes in inhibitory (I) and excitatory (E) lobster nerves

	I axons	E axons	I/E ratio
GABA concentration in axoplasm—M	0.105	0.0008	>100
Glutamate decarboxylase activity—p.mol/cm/hr	60	nil	>300
GABA-Glu transaminase activity—p.mol/cm/hr	32	23	1.5

Results obtained by assays of single axons, physiologically identified as having I or E motor function (Kravitz and Potter, 1965; Hall et al., 1970).

should be possible to demonstrate such a release directly in isolated nerve-muscle preparations. This indeed proved to be the case; Otsuka et al. (1966) found that the efflux of GABA from such preparations was increased during electrical stimulation of the I nerve, but not in response to stimulation of the E nerve (Table 4-2).

Thus the evidence that GABA is the inhibitory transmitter released at inhibitory terminals in lobster muscles is as complete as that for any other transmitter. To summarize: GABA mimics very precisely the actions of the naturally occurring inhibitory transmitter; GABA is present in high concentrations in I motor neurons but not in E neurons; the biosynthetic enzyme is present exclusively in I neurons; and GABA is released in response to I nerve stimulation but not to E nerve stimulation. It seems very probable that GABA serves a similar function at other inhibitory synapses in the lobster—for example, on the stretch receptor—and that GABA also plays a similar role in crustaceans other than the lobster.

Table 4-2   Release of GABA from lobster inhibitory neurons

Sample	GABA Content—10^{-10} of Collection Samples	Net Release of GABA—10^{-10} moles
Rest	1.7 ± 0.12 (46)	–
I nerve stimulation, 5/sec	3.2 ± 0.76 (8)	1.5
I nerve stimulation, 10/sec	4.9 ± 0.61 (5)	3.2
E nerve stimulation, 5 & 10/sec	1.7 ± 0.26 (10)	nil

Average amounts of GABA recovered in 25-minute rest and stimulation periods from superfused lobster opener muscle preparations. Inhibitory (I) or excitatory (E) nerve stimulation was applied at the stated frequency for the first 15 minutes of the 25-minute collection period. Values are means ± S.E.M. for number of determinations indicated in parentheses. From Iversen et al. (1966).

In Mammalian CNS

Interest in the effects of GABA on invertebrate receptors was first stimulated by the finding that GABA was probably identical with an important inhibitory substance present in extracts of mammalian brain, termed Factor I (Elliott and Jasper, 1959; Florey, 1964). The finding that GABA had extremely potent inhibitory effects on invertebrate stretch receptor neurons and muscles prompted considerable interest in the possibility that GABA might also be involved in inhibitory synaptic transmission in the mammalian CNS. It is only during the past five years, however, that persuasive evidence has become available to support this view. There are many reasons for the rather remarkable delay which occurred in obtaining such evidence. Perhaps the most important factor responsible for this delay was the fact that GABA was first investigated as a potential candidate for the major inhibitory transmitter in the mammalian spinal cord. It was soon found that although GABA had powerful inhibitory effects when applied locally onto spinal neurons by microiontophoresis, these effects did not exactly mimic those of the naturally occurring inhibitory transmitter for such neurons (for review see Curtis and Watkins, 1965). In particular, GABA usually failed to cause a hyperpolarization of spinal neurons, whereas naturally occurring IPSP's were hyperpolarizing. Furthermore, naturally occurring inhibitory transmission in the spinal cord was antagonized by strychnine, which usually failed to block the inhibitory actions of GABA on the same neurons (Curtis and Watkins, 1965; Curtis, 1969). Largely because of these discrepancies, GABA fell temporarily out of favor as a candidate for an inhibitory transmitter in mammalian CNS. It is now possible to explain the reason for these early findings in spinal cord, since it seems likely that glycine rather than GABA is the major inhibitory transmitter in the spinal cord (Aprison, Davidoff, and Werman, 1970; Curtis, 1969). On the other hand, GABA seems likely to be an important transmitter in other areas of the mammalian CNS, for example, in the cerebellum and cerebral cortex (for reviews see Krnjević, 1970; Hebb, 1970).

Interest in GABA was revived by the finding that micro-iontophoretically applied GABA caused hyperpolarization of Deiters' neurons (Obata et al., 1967) and in the cerebral cortex (Krnjević and Schwartz, 1966). The output of the cerebellum is inhibitory and is transmitted by Purkinje cell axons which terminate on Deiters' neurons. The effects of

GABA on Deiters' neurons were found to be similar to those evoked by stimulation of Purkinje cell axons, and both effects were unaffected by strychnine (Obata et al., 1967). Krnjević and his colleagues in an important series of studies were able to show that inhibitory synaptic transmission in the cerebral cortex was also strychnine-insensitive (Krnjević et al., 1966), and by intracellular recording techniques that the actions of the naturally occurring cortical inhibitory transmitter were closely similar to those produced by applied GABA (Krnjević and Schwartz, 1967). In both cases the hyperpolarizing response was due to a selective increase in the permeability of the neuron membrane to chloride ions; the response could be converted into a depolarizing one by the intracellular injection of chloride ions.

Recently it has been reported that the alkaloid bicuculline acts as a specific antagonist of the actions of GABA in the mammalian brain (Curtis et al., 1970a). Bicuculline antagonized the naturally occurring inhibitory transmitter and applied GABA at strychnine-insensitive neurons in the cerebral cortex, cerebelllum, and hippocampus (Curtis et al., 1970b). The discovery of bicuculline may mark a most important advance, since by this means it seems possible to establish a "pharmacological identity" between the actions of the naturally occurring inhibitory transmitter and GABA in various brain regions. So far, however, a conflicting claim has appeared in the literature concerning the usefulness of bicuculline in this respect (Godfraind et al., 1970).

Although there is little direct evidence that GABA is localized in inhibitory nerve terminals in the brain, the regional distribution of GABA in the mammalian CNS is consistent with the view that it serves an inhibitory transmitter role. Thus GABA concentrations are high in regions such as the cerebral cortex, in which strychnine-insensitive inhibition predominates, and lower in areas such as spinal cord, in which inhibition is mainly strychnine-sensitive, probably involving glycine as transmitter (Baxter, 1970; Fahn and Côté, 1968; Shank and Aprison, 1970). More detailed studies of the distribution of GABA in the layers of the cerebellar cortex (Kuriyama et al., 1966b) have shown that GABA is present in highest concentrations in the Purkinje cell layer. Similar studies in retina indicate that GABA may be associated with inhibitory interneurons in the amacrine cell layers of the retina (Kuriyama et al., 1968a) and with inhibitory interneurons in the hippocampus (Fonnum and Storm-Mathison, 1971). Microchemical analyses of individual neurons dissected from cerebellum and Deiters' nucleus suggest that GABA is present in high concentrations in Purkinje cells, and in the terminals of these neurons on Deiters' neurons. The amount of GABA associated with individual Deiters' neurons was found to be markedly reduced after lesions which caused degeneration of the Purkinje fiber input (Otsuka et al., 1971). Glutamate decarboxylase activity in Deiters' nucleus was also found to be reduced after cerebellar lesions which caused a degeneration of Purkinje axon terminals, suggesting that the GABA biosynthetic enzyme is also concentrated in these inhibitory nerve terminals (Fonnum et al., 1970).

A release of GABA has been detected by perfusion of the fourth ventricle in the cat during stimulation of the Purkinje axons (Obata and Takeda, 1969). In our own studies we have also been able to demonstrate a similar release of GABA from the surface of the cat visual cortex, during electrical stimulation of the surface of the cortex, or of the lateral geniculate nucleus under conditions which evoke cortical synaptic inhibition (Iversen et al., 1971). In these experiments stimulation caused a marked increase in the rate of efflux of GABA into a cortical superfusate (Table 4-3). Chemical analysis of the collected superfusate samples revealed that the release of GABA was highly specific—there were no significant changes in the efflux of any other amino acid or ninhydrin-positive substance. While these experiments are not as simple as those with the crustacean neuromuscular junction, in which a clearly defined neuronal pathway was stimulated, the results, nevertheless, add further weight to the view that GABA is an important inhibitory transmitter in the mammalian brain.

Table 4-3   Release of GABA from cat cerebral cortex by electrical stimulation

Type of stimulation	GABA release ($n.mole/7min/cm^2$)		
	Before stim. (A)	During stim. (B)	Increase on stim. (B/A)
Bipolar electrodes on cortical surface	0.30 ± 0.09	$2.19 \pm 0.61**$	7.4
Monopolar electrode on cortical surface	0.20 ± 0.05	$0.59 \pm 0.11*$	2.9
Lateral geniculate nucleus	0.22 ± 0.05	$1.26 \pm 0.24**$	5.7

GABA was collected and assayed in 7-minute cortical superfusate samples before and during stimulation. Results are means $\pm$ S.E.M. for six to twelve experiments for each type of stimulation (from Iversen et al., 1971). $* = P < 0.025$, $** = P < 0.01$ when compared with pre-stimulation value.

In summary, GABA mimics very precisely the effects of the naturally occurring inhibitory transmitter on certain neurons in the mammalian cerebellum and cerebral cortex; such neurons are strychnine-insensitive and may be bicuculline-sensitive. In at least one instance—the terminals of Purkinje axons on Deiters' neurons—there is evidence that GABA is present in high concentrations in inhibitory nerve terminals, and the biosynthetic enzyme GAD is also concentrated in these terminals. Finally, a release of GABA in response to stimulation of inhibitory pathways has been demonstrated. It thus seems very likely that GABA does act as a major inhibitory transmitter substance in the CNS, although it is also clear that it is not the only such transmitter.

This conclusion does not necessarily imply that a transmitter role represents the *only* physiological function of GABA in the mammalian CNS. The possibility that GABA is *also* involved in some way in the regulation of intermediary metabolism in the brain is one that has attracted biochemists, and this possible additional role of GABA must still be considered. However, the precise function which GABA might fulfill in intermediary metabolism remains unspecified, whereas its role in inhibitory synaptic transmission is now clearly delineated. The latter role thus seems likely to be the most fruitful area for further investigation.

Biochemistry and Pharmacology of GABA Synapses

Pharmacology of GABA Receptors

Invertebrates. Receptors for GABA in crustacean stretch receptors and neuromuscular junctions have been extensively studied pharmacologically (Edwards and Kuffler, 1959; Grundfest et al., 1959; McGeer et al., 1961; Dudel, 1965a,b). The relative potencies of various structural analogues of GABA in such preparations are summarized in Table 4-4. The results are generally consistent; in each case GABA was found to be the most potent inhibitory agonist. Shortening or lengthening the carbon chain of GABA greatly reduced agonist potency, with approximately a tenfold decrease for each carbon added or subtracted. Unsubstituted acidic and basic groups appeared to be essential, and substitutions on the carbon chain of GABA invariably reduced activity. Of the compounds substituted in this way, the β-hydroxy analogue of GABA retained the highest potency. Substitution of the amino group of GABA by a guanidino group

Table 4-4   Activity of GABA analogues at GABA receptors in crustaceans

Compound	Structure	Activity relative to GABA = 1000		
		(a)	(b)	(c)
glycine	$H_2N.CH_2.COOH$	1	1	1
β-alanine	$H_2N.CH_2CH_2.COOH$	50	41	3
GABA	*$H_2N.CH_2CH_2CH_2.COOH$*	*1000*	*1000*	*1000*
5-aminopentanoic acid	$H_2N.CH_2CH_2CH_2CH_2.COOH$	77	25	20
6-aminohexanoic acid	$H_2N.CH_2CH_2CH_2CH_2CH_2.COOH$	10	12	1
7-amino-n-caprylic acid	$H_2N.CH_2CH_2CH_2CH_2CH_2CH_2.COOH$	–	1	–
α-guanidinoacetic acid	$H_2N.C.NH.CH_2.COOH$ NH	715	290	333
β-guanidinoproprionic acid	$H_2N.C.NH.CH_2CH_2.COOH$ NH	715	990	1000*
γ-guanidinobutyric acid	$H_2N.C.NH.CH_2CH_2CH_2.COOH$ NH	125	6	10*
β-guanidinobutyric acid	$H_2N.C.NH.CH.CH_2.COOH$ NH CH_3	110	–	143*
γ-hydroxybutyric acid	$HO.CH_2CH_2CH_2.COOH$	14	–	–
2,4-diaminobutyric acid	$H_2N.CH_2CH_2CH.COOH$ NH_2	5	–	–
β-hydroxy-GABA	$H_2N.CH_2CH$ $CH_2.COOH$ OH	–	100	500
β-aminobutyric acid	$H_2N.CH_2CH$ $CH_2.COOH$ NH_2	–	4	1
taurine	$H_2N.CH_2CH_2CH_2SO_3H$	5	–	–

Results from (a) = Edwards and Kuffler (1959), crayfish stretch receptor; (b) = McGeer et al. (1961), crayfish stretch receptor, and c) = Dudel (1965a), crayfish muscle. In all cases GABA was effective at a concentration of approximately 10 μM. Asterisk * indicates that these drugs failed to cause a reduction in resistance of muscle membrane.

as in guanidinoacetic acid led to the retention of potent inhibitory actions. However, in crayfish muscle guanidino analogues other than guanidinoacetic acid showed interesting differences in their actions on presynaptic inhibitory receptors on excitatory nerve terminals, and postsynaptic inhibitory receptors on muscle fibers. The guanidino analogues, particularly β-guanidinopropionic acid, were potent agonists at the presynaptic receptor sites, but these compounds did not have direct inhibitory effects on the muscle membrane receptors. Thus, this group of compounds did not cause an increase in the conductance of the muscle membrane (Dudel, 1965a). On the contrary, β-guanidinopropionic acid acted as a competitive antagonist of the actions of GABA at such postsynaptic inhibitory receptors (Dudel, 1965b). These results thus suggest that there may be different types of GABA receptor at presynaptic and postsynaptic synapses in the crustacean neuromuscular system. Both types of receptor are potently stimulated by GABA, and at each, picrotoxin is the most effective antagonist drug. Recently it has been found that the alkaloid bicuculline will also antagonize the actions of GABA on crustacean stretch receptors (McLennan, 1970).

Mammalian Neurons. Information on the pharmacology of GABA receptors in the mammalian CNS has proved far more difficult to obtain. The technique of micro-iontophoretic application of drugs onto the surface of neurons in the CNS does not lend itself readily to quantitative studies of dose-dependent effects. Because of uncertainties about the exact position of the micro-electrode tip with respect to the neuron from which recordings are made, and because it is difficult to determine the exact amount of drug discharged from the electrode, it is impossible to ascertain precisely the concentration of drug to which the receptors are exposed. Another difficulty stems from the existence in the CNS of inhibitory receptors other than those for GABA. Thus, in the spinal cord, receptors for glycine are present in abundance and have to be distinguished from those at which GABA is the agonist drug. Fortunately, the latter distinction can be made fairly readily by the use of strychnine, which at low doses is a selective antagonist of the glycine receptors (Curtis, 1969). At high doses, however, strychnine also antagonizes the actions of GABA on, for example, cortical neurons (Johnson et al., 1970). GABA appears to be a very potent agonist for the strychnine-insensitive type of receptors, although the sulphonic acid analogue of GABA, 3-aminopropanesulphonic acid, may be slightly more potent than GABA on spinal cord GABA receptors (Curtis et al., 1968 a,b). Analogues of GABA with shorter carbon chains appear to be active only on glycine receptors, whereas longer chain analogues and substituted GABA analogues act only as agonists for

Table 4-5   Inhibition of spinal neurons by amino acids

Compound	Action	Strychnine-sensitive
glycine	—— Yes	
L-α-alanine	— Yes	agonists for glycine receptors?
L-serine	– Yes	
β-alanine	—— Yes	
taurine	— Yes	
GABA	—— No	
3-hydroxy-GABA	— No	agonists for GABA receptors?
3-aminopropanesulphonic acid	—— No	
5-aminopentanoic acid	— No	
6-aminohexanoic acid	– No	

(From Curtis, 1969)

the GABA receptors, with potencies lower than that of GABA itself (Curtis et al., 1968a,b).

Table 4-5 summarizes the actions of these compounds on receptors in the spinal cord. As mentioned above, the alkaloid bicuculline is reported to act as an antagonist at GABA receptors while having no effect on the actions of glycine (Curtis et al., 1970). An interesting analogue of GABA is the hallucinogenic isoxazole derivative muscimol (Fig. 4-2), which was reported to have an inhibitory potency comparable to that of GABA at strychnine-insensitive receptors on spinal neurons (Johnston et al., 1968).

In summary—rather little is yet known about the pharmacology of GABA receptors, particularly in the mammalian CNS. These is as yet insufficient evidence to determine whether the latter receptors are closely

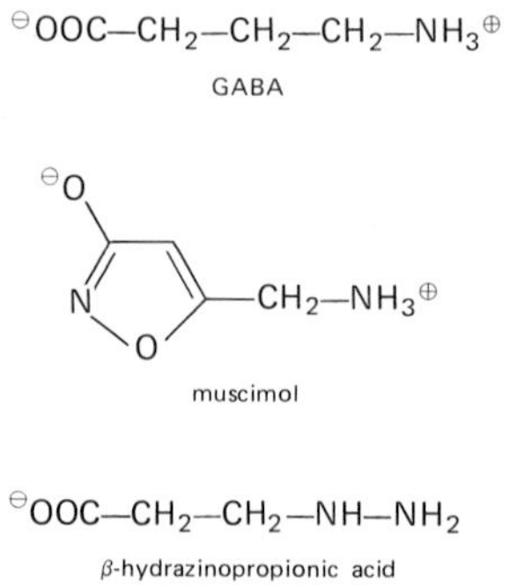

$$^{\ominus}OOC-CH_2-CH_2-CH_2-NH_3^{\oplus}$$

GABA

muscimol

$$^{\ominus}OOC-CH_2-CH_2-NH-NH_2$$

β-hydrazinopropionic acid

Figure 4-2

similar or even perhaps identical in their pharmacological properties to those in the crustacean nervous system. There are certain similarities: in each case, when structural analogues of GABA are tested, GABA is the most potent agonist; the effects of GABA in both systems are mediated by an increase in the chloride-ion permeability of the postsynaptic membrane; and bicuculline antagonizes both vertebrate and invertebrate GABA receptors.

Biosynthesis of GABA

Glutamate Decarboxylase (GAD I). GABA is formed in nervous tissues by the decarboxylation of L-glutamate, catalyzed by the enzyme L-glutamate decarboxylase (GAD I). The enzyme has been purified from mouse and calf brain (Susz et al., 1966; Jenny and Solberg, 1969; Roberts and Kuriyama, 1968) and from lobster CNS (Molinoff and Kravitz, 1968). The enzymes from mouse and calf brain seem to be similar in their properties, but the enzyme from lobster CNS differs in certain important respects from the mammalian enzymes. The lobster GAD is not strongly inhibited by chloride ions, and exhibits product inhibition with a Ki for GABA of 1.25 mM (Molinoff and Kravitz, 1968). Mammalian GAD I is strongly inhibited by chloride ions in the range 10 to 100 mM, but is insensitive to inhibition by GABA. The chloride effect is also found with other anions, with activity apparently related to the free energy of adsorption of various anions $(I^- > NO_3^- > Br^- > Cl^- > acetate^-)$ (Susz et al., 1966). The anion inhibition is reversible and competitive with GABA. The inhibition obtained with any anion is dependent on the pH, with the effect being greater at pH 5.0 to 5.5 than at pH 7.0 to 7.5 (Susz et al., 1966). These results suggest that the anionic inhibition may be due to an interaction with positively charged group(s) at the active site of the enzyme. Both invertebrate and mammalian enzymes require pyridoxal phosphate as cofactor, and are inhibited by a wide variety of pyridoxal antagonists, including various carbonyl trapping agents such as aminooxyacetic acid and various hydrazines (Baxter, 1970).

GAD II. A second mammalian glutamate decarboxylase, GAD II, has been described. This enzyme is distinguished from GAD I because it is insensitive to inhibition by chloride ions, and is stimulated rather than inhibited by carbonyl trapping agents (1 mM amino-oxyacetic) (Haber,

Kuriyama, and Roberts, 1970a,b). In contrast to GAD I, the GAD II enzyme has been found in various non-neuronal tissues, including mammalian kidney, cerebral and peripheral blood vessels, white matter of CNS and in human glial cells grown in tissue culture and gliomas removed at surgery (Haber et al., 1970a,b; Kuriyama et al., 1970). The physiological or metabolic significance of this second type of glutamate decarboxylase is at present unknown, but it seems unlikely to be involved in the biosynthesis of GABA at inhibitory nerve terminals.

Regulation of GABA Synthesis. The rate of biosynthesis of GABA in the mammalian brain has been the subject of many investigations, but the results available from studies using labelled precursors such as glucose are often conflicting. This is probably due to the complexities involved in interpreting metabolic studies in the CNS, where a multiplicity of "metabolic pools" exists for various intermediary metabolites. A recent study in which the rate of turnover of the GABA pool in cerebral cortex slices was measured after pulse-labelling with radioactive GABA, indicated that the GABA turnover was equivalent to about 8 per cent of the total carbon flux of the tricarboxylic acid cycle (Balazs et al., 1970). This would suggest a half-time for the GABA pool in brain of approximately 10 minutes. No comparable estimates are available for GABA turnover in the crustacean nervous system.

On the other hand, the mechanisms involved in the regulation of GABA synthesis are better understood in the crustacean system than in the mammalian. In detailed studies of GABA metabolism in isolated large inhibitory and excitatory motor axons of the lobster it has been found that GAD is present in high activity only in the axoplasm of the inhibitory fibers (Kravitz et al., 1965; Hall et al., 1970). GABA-Glu transaminase activity (GABA-T) is present in both inhibitory and excitatory axoplasm, but the maximum activity of this enzyme is less than that of GAD in the inhibitory nerve axoplasm. Consequently, since both types of axon contain a high concentration of L-glutamate, GABA will tend to accumulate in the inhibitory neurons. A steady state will then be reached regulated by negative feedback, since high concentrations of GABA inhibit lobster GAD. Measurements of the Ki for GABA inhibition of GAD, and the steady state concentrations of glutamate and GABA in the inhibitory nerve axoplasm are consistent with this proposed regulatory mechanism. (Kravitz et al., 1965; Hall et al., 1970).

Product inhibition, however, cannot be the mechanism by which GABA synthesis is regulated in the mammalian CNS, since here the GAD I is not inhibited by GABA. The marked inhibitory effects of chloride-ion concentration on mammalian GAD I seem more likely to be involved in the regulation of GABA synthesis in mammalian brain (Roberts and Kuriyama, 1968; Baxter, 1970). It has even been suggested that variations in the intracellular chloride-ion concentration might be sufficient to determine whether a given neuron synthesized and released GABA or glutamate as inhibitory or excitatory transmitter respectively (Roberts and Kuriyama, 1968). The concept that inhibitory neurons which utilize GABA and excitatory neurons which utilize glutamate might differ only by their intracellular anion content is intriguing, but so far lacks any direct confirmatory evidence. Since the chloride concentration of inhibitory nerve terminals is not known, it is also impossible to determine whether this is in fact important in regulating the activity of GAD I in the mammalian brain. Since there is evidence that neurons in the molluscan nervous system have widely different intracellular chloride-ion concentrations (Kerbut and Meech, 1966) this remains an attractive hypothesis.

Even less is known about the factors which control the rate of synthesis of the enzyme GAD. There have been reports that the activity of this enzyme changes during hibernation (Robinson and Bradley, 1963), after adrenalectomy (Pandolfo and Macaione, 1964), and after electroconvulsive shock treatment (Pfeifer et al., 1962). It has been suggested that GABA may act as a repressor for GAD synthesis, since elevated steady state levels of GABA inhibited the formation of GAD in developing chick and mouse brain (Haber et al., 1970c; Sze, 1970; Sze and Lovell, 1970b).

Cellular and Subcellular Location of GAD I. There are considerable regional differences in GAD activity within the mammalian CNS (Albers and Brady, 1959; Muller and Langemann, 1962). White matter has the lowest activity; and highest activity was found in monkey brain to be in the substantia nigra. More detailed studies using microchemical procedures have shown that GAD activity is particularly high in the Purkinje cell layer of the cerebellum (Kuriyama et al., 1966b), in dorsal gray matter of spinal cord (Graham and Aprison, 1969), and in the pyramidal layer of the hippocampus (Fonnum and Storm-Mathisen, 1971). A definite association between the GAD activity of Deiters' nucleus and the Purkinje nerve terminals in this region was indicated by the finding that the GAD activity of Deiters' nucleus was significantly reduced after cerebellar lesions which caused a specific degeneration of such terminals (Fonnum et al., 1970).

Several studies have examined the subcellular distribution of GAD in brain homogenates (Salganicoff and De Robertis, 1965; Balazs et al., 1966; Fonnum, 1968; Neal and Iversen, 1969). These results consistently indicate that GAD in brain homogenates is associated with synaptosomes, which may contain as much as 75 to 80 per cent of the total activity, the remaining enzyme being recovered in the supernatant fraction. GAD in homogenates of Deiters' nucleus was also recovered in a synaptosome fraction, a finding consistent with the hypothesis that the enzyme is contained mainly in Purkinje fiber terminals in this region (Fonnum et al., 1970). The subcellular distribution of GAD thus suggests that the enzyme is localized in nerve terminals in mammalian brain. The distribution of GAD closely resembles that of choline acetyl transferase (Whittaker, 1965). This suggests that it is unlikely that GAD I is associated in any important amounts with non-neuronal structures in the brain. The large amounts of GAD in nerve terminals indicate that these probably represent the most important sites for GABA synthesis. That nerve terminals are capable of GABA synthesis is clearly indicated by experiments which show that GABA is formed rapidly from labelled glucose in isolated synaptosome preparations incubated *in vitro* (Bradford and Thomas, 1969).

Within nerve terminals, GAD appears to be free within the axoplasm, since virtually all of the particle-bound enzyme associated with synaptosome fractions can be released by hyposmotic shock (Fonnum, 1968). Some enzyme may be recovered in association with particle fractions if the osmotic lysis is performed in the presence of low concentrations of Ca^{++} ions, but such association is thought to be artifactual (Fonnum, 1968). In the lobster inhibitory nerve axoplasm GAD is also present in a free form (Hall et al., 1970).

Inhibition of GABA Synthesis in vivo. A number of studies have sought to correlate the convulsant effects of various hydrazides with an inhibition of GABA synthesis caused by these compounds (Killam and Bain, 1957; Baxter and Roberts, 1959, 1961; Balzer et al., 1960; Tapia and Awapara,

1967, 1969). Unfortunately this attractive hypothesis has proved upon further investigation to be considerably more complex. While it is known that various convulsant hydrazides inhibit GAD in *in vitro* studies, it is not clear that such inhibition occurs *in vivo*. Even if it does, the hydrazides seem to act mainly as pyridoxal antagonists, and as such they are likely to interfere with the activity of many other pyridoxal enzymes *in vivo*. GAD inhibition *in vivo* is also difficult to assess, since such inhibition may not be apparent when the enzyme is assayed *in vitro* in a system with added pyridoxal phosphate. The hypothesis that convlusant hydrazides act by inhibition of GABA synthesis seemed to be supported by the finding that the concentration of GABA in the brain was reduced after the administration of these compounds (Balzer et al., 1960; Maynert and Kaji, 1962). However, the convulsions induced by thiosemicarbazide (20 mg/kg) were prevented by administration of pyridoxal (50 mg/kg), although there was still a decline in brain GABA concentration (Baxter, 1969). Thiosemicarbazide was also found to inhibit the conversion of labelled glutamate to GABA in brain homogenates, but it was ineffective in slices of intact brain (Sze and Lovell, 1970a). It must be concluded that no causal relation has yet been established between the convulsant effects of substances such as thiosemicarbazide and an inhibition of GABA synthesis. What is needed for future pharmacological studies is a systematic search for more specific inhibitors of GAD, perhaps among analogues of L-glutamate rather than pyridoxal antagonists. Whether L-glutamate-γ-hydrazide (Tapia and Awapura, 1967) or allylglycine (Alberici et al., 1968) represents such specific inhibitors is not clear; neither of these compounds seems to be entirely specific in its effects on GAD, although both have convulsant activity and are GAD inhibitors.

Catabolism of GABA

GABA-Glu Transaminase and SSA-dehydrogenase. The pathways of GABA metabolism are similar in the lobster nervous system and mammalian brain (Fig. 4-3). In each case GABA is metabolized by a pyridoxal-dependent transaminase, and the deaminated product succinic semialdehyde is oxidized to succinate by a specific NAD-dependent dehydrogenase. GABA-Glu transaminase (GABA-T) has been studied in purified preparations from mammalian brain (Waksman and Roberts, 1965; Sytinsky and Vasilijev, 1970) and in extracts of lobster nervous

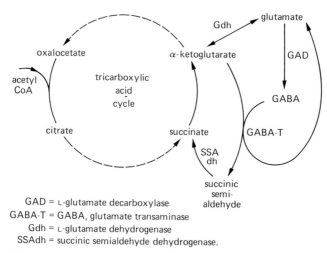

GAD = L-glutamate decarboxylase
GABA-T = GABA, glutamate transaminase
Gdh = L-glutamate dehydrogenase
SSAdh = succinic semialdehyde dehydrogenase.

Figure 4-3   Metabolism of GABA in nervous tissue.

system (Hall and Kravitz, 1967a). The lobster enzyme has a K_m for L-glutamate of 0.4 to 0.6 mM, and for α-ketoglutarate (α-KG) of 0.1 to 0.2 mM and a pH optimum of 8.5 to 9.0. The mammalian enzyme has a K_m for L-glutamate of 4 to 5 mM and K_m for α-KG of 2 to 5 mM, with a pH optimum of 8.0 to 8.5. Both invertebrate and mammalian transaminases will also act on other substrates related to GABA, including β-alanine, δ-aminovaleric acid, other ω-amino acids, and $\alpha\gamma$-diaminoglutaric acid. For both the lobster and mammalian enzyme, however, there seems to be an absolute specificity for α-KG.

Although the GABA-T reaction is reversible, the back reaction from succinic semialdehyde and glutamate probably does not occur to any important extent *in vivo,* since succinic semialdehyde (SSA)-dehydrogenase is present in high activity in conjunction with GABA-T (Miller and Pitts, 1967; Sheridan et al., 1967) and thus effectively removes succinic semialdehyde. SSA-dehydrogenase from mammalian brain (Kammeraat and Veldstra, 1968; Albers and Koval, 1961) has a high specificity for both succinic semialdehyde and NAD; the K_m values are 5 to 10 μM for SSA and about 0.1 mM for NAD. In contrast, the lobster enzyme will also act to some extent on acetaldehyde as substrate and can also utilize NADP (Hall and Kravitz, 1967b).

Alternative Pathways for GABA Metabolism. A variety of alternative metabolic pathways have been postulated for GABA metabolism in mammalian brain. These include the formation of γ-guanidinobutyric acid by transamidination with arginine; formation of GABA-containing peptides such as homocarnosine (GABA-histidine) and homoanserine (GABA-1-methyl histidine); formation of β-hydroxy-GABA, γ-butyrobetaine, γ-aminobutyrylcholine, or homopantothenic acid (for review see Baxter, 1970). A most interesting possibility is that SSA may under certain conditions become reduced to form γ-hydroxybutyric acid, instead of being oxidized in the normal manner. It has been reported that SSA can be converted to γ-hydroxybutyric by lactic dehydrogenase (Fishbein and Bessman, 1964). The presence of γ-hydroxybutyrate in brain has been confirmed by a gas chromatographic procedure (Roth and Giarman, 1970a,b), and the formation of small amounts of this substance from labelled GABA has also been demonstrated in this way (Roth and Giarman, 1970b). This pathway could be of considerable importance, since γ-hydroxybutyrate is known to have strong depressant activity in the CNS; it acts as a soporific and anesthetic when administered *in vivo* (Laborit, 1964; Roth et al., 1966). Nevertheless, there seems little doubt that the metabolism of GABA by GABA-T and SSA-dehydrogenase constitutes the *major* pathway for GABA metabolism in mammalian brain (Balazs et al., 1970).

Cellular and Subcellular Location of Catabolic Enzymes. The distribution of GABA-T has been studied by biochemical assay of the enzyme in dissected regions of CNS and other tissues, and in subcellular fractions. Unlike GAD, GABA-T is not restricted to CNS tissues, but occurs in peripheral organs also, particularly in liver and kidney (Caciappo et al., 1959). Within the CNS the enzyme is found in highest activity in gray matter, and there is considerable variation in activity among different regions of brain and spinal cord (Salvador and Albers, 1959; Sheridan, Sims, and Pitts, 1967); with high activity in caudate nucleus, hypothalamus, cortical gray, and certain cranial nerve nuclei. The cellular localization of this enzyme and SSA-dehydrogenase has also been studied by a specific histochemical method, in which the $NADH_2$ formed during the oxidation of GABA to succinate reduces a tetrazolium salt to an insoluble formazan derivative (van Gelder, 1965, 1966).

The results obtained with this method are in good agreement with those from biochemical analyses, and show that in mouse and rabbit brain stem and spinal cord the GABA metabolizing enzymes are present in particularly high activity in nerve cell bodies and nerve endings in the reticular system of the brain stem, in motor neurons of the ventral horn of spinal cord, in neurons of cranial nerve nuclei (vagus, hypoglossal, trigeminal), and in Purkinje cells in cerebellum. The histochemical method also reveals high activities of the GABA-metabolizing enzymes in a variety of non-neuronal elements in the CNS. There appears to be high activity in all cells in contact with the blood or cerebrospinal fluid, including ependymal cells lining the ventricular system, the choroid plexus, and cerebral blood vessels. It has been suggested that the localization of the enzymes in such sites may account for the blood-brain barrier for GABA (van Gelder, 1967). The occurrence of GAD II in similar sites, such as the cerebral blood vessels, may also constitute an enzymic barrier for the entry of glutamate into the brain, since glutamate would be converted by this enzyme into GABA which would then be degraded by the GABA-metabolizing enzymes. Since glutamate is a normal component of plasma and possesses powerful excitatory effects in the CNS, such a mechanism might be of more physiological importance than a barrier for GABA itself, which is not known to occur in plasma.

Subcellular distribution studies show that both GABA-T and SSA-dehydrogenase are mitochondrial enzymes (Salganicoff and De Robertis, 1965; Balazs et al., 1966). In homogenates of brain tissue the enzymes are recovered almost entirely in free mitochondria, with only minor amounts in fractions containing synaptosome particles (which contain GAD). However, there is evidence that several isozymes of GABA-T exist, which can be separated by electrophoresis; and the more anionic of these are recovered mainly in the supernatant fractions after subcellular fractionation of mouse and rat brain homogenates (Waksman and Roberts, 1965; Waksman and Bloch, 1968).

The distribution of the GABA metabolizing enzymes between inhibitory and excitatory motor axons of the lobster has also been examined (Kravitz et al., 1965; Hall et al., 1970). Both GABA-T and SSA-dehydrogenase were present in excitatory and inhibitory axons, and in each case GABA-T was the rate-limiting enzyme. The activity of GABA-T in excitatory axoplasm was about 50 per cent higher than in inhibitory nerves, and the enzyme had similar kinetic and electrophoretic properties in the two types of axon.

It would seem, therefore, that in the invertebrate and mammalian nervous system the enzymes responsible for GABA metabolism are widely distributed; they occur in neurons which store and release GABA (lobster inhibitory motor neurons; cerebellar Purkinje cells), but also in neurons which do not use GABA as a neurotransmitter (lobster excitatory motor neurons, spinal cord motor neurons) and in other non-neuronal tissues. The finding that the bulk of GABA-T activity in homogenates of mammalian brain is associated with free mitochondria would suggest that most of the enzyme is localized in structures other than nerve terminals. This pattern of distribution is similar to that observed for the catecholamine metabolizing enzymes monoamine oxidase and catechol-O-methyltransferase (Iversen, 1967).

Although there have been few studies of the distribution of SSA-dehydrogenase, it seems likely that this mitochondrial enzyme is distributed in a manner very similar to that of GABA-T (Miller and Pitts, 1967; Hall et al., 1970).

Inhibition of GABA Metabolism. A variety of carbonyl reagents, such as hydroxylamine (Baxter and Roberts, 1959), hydrazines (Medina, 1963), γ-glutamyl hydrazide (Massieu et al., 1964), cycloserine (Dann and Carter, 1964), amino-oxyacetic acid (Wallach, 1961; van Gelder, 1966), and other oxy-amino acids (Schumann et al., 1961), are potent inhibitors of GABA-T in *in vitro* systems, and many of these compounds are also effective inhibitors of the enzyme when administered *in vivo*. Although several of these substances are also inhibitors of GAD *in vitro,* they appear to inhibit GABA-T preferentially *in vivo,* with much less effect on GAD. One possible explanation for such selectivity may be that pyridoxal-inhibitor complexes may be bound with higher affinity by GABA-T than by GAD, thus making reactivation of the former enzyme by pyridoxal phosphate more difficult (Baxter, 1970). Alternatively, the differential effects of inhibitors on GAD and GABA-T may be related to differences in the cellular distribution of these enzymes and the inhibitors *in vivo*. The administration of GABA-T inhibitors *in vivo* leads to rises in the steady state concentration of GABA in the brain, which may increase by as much as 500 per cent after, for example, amino-oxyacetic acid (Wallach, 1961; van Gelder, 1966). After the administration of the latter compound inhibition of GABA-T is almost immediate, the rise in brain GABA occurs very rapidly, reaching a maximum after 3 to 4 hours (van Gelder, 1966); GABA-T inhibition persists for as long as 14 to 21 days after a large dose of amino-oxyacetic acid *in vivo* (Rubinstein and Roberts, 1967). The use of amino-oxyacetic acid thus represents one of the few pharmacological manipulations of the GABA system in brain which are currently possible. There have been several attempts to correlate the rise in GABA concentration induced by this compound and related reagents, with the anticonvulsant properties of these substances (see Baxter, 1970; Roberts and Kuriyama, 1968). However, there seems only a poor correlation. Kuriyama et al. (1966a), for example, found that normal susceptibility to electroconvulsive seizures in mice injected with AOAA was restored at a time when brain GABA levels remained very high. It now seems generally agreed that the convulsant or anticonvulsant properties of the drugs described above are not obviously correlated with their effects on the concentration of GABA in the brain. This is perhaps not surprising, since compounds such as hydroxylamine or AOAA are unlikely to be entirely specific inhibitors of GABA-T. Numerous other pyridoxal enzymes may also be inhibited by the administration of such compounds, so that they may interfere with the metabolism not only of GABA but possibly of other amino acids or amines in the CNS, including glycine, the catecholamines, and glutamic acid. Amino-oxyacetic acid, for example, acts as a powerful inhibitor of pyridoxal kinase *in vivo* (Da Vanzo et al., 1966).

It has been suggested that the preferential inhibition of GABA-T by compounds such as amino-oxyacetic acid, without inhibition of GAD, reflects the different cellular location of these two enzymes (Roberts and Kuriyama, 1968). However, if this is the case it is a little difficult to understand why the steady state concentration of GABA should increase after GABA-T inhibition. It would seem more likely that GABA can be synthesized and metabolized by GAD and GABA-T in inhibitory nerve terminals, and that it is the inhibition of the relatively small proportion of GABA-T associated with such terminals that is critical in causing elevated GABA levels. This would be analogous to the rise in intraneuronal catecholamine concentrations induced in adrenergic nerve terminals by the administration of MAO inhibitors (Iversen, 1967).

A useful indication of the dynamic aspects of GABA metabolism may be derived from studies with amino-oxyacetic acid and related compounds. The rate of rise in brain GABA after inhibition of GABA-T can be used to indicate the rate of biosynthesis of GABA, in the same way that the rate of monoamine biosynthesis has been estimated after administration of monoamine oxidase inhibitors (Costa, 1970). From such data van Gelder (1966) has estimated a rate of GABA synthesis in the mouse brain of 5 to 6 μmoles/g/hr, a value not inconsistent with the estimates made by pulse-labelling experiments in brain slices *in vitro* quoted above (Balazs et al., 1970).

Recently, β-hydrazinopropionic acid has been reported to be a potent inhibitor of GABA-T with long-lasting effects when administered *in vivo* (van Gelder, 1968). This compound also leads to elevations in brain GABA, and is of particular interest since the structure of β-hydrazinopropionic acid (Fig. 4-5) is isosteric with that of GABA, and it may thus prove to be a more specific inhibitor of the GABA-T enzyme than those previously described.

Storage of GABA

The distribution of GABA in inhibitory neurons of the lobster and within the mammalian CNS has already been described on pp. 23-24 above. Within the mammalian CNS the cellular localization of the GABA stores remains obscure. Although there is evidence that GABA may be specifically concentrated in certain inhibitory neurons, such as the Purkinje cell terminals in the cerebellar nuclei (Otsuka et al., 1971), in most regions of the brain such evidence is lacking. Subcellular distribution studies have also provided only equivocal evidence of the cellular localization of the amino acid. Under certain conditions as much as 60 per cent of the total GABA in brain homogenates can be recovered in a particle-bound form, mainly accounted for by synaptosome particles (Elliott, 1965; Neal and Iversen, 1969). The recovery of GABA in such experiments, however, is very variable and is dependent on the technique employed. Subcellular fractionation procedures which are lengthy and involve several manipulative stages generally lead to very low recoveries of GABA in the synaptosome fraction (Mangan and Whittaker, 1966); whereas simplified procedures can give rise to recoveries of as much as 40 to 60 per cent of total GABA in such particles (Neal and Iversen, 1969). This is in contrast to the consistently high recoveries of GAD in synaptosome fractions (Section II above). We have concluded (Neal and Iversen, 1969) that GABA is probably easily lost from synaptosomes during subcellular fractionation experiments. The results of such experiments, therefore, can only be regarded as approximate indicators of the actual distribution of the amino acid in the intact itssue. There is little doubt, however, that at least some of the endogenous GABA in mammalian CNS is stored in nerve terminals.

Within the nerve terminals there is little information available on the possible mechanisms involved in the storage of GABA prior to its release as a neurotransmitter substance. On osmotic lysis most of the GABA contained in synaptosome fractions is released into the supernatant (Mangan and Whittaker, 1966). It has been reported, however, that small amounts of GABA are associated with synaptic vesicle fractions obtained after osmotic lysis of synaptosomes (Whittaker, 1968; Kuriyama et al., 1968b). Electron microscopy shows that inhibitory nerve terminals in the crustacean and mammalian nervous systems contain large numbers of synaptic vesicles, and one might expect such vesicles to represent the major storage sites for GABA, by analogy with the situation in adrenergic and cholinergic nerve terminals. On the other hand, in inhibitory nerve axoplasm in the lobster, very high concentrations of GABA (0.1M) exist in a free form (Kravitz et al., 1965). It is thus, *a priori,* not necessary to invoke vesicle storage mechanisms in order to explain the high concentrations of GABA which exist in inhibitory neurons. It may be that GABA is stored in synaptic vesicles at storage sites which have only a low affinity for the amino acid, so that vesicle-bound GABA is in equilibrium with a large fraction of free axoplasmic amino acid.

Uptake of GABA

A variety of specific transport systems are associated with neurons in which noradrenaline, dopamine, 5-hydroxytryptamine, and acetylcholine act as neurotransmitters (Iversen, 1970). GABA-inhibitory neurons are no exceptions to this general phenomenon, since they also have a specific GABA uptake mechanism associated with them. It has been known for some time that mammalian brain slices actively accumulate exogenous GABA (Elliott and van Gelder, 1956; Tsukada et al., 1963; Blasberg and Lajtha, 1966; Nakamura and Nagayama, 1966). In our own studies of this uptake system (Iversen and Neal, 1968) we confirmed and extended these observations, using the uptake of ^{3}H-GABA by small slices of rat cerebral cortex as the model system. Such slices accumulated

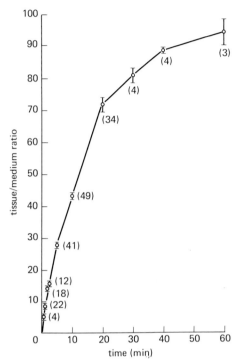

Figure 4-4   Uptake of ³H-GABA by slices of rat cerebral cortex incubated with the labelled amino acid (0.05μM) at 25°C *in vitro*. Values are means ± S.E.M. for number of determinations in parentheses (Iversen and Neal, 1968).

³H-GABA very rapidly when incubated in a low concentration of the labelled amino acid, giving rise to tissue-medium ratios as high as 100 to 1 (Fig. 4-4). Only the unchanged amino acid accumulated in the tissue slices, although some labelled metabolites of ³H-GABA were formed and lost to the incubation medium. The uptake of ³H-GABA was a temperature-dependent process which required the presence of sodium ions in the external medium. The rates of GABA uptake at various external GABA concentrations could be described by saturation kinetics, with a K_m of 22 μM and V_{max} = 0.116 μmoles/g/min (Iversen and Neal, 1968). A variety of GABA analogues and other compounds has been tested as inhibitors of ³H-GABA uptake by rat cortical slices (Iversen and Johnston, 1971) (Table 4-6). These results emphasize the high degree of specificity of the GABA uptake process; among the GABA analogues

Table 4-6   Inhibitors of ^{3}H-GABA uptake by slices of rat cerebral cortex

Inhibitor	IC50 value—μM
para-chloromercuriphenylsulphonic acid	30
chlorpromazine	32
DL-2-fluoro-GABA	35
L-2,4-diaminobutyric acid	50
DL-2,4-diaminobutyric acid	108
DL-3-hydroxy-GABA	100
haloperidol	200
2-guanidinopropionic acid	220
5-aminopentanoic acid	230
2-hydrazinopropionic acid	500

IC50 value = concentration of inhibitor required to produce 50 per cent inhibition of ^{3}H-GABA uptake. Data from Iversen and Johnston (1971).

tested only 3-hydroxy-GABA, 2-fluoro-GABA, L-2,4-diaminobutyric acid, and 2-guanidinopropionic acid had affinities for uptake comparable to that of GABA. The most potent inhibitors proved to be para-chloro-mercuriphenylsulphonate (and other thiol reagents), chlorpromazine, and imipramine. None of these are specific in their actions on GABA uptake (Johnston and Iversen, 1971). So far, we have not succeeded in discovering a suitable specific inhibitor of GABA uptake which could be used to investigate the possible physiological functions of this process. The hypothesis that the uptake of GABA may be important as a mechanism for terminating the actions of GABA in the brain after its release at inhibitory synapses is attractive, but remains unsubstantiated.

In lobster nerve-muscle and crayfish stretch receptor preparations there is also an uptake of exogenous GABA (Sisken and Roberts, 1963; Iversen and Kravitz, 1968) which has properties similar to that of the system in mammalian brain.

It has recently proved possible to obtain further information on the cellular localization of GABA uptake sites in both crustacean and mammalian tissues. In rat cortical slices the subcellular distribution of ^{3}H-GABA was found to be very similar to that of endogenous GABA and the enzyme GAD (Neal and Iversen, 1969). About 40 per cent of the ^{3}H-GABA in homogenates of labelled cortical slices could be recovered in synaptosome fractions after density gradient centrifugation. More recently the sites of ^{3}H-GABA uptake in lobster muscle preparations and rat cortical slices have been investigated directly by electron microscope au-

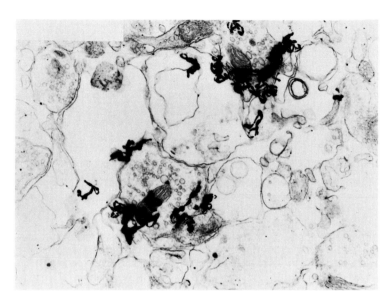

Figure 4-5   Electron microscope autoradiogram showing localization of ³H-GABA over two nerve terminals in a slice of rat cerebral cortex previously incubated with the labelled amino acid *in vitro* (Bloom and Iversen, 1971).

toradiography. Orkand and Kravitz (1971) found that sufficient ³H-GABA was retained (about 40 per cent) in lobster nerve-muscle preparations by glutaraldehyde fixation to permit such investigations. They found that ³H-GABA was accumulated mainly in connective tissue and Schwann cell elements in association with the terminal motor innervation of the lobster muscles, there was no indication that any ³H-GABA was taken up by the nerve terminals themselves. In slices of rat cerebral cortex, however, where glutaraldehyde fixation led to the retention of more than two-thirds of the accumulated ³H-GABA, we have obtained different results (Bloom and Iversen, 1971) (Fig. 4-5). In such slices statistical analysis of several autoradiograms showed nerve terminals and preterminal axons were the primary sites of ³H-GABA uptake, with only small amounts of labelled amino acid associated with neuron cell bodies and dendrites or glial cells (Table 4-7). Furthermore, not all nerve terminals were labelled by ³H-GABA, but only a distinct population accounting for approximately 30 per cent of all terminals in the rat cortex. These results provide the first direct evidence that GABA uptake sites are asso-

Table 4-7   Localization of ^{3}H-GABA in slices of rat cerebral cortex

Tissue Component	Mean percentage of surface area occupied[1]	Mean percentage of total silver grains[2]
GLIAL CELLS	13.0 ± 1.1	2.1 ± 0.1
NEURON CELL BODIES + DENDRITES	38.9 ± 3.0	11.3 ± 1.8
NERVE TERMINALS	23.5± 3.6	70.7 ± 2.3
MYELINATED AXONS	5.0 ± 1.7	1.0 ± 0.05
UNMYELINATED AXONS	14.5 ± 1.3	11.2 ± 1.5
UNIDENTIFIED AND EXTRACELLULAR SPACE	5.3 ± 1.1	3.2 ± 1.1

[1] Percentage of total area occupied by various tissue components was estimated by application of a 220-point grid to randomly selected low-power electron micrographs of cortical tissue. The area of tissue in each micrograph was 275 μ^2, and the results are means + S.E. for five analyses of this type.
[2] The distribution of silver grains was analyzed in the same electron micrographs; results are expressed as the mean percentage (± S.E.M.) of total grain population in each micrograph located over the various tissue components (from Bloom and Iversen, 1971).

ciated with nerve terminals in the mammalian CNS, and we believe that this method may permit the identification of those synaptic terminals which normally store and use GABA as a transmitter in the mammalian CNS.

Exogenous GABA is also taken up *in vitro* by particles in brain homogenate and this process is mediated by a carrier transport mechanism similar or identical to that described in tissue slices (Sano and Roberts, 1963; Weinstein et al., 1965; Varon et al., 1965; Iversen and Johnston, 1971). In the latter study we have established, by density gradient centrifugation (Fig. 4-6) that the particles responsible for this uptake of GABA are probably synaptosomes, and this conclusion is also confirmed by electron microscope autoradiographic experiments (Bloom and Iversen, 1971). As much as two-thirds of the ^{3}H-GABA uptake sites in slices of rat brain or spinal cord survive homogenization of the tissue, and are retained in synaptosome particles (Iversen and Johnston, 1971). The uptake of ^{3}H-GABA by such particles is sodium-dependent (Weinstein et al., 1965) and has kinetic properties and a drug sensitivity similar to that in intact slices (K_m for GABA $= 18.5\ \mu$M).

It seems, therefore, that most of the uptake of exogenous GABA observed in slices of mammalian brain can be accounted for by GABA uptake sites which are predominantly localized at inhibitory nerve terminals.

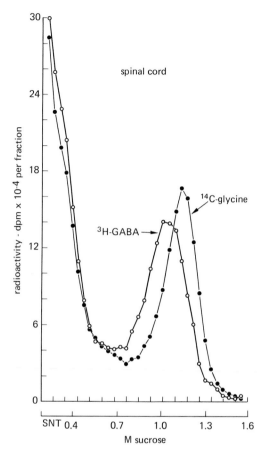

Figure 4-6   Distribution of ^{3}H-GABA and ^{14}C-glycine on a sucrose density gradient after centrifugation of a sample of spinal cord homogenate labelled by incubation with a mixture of the two amino acids *in vitro*. Both labelled amino acids appear in the supernatant fractions at the top of the centrifuge tube, and also in particle fractions whose equilibrium density corresponds to that of synaptosomes. The two amino acids appear to be taken up by different populations of such particles (Iversen and Johnston, 1971).

As mentioned above, the physiological role of this uptake mechanism remains obscure; however, the existence of such a specific uptake system offers a most useful research tool. By exposing mammalian CNS tissue to exogenous radioactively labelled GABA it appears to be possible to introduce selectively the labelled amino acid into the endogenous

GABA stores in inhibitory nerve terminals, in much the same way that labelled catecholamines can be introduced selectively into adrenergic nerve terminals (Axelrod and Kopin, 1969; Iversen, 1970). In keeping with this hypothesis, we have been able to show that different populations of nerve terminals are responsible for the uptake of GABA and labelled catecholamines or glycine in rat brain or spinal cord (Iversen and Snyder, 1968; Iversen and Johnston, 1971) (Fig. 4-6).

Release of GABA

An increased efflux of GABA has been demonstrated in response to stimulation of inhibitory synaptic transmission on both crustacean and mammalian systems (pp. 23-24). In the lobster nerve-muscle preparation we were able to demonstrate a release of GABA in response to stimulation of the inhibitory motor nerve (Otsuka et al., 1966). Stimulation of the excitatory motor nerve in the same preparations, however, failed to evoke any release of GABA. The amount of GABA released during inhibitory nerve stimulation was proportional to the frequency of stimulation (Table 4-2), that is, it was related to the total number of stimuli delivered. Both inhibitory junctional potentials and GABA release were reversibly abolished if the muscles were superfused with a medium in which the calcium-ion concentration was reduced, although this had no effect on the spontaneous efflux of GABA (Otsuka et al., 1966). These results are, thus, similar to those obtained for other neurotransmitters, such as acetylcholine or noradrenaline, where it has been shown that the release of transmitter evoked by depolarization of the presynaptic nerve terminals is calcium-dependent, whereas the spontaneous release of transmitter during rest is not calcium-dependent (Rubin, 1970).

In the mammalian CNS a release of GABA has been demonstrated from the perfused fourth ventricle of the cat in response to stimulation of Purkinje fibers (Obata and Takeda, 1969). A similar release also occurs from the surface of the cerebral cortex of the cat in response to electrical stimulation of either the surface of the cortex or a remote nucleus (lateral geniculate nucleus) (Iversen et al., 1971). In these experiments the stimulation parameters were chosen to mimic those used by Krnjević et al. (1966), and produced mainly inhibitory synaptic activity of long duration in the cerebral cortex. The release of GABA and the inhibition of cortical activity evoked by stimulation were abolished if the cortex was exposed to a calcium-free medium, and this effect was reversible (Iversen et al., 1971). In similar experiments by using an amino acid analyzer we were able to show that GABA was the only amino acid whose efflux was significantly changed during stimulation.

Jasper et al. (1965), Crowshaw et al. (1967), and Jasper and Koyama (1969) have also measured the release of small amounts of GABA from the surface of the cerebral cortex. Jasper et al. (1965) and Jasper and Koyama (1969) reported that the rate of efflux of GABA was related to the state of neuronal activity in the cortex, as measured by the EEG; GABA release was highest under conditions in which inhibitory synaptic activity might be assumed to be greatest (low frequency large amplitude EEG activity).

Mitchell and Srinivasan (1969) have also shown that stimulation under similar conditions leads to a release of ^{3}H-GABA from the surface of the cat cerebral cortex previously exposed to the labelled amino acid. A release of ^{3}H-GABA from slices of rat cerebral cortex was also demonstrated during electrical stimulation (Srinivasan et al., 1969). This process was partially calcium-dependent and was antagonized by magnesium ions. Stimulation of cerebral cortical slices under similar conditions failed to evoke any significant increase in the rate of efflux of other labelled amino acids, such as valine or leucine. The finding that exogenous ^{3}H-GABA can be released by stimulation is consistent with the evidence, summarized above, that the labelled amino acid is selectively taken up and accumulated in inhibitory nerve terminals which contain endogenous GABA. The use of ^{3}H-GABA thus offers a simple method for studying the release of GABA from inhibitory terminals in the brain, and the effects of drugs on this process. Nevertheless, it remains technically difficult to demonstrate the release of GABA from inhibitory synapses in the mammalian brain. Unlike the studies with the crustacean nerve-muscle preparation, the collection of GABA from the mammalian CNS necessitates stimulation of ill-defined neuronal pathways, and most of the inhibitory synapses in the brain are not accessible for such collection experiments. Even in successful experiments, the amounts of endogenous or ^{3}H-GABA released during stimulation are small. There is, furthermore, no means of preventing the normal inactivation of the released transmitter at GABA synapses, so that the amount collected probably represents only a small proportion of that actually released from presynaptic terminals.

Summary—The GABA Synapse

To summarize—there is convincing evidence that GABA is an inhibitory transmitter at synapses in the crustacean and mammalian nervous systems. Nerve terminals which store and release GABA (Fig. 4-7) resemble those using other transmitters in that (1) they contain the biosynthetic enzyme (GAD) and are thus capable of a local biosynthesis of the transmitter, GABA; (2) they contain enzymic machinery for GABA catabolism, so that a steady state storage level of GABA in the terminal is probably maintained by continuous synthesis and catabolism of the transmitter; the catabolic enzymes are also found in cellular sites other than the GABA-containing nerves (compare acetylcholinesterase, monoamine oxidase); (3) GABA-containing nerve terminals also contain large numbers of synaptic vesicles, although it has not yet been established that these represent the major storage sites for GABA; (4) the release of GABA from inhibitory nerve terminals by nerve stimulation is a calcium-dependent process; (5) in the mammalian CNS, but not in the lobster,

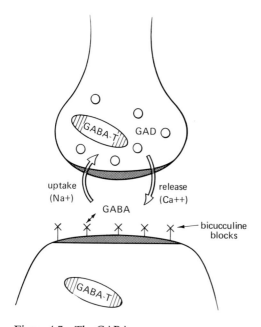

Figure 4-7   The GABA synapse.

GABA-containing nerve terminals possess an active uptake system for GABA, which may serve to terminate the actions of the released transmitter by a recapture process; (6) specific receptor sites for GABA exist on the surface of the postsynaptic cells innervated by GABA neurons.

As yet we know of only a few drugs which have specific actions on GABA synapses. Compounds which interfere with GABA metabolism, notably those that impair the catabolism of GABA *in vivo,* produce marked changes in the steady state storage concentration of GABA in the mammalian CNS. However, it is not clear that such changes occur only in neuronal storage sites, or whether they can lead to changes in the amount of GABA released at inhibitory synapses. In addition, most compounds of this type are relatively nonspecific in their actions, and probably interfere with various other aspects of amino acid metabolism in the CNS. A variety of drugs and conditions have been shown to influence the steady state concentration of GABA in the mammalian brain; these include compounds generally thought to act on aminergic transmission such as reserpine (which leads to a reduction in cerebral GABA concentration, Balzer et al., 1961) and monoamine oxidase inhibitors (some of which act as inhibitors of GABA-T and cause rises in cerebral GABA Popov et al., 1968); cerebral GABA is also influenced by other factors such as hyperbaric oxygen (Wood and Watson, 1963; Wood, 1967). However, changes in GABA concentrations may be the result of many different mechanisms of action, including displacement from storage sites, inhibition of biosynthesis, or catabolism. Furthermore, such changes need not necessarily imply a direct action of the drug on GABA neurons, but might be indirect consequences of drug actions on other types of neuron. The literature on drug effects on adrenergic systems should teach us that rather little insight has been gained into drug actions by examination of effects on the steady state concentrations of noradrenaline or dopamine in the CNS.

We also know very little of the physiological or pharmacological interactions between GABA neurons and those using other transmitters. That such interactions may be of considerable interest is illustrated by the finding that γ-hydroxybutyrate, which may be a metabolite of GABA, has a dramatic effect on dopamine-containing neurons in the basal ganglia. Administration of γ-hydroxybutyrate leads to a marked elevation in striatal dopamine, apparently due to an inhibition of dopamine release (Gessa et al., 1968; Roth and Suhr, 1970).

We may hope that recent advances in our understanding of the role of GABA in the physiological functions of the nervous system will encourage rapid advances in our understanding of the biochemistry and pharmacology of GABA neurons in the next few years. We know by analogy with adrenergic and cholinergic mechanisms at least some of the questions that should be asked.

References

Alberici, M., De Lores Arnaiz, G. R., and De Robertis, E. 1968. *Biochem. Pharmacol.* 18:137.
Albers, R. W., and Brady, R. O. 1959. *J. Biol. Chem.* 234:926.
Albers, R. W., and Koval, G. J. 1961. *Biochim. Biophys. Acta* 52:29.
Aprison, M. H., Davidoff, R. A., and Werman, R. 1970. In *Handbook of Neurochemistry* A. Lajtha (Ed.), vol. 3, Plenum Press, New York, p. 381.
Balazs, R., Dahl, D., and Harwood, J. R. 1966. *J. Neurochem.* 13:897.
Balazs, R., Machiyama, Y., Hammond, B. J., Julian, T., and Richter, D. 1970. *Biochem. J.* 116:445.
Balzer, H., Holtz, P., and Palm, D. 1960. *Arch. exp. Path. u. Pharmakol.* 239:520.
Balzer, H., Holtz, P., and Palm, D. 1961. *Experientia* 17:38.
Baxter, C. F. 1969. *Ann. N.Y. Acad. Sci.* 166:267.
Baxter, C. F. 1970. In *Handbook of Neurochemistry,* A. Lajtha (Ed.), vol. 3, Plenum Press, New York, p. 289.
Baxter, C. F., and Roberts, E. 1959. *Proc. Soc. Exp. Biol. Med.* 101:811.
Baxter, C. F., and Roberts, E. 1961. *J. Biol. Chem.* 236:3287.
Bazemore, A., Elliott, K. A. C., and Florey, E. 1957. *J. Neurochem.* 1:334.
Blasberg, R., and Lajtha, A. 1966. *Brain Res.* 1:86.
Bloom, F. E., and Iversen, L. L. 1971. *Nature* 229:628.
Boistel, J., and Fatt, P. 1958. *J. Physiol.* (Lond.) 144:176.
Bradford, H. F., and Thomas, A. J. 1969. *J. Neurochem.* 16:1495.
Capiappo, F., Pandolfo, L., and Di Chiara, C. 1959. *Boll. Soc. Ital. Biol. Sper.* 36:465.
Costa, E. 1970. *Adv. Biochem. Psychopharmacol.* 2:169.
Crowshaw, K., Jessup, S. J., and Ramwell, P. W. 1967. *Biochem. J.* 103:79.
Curtis, D. R. 1969. *Recent Prog. in Brain Res.* 31:171.
Curtis, D. R., and Watkins, J. C. 1965. *Pharmacol. Rev.* 17:347.
Curtis, D. R., Hösli, L., and Johnston, G. A. R. 1968a. *Exp. Brain Res.* 6:1.
Curtis, D. R., Hösli, L., Johnston, G. A. R., and Johnston, I. H. 1968b. *Exp. Brain Res.* 5:235.
Curtis, D. R., Duggan, A. W., Felix, D., and Johnston, G. A. R. 1970a. *Nature* 226:1222.
Curtis, D. R., Felix, D., and McLennan, H. 1970b. *Brit. J. Pharmac.* 40:881.
Dann, O. T., and Carter, C. E. 1964. *Biochem. Pharmacol.* 13:677.
Da Vanzo, J. P., Kang, L., Ruckart, R., and Daugherty, M. 1966. *Biochem. Pharmacol.* 15:124.

Dudel, J. 1965a. *Pflugers Archiv.* 283:104.

Dudel, J. 1965b. *Pflugers Archiv.* 284:81.

Dudel, J., and Kuffler, S. W. 1961. *J. Physiol.* (Lond.) 155:543.

Dudel, J., Gryder, R., Kaji, A., Kuffler, S. W., and Potter, D. D. 1963. *J. Neurophysiol.* 26:721.

Edwards, C., and Kuffler, S. W. 1959. *J. Neurochem.* 4:19.

Elliott, K. A. C. 1965. *Brit. Med. Bull.* 21:70.

Elliott, K. A. C., and Jasper, H. H. 1959. *Physiol. Rev.* 39:383.

Elliott, K. A. C., and Van Gelder, N. M. 1958. *J. Neurochem.* 3:28.

Fahn, S., and Côté, L. J. 1968. *J. Neurochem.* 15:209.

Fatt, P., and Katz, B. 1953. *J. Physiol.* (Lond.) 131:374.

Fishbein, W. N., and Bessmann, S. P. 1964. *J. Biol. Chem.* 239:357.

Florey, E. 1957. *Naturwissensch.* 44:424.

Florey, E. 1964. In *Neuroendocrinology,* E. Bajusz and G. Jasmin (Eds.), S. Karger, Basel, p. 1741.

Fonnum, F. 1968. *Biochem. J.* 106:401.

Fonnum, F., Storm-Mathisen, J., and Walberg, F. 1970. *Brain Res.* 20:259.

Fonnum, F., and Storm-Mathisen, J. 1971. *J. Neurochem.* (in press).

Furshpan, E. 1959. In *Handbook of Physiology,* vol. 1, American Physiological Society, Washington, D.C., p. 239.

Gessa, G. L., Crabai, F., Vargiu, L., and Spano, P. F. 1968. *J. Neurochem.* 15:377.

Godfraind, J. M., Krnjević, K., and Pumain, R. 1970. *Nature* 228:675.

Graham, L. T., and Aprison, M. H. 1969. *J. Neurochem.* 16:559.

Grundfest, J., Reuben, J. P., and Rickles, W. H. 1959. *J. Gen. Physiol.* 42:1301.

Haber, B., Kuriyama, K., and Roberts, E. 1970a. *Biochem. Pharmacol.* 19:1119.

Haber, B., Kuriyama, K., and Roberts, E. 1970b. *Science* 168:598.

Haber, B., Sze, P. Y., Kuriyama, K., and Roberts, E. 1970c. *Brain Res.* 18:545.

Hall, Z. W., and Kravitz, E. A. 1967a. *J. Neurochem.* 14:45.

Hall, Z. W., and Kravitz, E. A. 1967b. *J. Neurochem.* 14:55.

Hall, Z. W., Bownds, M. D., and Kravitz, E. A. 1970. *J. Cell. Biol.* 46:290.

Hebb, C. 1970. *Ann. Rev. Physiol.* 32:165.

Iversen, L. L. 1967. *The Uptake and Storage of Noradrenaline in Sympathetic Nerves,* Cambridge University Press, London and New York.

Iversen, L. L., 1970. *Adv. Biochem. Psychopharmacol.* 2:109.

Iversen, L. L., and Johnston, G. A. R. 1971. *J. Neurochem.* 18:1939.

Iversen, L. L., and Kravitz, E. A. 1968. *J. Neurochem.* 15:609.

Iversen, L. L., and Neal, M. J. 1968. *J. Neurochem.* 15:1141.

Iversen, L. L., and Snyder, S. H. 1968. *Nature* 220:796.

Iversen, L. L., Kravitz, E. A., and Otsuka, M. 1966. *J. Physiol.* (Lond.) 188:21P.

Iversen, L. L., Mitchell, J. F., and Srinivasan, V. 1971. *J. Physiol.* (Lond.) 212:519.

Jasper, H. H., and Koyama, I. 1969. *Canad. J. Physiol. Pharmacol.* 47:889.

Jasper, H. H., Khan, R. T., and Elliott, K. A. C. 1965. *Science* 147:1448.

Jenny, E., and Solberg, R. 1969. *Helv. Physiol. Pharmacol. Acta* 26:270.

Johnson, E. S., Roberts, M. H. T., and Straughanm, D. W. 1970. *Brit. J. Pharmacol.* 38:659.

Johnston, G. A. R., and Iversen, L. L. 1971. *J. Neurochem.* 18:1951.

Johnston, G. A. R., Curtis, D. R., de Groat, W. C., and Duggan, W. 1968. *Biochem. Pharmacol.* 17:2488.

Kammeraat, C., and Veldstra, H. 1968. *Biochim. Biophys. Acta* 151:1.

Kerkut, G. A., and Meech, R. W. 1966. *Life Sci.* 5:453.

Killam, K. F., and Bain, J. A. 1957. *J. Pharmac. Exp. Ther.* 119:255.

Kravitz, E. A., and Potter, D. D. 1965. *J. Neurochem.* 12:323.

Kravitz, E A., Molinoff, P. B., and Hall, Z. W. 1965. *Proc. Nat. Acad. Sci. U.S.* 54: 778.

Kravitz, E. A., Kuffler, S. W., Potter, D. D., and Van Gelder, N. M. 1963. *J. Neurophysiol.* 26:729.

Krnjević, K. 1970. *Nature* 228:119.

Krnjević, K., and Schwartz, S. 1966. *Nature* 211:1372.

Krnjević, K., and Schwartz, S. 1967. *Exp. Brain Res.* 3:320.

Krnjević, K., Randic, M., and Straughan, D. W. 1966. *J. Physiol.* (Lond.) 184:16, 49, 78.

Kuffler, S. W. 1960. *Harvery Lectures, 1958/59,* 176.

Kuriyama, K., Roberts, E., and Rubinstein, M. K. 1966a. *Biochem. Pharmacol.* 15: 221.

Kuriyama, K., Haber, B., Sisken, B., and Roberts, E. 1966b. *Proc. Nat. Acad. Sci. U.S.* 55:846.

Kuriyama, K., Sisken, B., Haber, B., and Roberts, E. 1968a. *Brain Res.* 9:165.

Kuriyama, K., Roberts, E., and Kakefuda, T. 1968b. *Brain Res.* 8:132.

Kuriyama, K., Haber, B., and Roberts, E. 1970. *Brain Res.* 23:121.

Laborit, H. 1964. *Int. J. Neuropharmacol.* 3:433.

Mangan, J. L., and Whittaker, V. P. 1966. *Biochem. J.* 98:128.

Massieu, G. H., Tapia, R. I., Pasantes, H. O., and Ortega, B. G. 1964. *Biochem. Pharmacol.* 13:118.

Maynert, E. W., and Kaji, H. K. 1962. *J. Pharmac. Exp. Ther.* 137:114.

McGeer, E. G., McGeer, P. L., and McLennan, H. 1961. *J. Neurochem.* 8:36.

McLennan, H. 1970. *Nature* 228:674.

Medina, M. A. 1963. *J. Pharmac. Exp. Ther.* 140:133.

Miller, A. L., and Pitts, F. N. 1967. *J. Neurochem.* 14:579.

Mitchell, J. F., and Srinivasan, V. 1969. *Nature* 224:663.

Molinoff, P. B., and Kravitz, E. A. 1968. *J. Neurochem.* 15:391.

Muller, P. B., and Langemann, H. 1962. *J. Neurochem.* 9:399.

Nakamura, R., and Nagayama, M. 1966. *J. Neurochem.* 13:305.

Neal, M. J., and Iversen, L. L. 1969. *J. Neurochem.* 16:1245.

Obata, K., and Takeda, K. 1969. *J. Neurochem.* 16:1043.

Obata, K., Ito, M., Ochi, R., and Sato, N. 1967. *Exp. Brain Res.* 4:43.

Orkand, P., and Kravitz, E. A. 1971. *J. Cell. Biol.* 49:75.

Otsuka, M., Iversen, L. L., Hall, Z. W., and Kravitz, E. A. 1966. *Proc. Nat. Acad. Sci. U.S.* 56:1110.

Otsuka, M., Kravitz, E. A., and Potter, D. D. 1967. *J. Neurophysiol.* 30:757.

Otsuka, M., Obata, D., Miyata, Y., and Tanaka, Y. 1971. *J. Neurochem.* (in press).

Pandolfo, L., and Macaione, S. 1964. *Giorn. Biochim.* 13:256.

Pfeifer, A. K., Satory, E., and Vizi, E. S. 1962. *Arch. Intern. Pharmacodyn.* 138:230.

Popov, N., Pohle, W., and Matthies, H. 1968. *Acta Biol. Med. Ger.* 20:509.

Roberts, E., and Kuriyama, K. 1968. *Brain Res.* 8:1.

Robinson, J. B., and Bradley, R. M. 1963. *Nature* 197:389.

Roth, R. H., Delgado, J. M. R., and Giarman, N. J. 1966. *Int. J. Neuropharmacol.* 5:421.

Roth, R. H., and Giarman, N. J. 1970a. *Biochem. Pharmacol.* 19:1087.

Roth, R. H., and Giarman, N. J. 1970b. *Biochem. Pharmacol.* 19:3013.
Roth, R. H., and Suhr, Y. 1970. *Biochem. Pharmacol.* 19:3001.
Rubin, R. P. 1970. *Pharmacol. Rev.* 22:389.
Rubinstein, M. K., and Roberts, E. 1967. *Biochem. Pharmacol.* 16:1138.
Salganicoff, L., and De Robertis, E. 1965. *J. Neurochem.* 12:287.
Salvador, R. A., and Albers, R. W. 1959. *J. Biol. Chem.* 234:922.
Sano, K., and Roberts, E. 1963. *Biochem. Pharmacol.* 12:489.
Schumann, E. L., Paquette, L. A., Heinzelman, R. V., Wallach, D. P., Da Vanzo, J. P., and Greig, M. E. 1961. *J. Med. Chem.* 5:464.
Shank, R. P., and Aprison, M. H. 1970. *J. Neurochem.* 17:1461.
Sheridan, J. J., Sims, K. L., and Pitts, F. N. 1967. *J. Neurochem.* 14:571.
Sisken, B., and Roberts, E. 1963. *Biochem. Pharmacol.* 13:95.
Srinivasan, V., Neal, M. J., and Mitchell, J. F. 1969. *J. Neurochem.* 16:1235.
Susz, J. P., Haber, B., and Roberts, E. 1966. *Biochemistry* 5:2870.
Sytinksy, I. A., and Vasilijev, V. Y. 1970. *Enzymologia* 39:1.
Sze, P. Y. 1970. *Brain Res.* 19:322.
Sze, P. Y., and Lovell, R. A. 1970a. *Life Sci.* 9:889.
Sze, P. Y., and Lovell, R. A. 1970b. *J. Neurochem.* 17:1657.
Takeuchi, A., and Takeuchi, N. 1965. *J. Physiol.* (Lond.) 177:225.
Tapia, R., and Awapara, J. 1967. *Proc. Soc. Exp. Biol. Med.* 126:218.
Tapia, R., and Awapara, J. 1969. *Biochem. Pharmacol.* 18:145.
Tsukada, Y., Nagata, Y., Hirano, S., and Matsutani, T. 1963. *J. Neurochem.* 10:241.
Van Gelder, N. M., 1965. *J. Neurochem.* 12:231.
Van Gelder, N. M. 1966. *Biochem. Pharmacol.* 15:533.
Van Gelder, N. M., 1967. *Recent Prog. Brain Res.* 29:259.
Van Gelder, N. M. 1968. *J. Neurochem.* 15:747.
Varon, S., Weinstein, H., Baxter, C. F., and Roberts, E. 1965. *Biochem. Pharmacol.* 14:1755.
Wallach, D. P. 1961. *Biochem. Pharmacol.* 5:323.
Waksman, A., and Bloch, M. 1968. *J. Neurochem.* 15:99.
Waksman, A., and Roberts, E .1965. *Biochemistry* 4:2132.
Weinstein, H., Varon, S., Muhleman, D. R., and Roberts, E. 1965. *Biochem. Pharmacol.* 14:273.
Whittaker, V. P. 1965. *Progr. Biophys. Mol. Biol.* 15:39.
Whittaker, V. P. 1968. In *Structure and Function of Inhibitory Neuronal Mechanisms,* Pergamon Press, Oxford, p. 487.
Wood, J. D., 1968. *Exp. Brain. Res.* 4:81.
Wood, J. D., and Watson, W. J. 1963. *Van J. Biochem. Physiol.* 41:1970.

5

Interaction of Estrogens, Progestational Agents, and Androgens with Brain and Pituitary and Their Role in the Control of Ovulation

ARNOLD JOEL EISENFELD

In 1964 I had the good fortune to join the laboratory of Dr. Julius Axelrod. While discussing various areas of research Dr. Axelrod indicated his interest in the observation that estrogens concentrate in the uterus. He suggested that this might represent binding of the estrogens. Review of the literature indicated that the oral contraceptives containing an estrogen and progestational agent prevented pregnancy predominantly by inhibiting ovulation. This inhibition of ovulation appeared to be due to modulation of gonadotrophin secretion at either the hypothalamic or anterior pituitary level. Since little was known then about steroid interaction in the brain and pituitary and since this interaction was of potential therapeutic importance, Dr. Axelrod and I initiated investigations into possible binding mechanisms for estrogens in the hypothalamus and anterior pituitary.

In this chapter I shall first present in some detail the evidence that there is binding of estrogens in the brain and pituitary. To place this information in a somewhat broader perspective the following related concepts will also be discussed briefly: male-female differentiation of the brain, radioactive progesterone and androgen interaction with the brain and pituitary, the mechanism of sex steroid action at a molecular level, the regulation of pituitary function, and the role of estrogens and progestational agents in promoting ovulation in the normal cycle and in inhibition of ovulation with administration of the oral contraceptives.

Radioactive Estrogen Interaction with the Brain

Extraction of Radioactivity after Systemic Administration

After systemic administration to animals, radioactive estradiol concentrates in the uterus (Glascock and Hoekstra, 1959; Jacobson and Jensen, 1962). This observation suggested that we might study the interaction of estrogens with the brain with the aid of tracer doses of radioactive estradiol of high specific activity. We found high accumulation of ^{3}H-estradiol in the anterior pituitary; one hour after intravenous administration to rats of ^{3}H-17β-estradiol (6, 7-^{3}H), 0.1 μg per 100 g body weight, its concentration in the anterior pituitary is about one hundred times greater than in plasma (Eisenfeld and Axelrod, 1965, 1966) (Fig. 5-1). The anterior pituitary retains high levels of radioactivity for as long as 16 hours after administration (Attramadal, 1964). Demonstrating concentration of estradiol in the hypothalamus proved more difficult. One hour after intravenous administration of 0.1 μg/100 g the levels in the brain are much lower than in either pituitary or uterus. However, the concentration of unconjugated estradiol in the hypothalamus is twice that found in the cerebrum and four times that in plasma (Eisenfeld and Axelrod, 1966). (Unless otherwise specified the hypothalamic section includes the medial preoptic region and the pituitary stalk with pars tuberalis.) The difference between hypothalamus and cerebrum is due to longer retention in the hypothalamus (Eisenfeld, 1967a; McGuire and Lisk, 1968). The hypothalamic retention is not higher because of a difference in initial delivery via the bloodstream; at two minutes after intravenous administration the concentration in hypothalamus equals that of cerebrum and exceeds that of plasma (Eisenfeld, 1967a).

Digital computer analysis of the kinetics of distribution is consistent with the concept that there are two hypothalamic pools of estradiol; one attached to a limited concentration of binding molecules and a second nonspecific pool in which concentration of estradiol parallels that of plasma (Eisenfeld, 1967a). The concentration of estradiol in the hypothalamic nonspecific pool is approximated by the concentration of radioactivity measured in the cerebrum. Thus, the concentration of estradiol which behaves as if attached to binding molecules (bound pool) in the hypothalamus can be estimated by subtraction of the cerebral concentration from the hypothalamic concentration. With a slight increase in es-

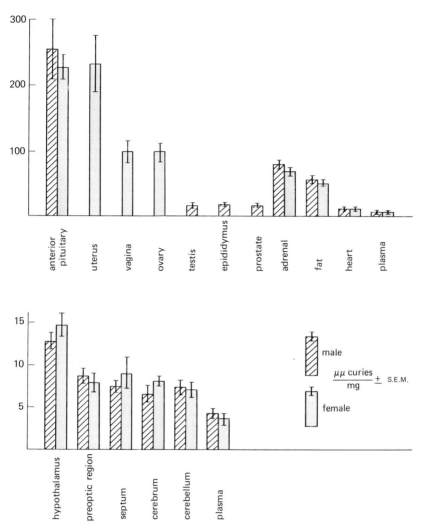

Figure 5-1   Distribution of ³H-estradiol in male and female rats. ³H-estradiol (0.1μ g/100 g, 38 c/mmole) was injected intravenously and tissues removed one hour later. The tissues were homogenized in water and unconjugated radioactivity extracted into toluene and measured. (Reproduced from *Endocrinology 79*, 38, 1966, by permission of the publisher).

*p < .05, **p < .001 compares to control concentrations

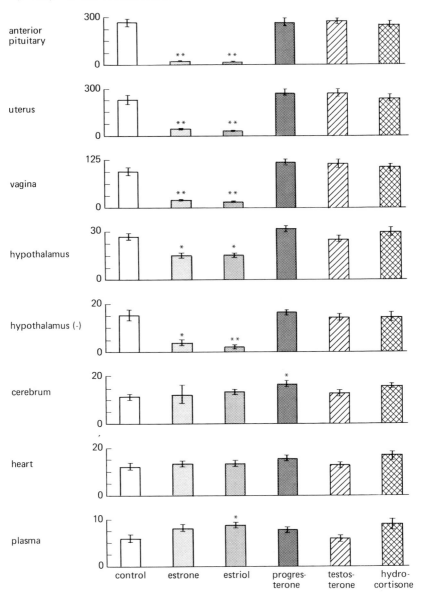

Figure 5-2   Effect of steroid hormones on the distribution of ^{3}H-estradiol. ^{3}H-estradiol (38c/mmole) was injected i.v. 30 seconds after 25 μg/100 g of nonradioactive estrone or estriol or 1 mg/100 g of progesterone, testosterone, or hydrocortisone. Subtraction of the cerebral concentration from the hypothalamic concentration is expressed by the symbol (—). Results are expressed as $\mu\mu$c/mg ± the standard error of the mean. (Reproduced from *Endocrinology 79,* 38, 1966, by permission of the publisher.)

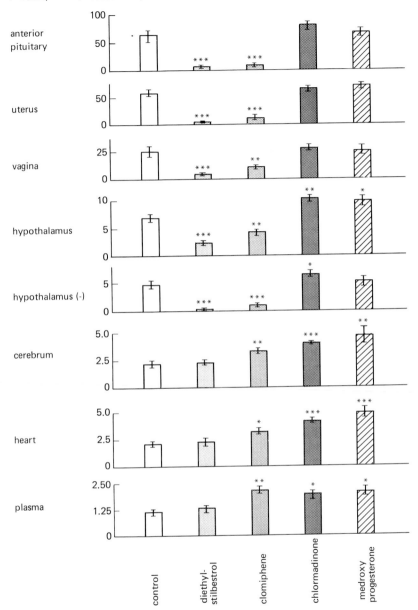

*: P<0.05, **
P<0.01, *** P<0.001 compared to concentrations in the controls.

Figure 5-3 Effect of drugs on the distribution of ^{3}H-estradiol. Diethylstilbestrol (25 μg/100 g), clomiphene (5 mg/100 g), chlormadinone (1 mg/100 g), or medroxyprogesterone (1 mg/100 g) was injected i.v. 30 seconds before 0.1 μg ^{3}H-estradiol/100 g (9.7c/mmole). Tissues were analyzed for ^{3}H-estradiol concentrations one hour later. Results are expressed as $\mu\mu$c/mg $\pm$ S.E.M. (Reproduced from *Biochemical Pharmacology 16*, 1781, 1967, by permission of the publisher).

specific; prior administration of either estriol, estrone, or diethylstilbestrol (a nonsteroidal synthetic estrogen with high potency) reduces the concentration of radioactive estradiol in the hypothalamus, anterior pituitary, and uterus while even large doses of either testosterone, progesterone or its derivatives, or hydrocortisone do not (Eisenfeld and Axelrod, 1966, 1967) (Fig. 5-2 and Fig. 5-3). Clomiphene, a fertility drug in women and partial estrogen agonist, reduces estradiol accumulation in the hypothalamus (Eisenfeld and Axelrod, 1967) as well as in the pituitary and uterus (Roy, Mahesh, and Greenblatt, 1964; Eisenfeld and Axelrod, 1967) (Fig. 5-3). Studies with drugs such as dimethylstilbestrol or U11100 (1-(2-(p-(3,4 dihydro-6-methoxy-2-phenyl-1-naphthyl) phenoxy) ethyl)-pyrrolidine hydrochloride) provide strong support for the concept that the retention of ^{3}H-estradiol in organs concerned with reproduction represents interaction with receptors. These drugs, which antagonize some of the effects of coadministered estradiol, reduce estradiol accumulation in hypothalamus and pituitary (Eisenfeld and Axelrod, 1967) and uterus (Jensen et al., 1966; Eisenfeld and Axelrod, 1967) (Fig. 5-4).

Estrogen accumulation has been studied in subdivisions of the hypothalamus separated by gross dissection. In the hypothalamus the region of the median eminence has the highest concentration of ^{3}H-estradiol with the anterior hypothalamus next highest (Kato and Villee, 1967a). The ratio of radioactivity in the middle or anterior hypothalamus to that in cerebrum increases with time after injection (Kato and Villee, 1967a; McGuire and Lisk, 1969a). Chronic administration of clomiphene or acute administration of 10 μg of 17β-estradiol, but not the weak estrogen 17α-estradiol, reduces this accumulation in the anterior and middle hypothalamus (Kato, Kobayashi, and Villee, 1968; Kato and Villee, 1967b).

With respect to subcellular localization, differential centrifugation has shown that some of the radioactivity in the hypothalamus and anterior pituitary is retained in the nuclear fraction. One hour after *in vivo* administration more than 50 per cent of the radioactivity from the hypothalamus and anterior pituitary is found in the 600 × g crude nuclear pellet after homogenization and centrifugation (Eisenfeld, 1967b). Highly purified nuclei contain 40 per cent of the estradiol from the hypothalamus (Zigmond and McEwen, 1970). The nuclear radioactivity per milligram of protein is 13 times that of the whole homogenate for the hypothalamus; the corresponding figure for the cerebrum is 0.8. ^{3}H-estradiol concentration in this highly purified nuclear fraction is reduced by low doses of 17β-

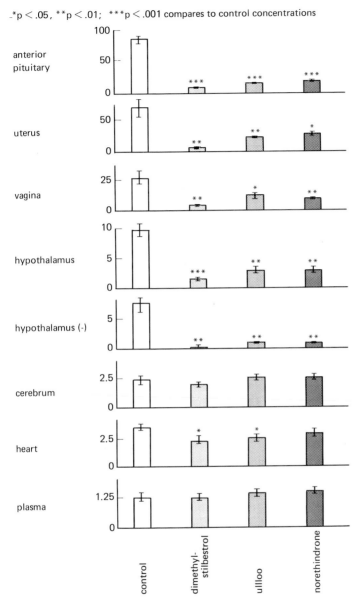

Figure 5-4   Distribution of ^{3}H-estradiol after administration of dimethylstilbesterol, U11100 or norethindrone. Dimethylstilbesterol (100 μ/100 g), U11100 (1 mg/100 g) or norethindrone (800 μg/100 g) was administered by tail vein 30 sec before 0.1 μg ^{3}H-estradiol/100g (9.7c/mmole). The concentration of 3H-estradiol in tissues 1 hr later is indicated as $\mu\mu$c/mg $\pm$ S.E.M. (Reproduced from *Biochemical Pharmacology* *16*, 1781, 1967, by permission of the publisher.)

estradiol but not by high doses of testosterone. The accumulation of radioactivity in the nuclear pellet is abolished almost completely by 1 mg of unlabelled estradiol while the accumulation in the whole tissue is reduced to 35 per cent of control. Nuclear retention in the anterior hypothalamus and pituitary is also depressed by chronic administration of clomiphene (Mowles, Ashkanazy, and Mix, 1970).

Autoradiographic Studies

A second approach to studying the interaction of labelled estrogens with the brain *in vivo* consists of autoradiography. It was necessary to modify the usual autoradiographic techniques in order to reduce the loss of estrogens into solvents and movement within the cells. Using frozen unfixed and unembedded sections dipped into photographic emulsion, the hypothalamus has a high concentration of silver grains in some neurons after local implantation of ^{14}C-diethylstilbestrol diacetate (Michael, 1962). After systemic administration of ^{3}H-hexestrol the grain counts are higher in the anterior pituitary than in uterine glands and 8 to 80 times greater in the region of the midline hypothalamus and lateral septum of the limbic system than in the lateral hypothalamus, cerebral cortex, cerebellum, caudate, or cervical cord (Michael, 1965a). Furthermore, after this systemic administration some neurons in the hypothalamus have the capacity to accumulate the radioactivity (Michael, 1965b).

In a modified technique described as dry mount autoradiography, tissue sections are freeze-dried and the section is applied to a dry emulsion (Stumpf, 1968a). With dry mount autoradiography, labelled neurons are found in the nucleus arcuatus, pars lateralis of the nucleus ventromedialis, anterior portion of the nucleus paraventricularis with its outgrowth of nucleus paraventricularis parvicellularis, a group of cells ventral to the magnacellular portion of nucleus paraventricularis, nucleus preopticus medialis, nucleus preopticus suprachiasmatis, and nucleus interstitialis striae terminalis. In addition labelled neurons are also found in the nucleus accumbens and nucleus septi lateralis, nucleus triangularis septi and the organon subfornicale. This radioactivity is concentrated in the nuclear subcellular fraction. It has been noted that this distribution pattern of labelled neurons is largely identical to regions of termination of the stria terminalis which originate in the nuclei of the amygdala (Stumpf,

1968). Unlabelled regions are nucleus supraopticus, suprachiasmatis, ventromedialis (part ventralis, centralis, dorsalis, and medialis), dorsomedialis, hypothalamicus lateralis, hypothalamicus posterior, and mammillaris. In general this localization in the hypothalamic and preoptic neurons has been confirmed using frozen sections melted onto slides covered with emulsion (Anderson and Greenwald, 1969) or freeze-dried sections, fixed with osmium vapor, epon-embedded and coated with stripping film (Attramadal, 1970a). The only differences have been the failure to find labelled neurons in the nucleus triangularis septi and in the organon subfornicale (Anderson and Greenwald, 1969). The grain count is reduced in the preoptic area and ventromedial arcuate nucleus region by pretreatment with 2 μg of estradiol or 2.5 mg of progesterone one hour before the ^{3}H-estradiol. Another brain region with neuronal concentration of radioactive grains is the medial amygdaloid nucleus (dorsal part of the posterior third) (Anderson and Greenwald, 1969).

In the anterior pituitary radioactive grains are concentrated in the nuclei of acidophiles, basophiles, and chromophobes (Stumpf, 1968b; Attramadal, 1970b). Grains in the anterior pituitary are reduced by pretreatment with estradiol but not significantly by progesterone (Anderson and Greenwald, 1969).

A different hypothalamic localization has been described in the only report of autoradiography on a primate. Twelve hours after intramuscular administration of ^{3}H-estradiol to a monkey the hypothalamus was sectioned by freezing microtomy and examined by autoradiography. In this study silver grains were found concentrated in an area of specialized ependymal cells (situated anteriolaterally in the tuber cinereum and distinguished by having long processes which extend to the region of the pars tuberalis); grains were not concentrated elsewhere (Anand-Kumar and Knowles, 1967). Additional studies of the primate brain are indicated.

Macromolecular Interactions

Estrogens attach to protein containing macromolecules prepared from the supernatant fraction of the uterus (Toft and Gorski, 1966). In solutions of low ionic strength the estrogen-binding macromolecules have sedimentation coefficients of approximately 8 to 9.5S with ultracentrifugation in sucrose gradients (Toft and Gorski, 1966; Jensen et al., 1969). These uterine-binding molecules have high specificity for estrogens (Korenman, 1969) and have sulfhydryl groups that are important for the estrogen binding (Jensen et al, 1967). The current concept is that the initial interaction of estradiol with a protein in the uterus occurs in the cytoplasm. The entire estradiol cytoplasmic protein complex then enters the nucleus (Jensen et al., 1968) and attaches to chromatin (Maurer and Chalkley, 1967). (Alternatively the estradiol may be transferred from the cytoplasmic protein to a different nuclear protein.) This concept is based on the observation that cytoplasmic-binding molecules appear to be required to demonstrate subsequent macromolecular binding in the nucleus (Jensen et al., 1968; Shyamala and Gorski, 1969).

Estrogen-binding macromolecules have been sought in supernatant fractions from the hypothalamus and pituitary. Tissues from chronically ovariectomized rats were homogenized by Tris HCl containing .0015 M EDTA and the supernatant fraction obtained by ultracentrifugation. Low concentrations of ^{3}H-estradiol were mixed with the supernatant fractions. After incubation radioactivity associated with macromolecules was separated from unbound estradiol by small polyacrylamide gel filtration columns at room temperature (Eisenfeld, 1969). Average values in the macromolecular fraction are uterus 18,000, anterior pituitary 11,000, hypothalamus 1500, cerebrum 300, cerebellum 250, heart 200, and plasma 50 dpm per milligram protein (Eisenfeld, 1970). The radioactivity in the macromolecular fraction from the hypothalamus and anterior pituitary chromatographs identically with authentic estradiol. Approximately equal concentrations of estrogen-binding macromolecules are found in the anterior and middle hypothalamus (Eisenfeld, unpublished).

Steroid specificity for these estrogen-binding macromolecules has been examined by mixing various nonradioactive steroids with ^{3}H-estradiol before adding the tissue supernatant (Eisenfeld, 1970). Nonradioactive estradiol (10^{-7}M) markedly reduces ^{3}H-estradiol concentrations while progesterone or testosterone (10^{-5}M) do not (Fig. 5-5).

The two estrogens in use in the combination or sequential oral contraceptives are 17α-ethinyl estradiol and mestranol (3-methoxy-17α-ethinyl estradiol). Each tablet contains 50 to 125 μg of one of these estrogens. 17α-ethinyl estradiol appears to bind well to the hypothalamic and anterior pituitary estrogen-binding macromolecules. In contrast, high concentrations of mestranol compete poorly with ^{3}H-estradiol for the hypotha-

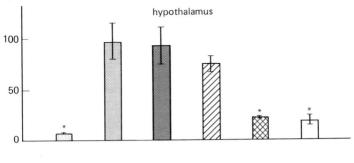
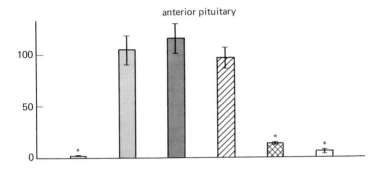
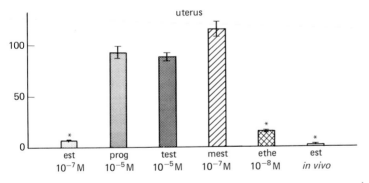

hypothalamus

anterior pituitary

uterus

| est | prog | test | mest | ethe | est |
| 10^{-7}M | 10^{-5}M | 10^{-5}M | 10^{-7}M | 10^{-8}M | *in vivo* |

Figure 5-5 ^{3}H-estradiol was mixed with estradiol (est), progesterone (prog), testosterone (test), mestranol (mest) or 17α-ehtinylestradiole (ethe) or their vehicle (5μl ethanol) and then 0.2 ml of tissue supernatants added. One group of animals was pretreated with 10 μg of estradiol per 100 g 75 minutes before removing their organs est *in vivo*). The final concentration of ^{3}H-estradiol was 2×10^{-9}M (48C/mmole); the final concentrations of the drugs are indicated in the graph. After one hour in ice with estradiol, progesterone, testosterone, or estrogen *in vivo* or 24 hours with mestranol or 17α-ethinyl-estradiol, macromolecular-bound ^{3}H-estradiol was measured by gel filtration. The results are expressed as the percentage of respective controls ± S.E.M.

lamic and anterior pituitary binding macromolecules (Fig. 5-5). This suggests that mestranol must be metabolized in the body to form 17α-ethinyl estradiol to be involved in inhibition of ovulation.

Macromolecular binding may also occur *in vivo*. Rats in one group were pretreated with nonradioactive estradiol before removing their organs (Fig. 5-5). When ^{3}H-estradiol is then mixed with the supernatant fraction of hypothalamus and anterior pituitary the radioactivity in the macromolecular fraction from these pretreated animals is less than 20 per cent of that found in control animals (Eisenfeld, 1970).

In order to characterize partially the chemical composition of the binding molecules, supernatants were incubated with ^{3}H-estradiol in the presence of various degradative enzymes (Eisenfeld, 1970). The hypothalamic and pituitary binding are markedly reduced by chymotrypsin (Fig. 5-6). This indicates that the binding molecules contain protein. In contrast, binding in the hypothalamus and pituitary is not reduced by either DNase or RNase. Para-chloromercuriphenylsulfonate, a reagent that reacts with free sulfhydryl groups, reduces macromolecular binding in hypothalamus and anterior pituitary.

Some radioactive estradiol sediments at about 9.5S after *in vitro* incubation of the supernatant from the bovine anterior pituitary, median eminence, and possibly the anterior and posterior hypothalamus but not from the cerebral cortex. No binding of ^{3}H-progesterone or ^{3}H-testosterone is found (Kahwanago, Heinrichs, and Herrmann, 1969). Incubation with high concentrations of either clomiphene or p-chloromercuriphenylsulfonate reduces 9S binding to approximately 50 per cent of control in the anterior hypothalamus, 20 per cent in the median eminence plus pars tuberalis, and 10 per cent in the anterior pituitary (Kahwanago, Heinrichs, and Herrmann, 1970). In the 9S regions of the sucrose gradient the pituitary supernatant can bind about 2×10^{-8} moles of estradiol per kg of wet weight (Jensen et al., in press).

Several *in vitro* binding properties of the hypothalamic and anterior pituitary supernatant thus are similar to those for the uterus. In addition a close parallel is found with respect to the properties of *in vitro* macromolecular binding and *in vivo* accumulation in the hypothalamus and anterior pituitary. The same relative concentration among organs, a finite capacity, and high specificity for estrogens are shown with both approaches.

In the *in vitro* studies very low concentrations of radioactivity have

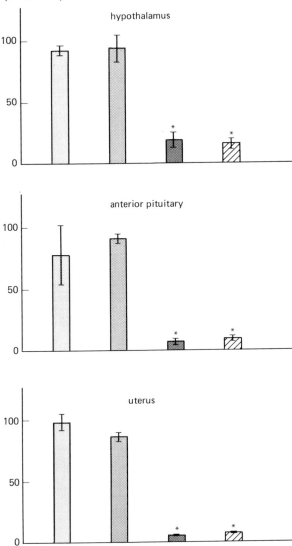

Figure 5-6 Supernatant fractions were shaken at 24° C with 2×10^{-9} M ^{3}H-estradiol (48 c/mmole) and 250 μg/ml of deoxyribonuclease (DNase), ribonuclease (RNase), or chymotrypsin (CHYMO). In another experiment sodium p-chloromercuriphenylsulfonate (PCMPS) $(1 \times 10^{-3}$ M) was added to the supernatant in ice half an hour before adding ^{3}H-estradiol. Macromolecular-bound estradiol was measured one hour after the addition of ^{3}H-estradiol. The results depict the mean ± S.E.M. expressed as the percentage of respective controls.

been found in the macromolecular fraction, using the supernatants of organs such as the cerebrum, cerebellum, or heart, which are not known to be affected directly by estrogens. This radioactivity is decreased to about half by 10^{-7}M estradiol, chymotrypsin, or p-chloromercuriphenyl-sulfonate (Eisenfeld, 1970). The possibility does exist, therefore, that the difference with respect to supernatant-binding macromolecules between hypothalamus, pituitary, and uterus, on the one hand, and organs such as cerebrum and heart, on the other, is not qualitative but quantitative. The hypothalamus has at least a 10-fold, and the anterior pituitary a 60-fold, higher concentration of specific binding macromolecules than either cerebrum or cerebellum.

In the hypothalamus it appears that estrogen binding is concentrated in highly selective groups of neurons. Other neurons, axons with myelin sheaths, and glia do not appear to concentrate estradiol highly. These latter components constitute the large bulk of the hypothalamus. In contrast, most cells in the anterior pituitary and uterus concentrate estradiol. When this difference is taken into consideration it is likely that for those neurons in the hypothalamus that do concentrate estradiol, the number of estradiol-binding molecules per cell may be in the same range as that in anterior pituitary or uterus.

Although the initial interaction of estrogen in the hypothalamus and anterior pituitary appears to be with cytoplasmic proteins, the ultimate cellular locus *in vivo* is predominantly nuclear as shown by either differential centrifugation or autoradiography. Nuclear retention of estradiol has now been shown after *in vitro* incubation of tissue fragments of hypothalamus and anterior pituitary. After incubation of tissue pieces with ^{3}H-estradiol, retention of the estradiol in purified nuclei is four times greater in hypothalamus than in cerebellum. The nuclear accumulation of radioactive estradiol is reduced by estradiol but not by cortisol, testosterone, or progesterone (Chader and Villee, 1970). Homogenates of anterior pituitary incubated with ^{3}H-estradiol have 8-fold higher nuclear uptake than liver; this accumulation of radioactivity in nuclei is not seen with incubation of anterior pituitary homogenates with ^{3}H-corticosterone, ^{3}H-progesterone, or ^{3}H-testosterone (Leavitt, Friend, and Robinson, 1969).

There is also some evidence for cytoplasmic to nuclear transfer in the hypothalamus and pituitary. If isolated nuclei are incubated with ^{3}H-estradiol in buffer the nuclear retention of radioactivity is low in both hypothalamus and cerebellum. If the supernatant and nuclear fractions are both mixed with ^{3}H-estradiol *in vitro* and the nuclei then reisolated, the nuclear retention in hypothalamus is increased to about three times cerebellar (Chader and Villee, 1970). With anterior pituitary nuclei incubated with ^{3}H-estradiol in either pituitary supernatant or buffer the nuclear pellet contains a 5-fold higher concentration of radioactivity from the samples suspended in the supernatant relative to those suspended in buffer (Leavitt, Friend, and Robinson, 1969).

In the uterus the transformation from cytoplasmic-binding molecule–estradiol complex to nuclear-binding molecule–estradiol complex may involve some change in the cytoplasmic-binding molecule. When estradiol is extracted with solutions of high ionic strength from the nucleus it remains attached to proteins with a sedimentation coefficient of 5S (Jensen et al., 1969). The cytoplasmic-binding molecules in solutions of high ionic strength sediment at 4S. It has been reported that the uterine cytoplasmic and nuclear macromolecules can be distinguished by using albumin (4.5S) as a sedimentation marker. An attempt has been made to determine the sedimentation coefficients for the supernatant- and nuclear-binding macromolecules from the hypothalamus and pituitary. After incubation of ^{3}H-estradiol with blocks of either anterior hypothalamic or pituitary tissue estradiol is bound to supernatant macromolecules which sediment at 8.5S in solutions of low ionic strength. The nuclear fraction, extracted with a solution of high ionic strength, from the pituitary and hypothalamic portions has some radioactivity sedimenting as 4.5S (Vertes and King, 1969). After *in vivo* administration the major part of the radioactivity in the nuclear fraction of the pituitary is macromolecular-bound (Mowles, Ashkanazy, and Mix, 1970).

In summary of estrogen interaction with the brain, estrogens are concentrated in the anterior pituitary and in discrete portions of both the hypothalamus and the limbic system. This accumulation has specificity for estrogens. In the rat, estradiol is concentrated highly in the nuclei of selected neurons and of all types of anterior pituitary cells. Protein-containing macromolecules prepared from the supernatant fractions of anterior pituitary and hypothalamus have a marked affinity and specificity for estrogens. Cytoplasmic binding may be required for nuclear binding. In later portions of this chapter the role of estrogens in the regulation of ovulation will be discussed. It may be that these hypothalamic and pituitary estrogen-binding proteins are involved in this regulation.

Estrogen Binding and Sexual Differentiation of the Brain

The possibility has been suggested that the male brain may be less responsive to estrogens than the female brain because of a deficiency of the
estrogen-binding mechanism in the male brain.

The male brain differs from the female with respect to gonadotrophin
regulation and behavior. The male pattern of gonadotrophin is thought
to be characterized by a constant secretion of FSH and LH; by contrast
there is cyclic discharge in the female. In rodents, the male pattern is due
to the presence of androgens within the first few days after birth. Castration of males within this period produces cyclic gonadotrophin secretion
so that ovaries transplanted into these males will ovulate cyclically. Males
will also ovulate transplanted ovaries if the androgen antagonist cyproterone is injected during their fetal and neonatal life (Neumann and Elger, 1966). Conversely, administration of testosterone to females in this
period prevents ovulation at maturity; the ovaries contain developed follicles but no corpora lutea (Harris, 1964). Aggression also seems to be
modulated by androgen early in life. After testosterone treatment when
adult, normal males or neonatally testosterone-treated female mice are
more likely to fight than are normal females or neonatally castrate males
(Edwards, 1968).

There is some evidence that neonatally androgen-treated females do not
respond to estrogens as well as normal females. As will be discussed later,
ovulation, which is missing in the neonatally androgen-treated female, is
thought to be promoted by a positive feedback estrogen effect leading to
the discharge of high concentrations of LH. Administration of estrogens
to castrate adult female rats promotes a characteristic behavior pattern—
assuming a lordotic position when mounted by a male. This response occurs less frequently if the females were androgen-treated neonatally (Gerall and Kenney, 1970). In this regard, normal males untreated at birth
and given estrogens after castration in adulthood will assume a lordotic
position when mounted by another male but only with doses of estrogen
many times higher than that required in castrate females (Davidson,
1969). The brain locus which appears responsible for estrogen-induced
lordosis is the preoptic-anterior hypothalamic region. Implants of estrogens in this region will promote lordosis in female castrates. Lesions of
this region abolish lordosis, and lordosis cannot be restored by estrogen
administration (Lisk, 1969). Finally, estrogen hypertrophy to neonatally

androgen-treated females results in subnormal pituitary hypertrophy (Harris and Levine, 1965) and less vaginal cornification with low doses administered (Gerall and Kenney, 1970).

Accordingly, investigation has begun concerning the possibility that this reduced responsiveness is due to a defective estrogen-binding mechanism in the normal male or neonatally testosterone-treated female. In comparing adult males and females no substantial difference has been found in estrogen accumulation in the hypothalamus, preoptic region, or pituitary (Eisenfeld and Axelrod, 1966; McEwen and Pfaff, 1970). Conflicting results have been obtained when neonatally androgen-treated females have been compared with normal females. Other investigators have found a partial decrease in accumulation of estrogens in the anterior and middle hypothalamus, pituitary, and uterus with no change in the posterior hypothalamus or cortex (Flerko, 1969); a decrease in pituitary concentration but not in portions of the hypothalamus (McGuire and Lisk, 1969b); and a slight decrease in the hypothalamus but not the pituitary (McEwen and Pfaff, 1970). An autoradiographic study found that neonatally androgenized females have half of the normal number of labelled cells in the preoptic and ventromedial-arcuate regions and a significant decrease in grain concentration in the pituitary (Anderson and Greenwald, 1969).

Radioactive Progesterone Interaction with the Brain

There has been little work reported concerning the interaction of radioactive progesterone with the brain. One hour after the administration of ^{3}H-progesterone to chronically castrate mature rats the radioactivity extractable into methylene chloride is slightly higher in the anterior, middle, and posterior hypothalamus than in cerebrum or blood but not cerebellum (Seiki et al., 1968). After incubation of bovine hypothalamic supernatant with ^{3}H-progesterone, no macromolecular bound radioactivity has been found after sucrose gradient ultracentrifugation (Kahwanago, Heinrichs, and Hermann, 1969). No nuclear accumulation has been found after incubation of the castrate rat anterior pituitary in vitro with ^{3}H-progesterone (Leavitt, Friend, and Robinson, 1969).

Specific progesterone interaction has not been clearly demonstrated in any target organ of the castrate rat. Perhaps progesterone interaction with the brain could be more readily shown in other animals. For example, ³H-progesterone concentrates in the guinea pig uterus. This accumulation in the guinea pig uterus appears to have specificity for progesterone and is increased in magnitude by estrogen pretreatment (Falk and Bardin, 1970).

Radioactive Androgen Interaction with the Brain

In the castrate male guinea pig one hour after administration of ³H-testosterone in oil, the level of radioactivity with the chromatographic mobility of testosterone is slightly higher in both hypothalamus and pituitary than in either cerebellum or plasma (Resko, Goy, and Phoenix, 1967). In another study in both male and female rats, methylene chloride extractable radioactivity is higher in the pituitary and slightly higher in the hypothalamus, preoptic region, and septum relative to cerebral cortex or blood (McEwen, Pfaff, and Zigmond, 1970). Total radioactivity in the hypothalamic and preoptic areas is not higher than in cortex one hour after intravenous administration of ³H-testosterone to castrate male rats while the pituitary concentration is five times greater than plasma (Whalen, Luttge, and Green, 1969).

Unlike estradiol, which is retained unchanged in female reproductive organs, testosterone is substantially metabolized to a specific derivative dihydrotestosterone (5-α-androstan-17β-ol-3-one) in male sexual accessory glands. Both testosterone and dihydrotestosterone are bound *in vivo* to macromolecules in the cytoplasmic and nuclear fractions (Bruchovsky and Wilson, 1968). Cyproterone, an androgen antagonist, is a competitive inhibitor of the cytoplasmic binding of testosterone (Stern and Eisenfeld, 1969). Formation of dihydrotestosterone may also occur in the pituitary and hypothalamus. At one hour after intravenous administration of ³H-testosterone, pituitary radioactivity with the chromatographic mobilities of testosterone and dihydrotestosterone is three times and thirty times plasma levels respectively. In the rat hypothalamus, radioactivity with the mobility of dihydrotestosterone is present in higher concentration than in the cerebrum while testosterone concentrations are equal. (In the ring dove both testosterone and dihydrotestosterone are several times higher in the hypothalamus than in cerebrum.) In the rat pituitary and hypothalamus but not in the cerebrum, the concentration of radioactivity with the mobility of testosterone and dihydrotestosterone relative to plasma is reduced by prior administration of cold testosterone, cyproterone, or progesterone (Stern and Eisenfeld, 1971).

Macromolecular binding of androgens by the pituitary and hypothalamus has been reported. Following intracarotid administration of ³H-testosterone to intact or castrate male rats or addition of ³H-testosterone to homogenates or tissue sections, some radioactivity is found in the macromolecular fraction after gel filtration (Samparez, Thieulant, and Jouan, 1969).

Mechanism of Action

The mechanism of action of sex steroids in the brain at the molecular level is unknown. The ultimate cellular modifications promoted by the sex steroids appear quite different in the brain in comparison with peripheral reproductive organs. For example, estradiol promotes uterine growth and secretion, vaginal epithelium cornification, pituitary hypertrophy and may act at the hypothalamic level by influencing neuronal function. However, the early steps in the sequence of action could be similar, with tissue differentiation expressed at a later point. With this possibility in mind the current thought of the mechanism of action in peripheral reproductive organs will be presented. It is thought that the initial interaction is with a cytoplasmic protein for estrogens in uterus (Toft and Gorski, 1966), progesterone in chick oviduct (O'Malley, Sherman, and Toft, 1970), and androgens in prostate (Fang, Anderson, and Liao, 1969). If the radioactive steroids are added to these respective target organs *in vitro* at a low temperature supernatant binding occurs. If the temperature is then raised supernatant binding decreases and most of the radioactive steroid is then found in the nucleus attached to protein with similar properties to those of the supernatant-binding molecules (Jensen et al., 1968; O'Malley, Sherman, and Toft, 1970; Fang, Anderson, and Liao, 1969). Estrogens (Maurer and Chalkley, 1966) and androgens (Bruchovsky and Wilson, 1968) while still attached to protein associate with chromatin. With estrogens the evidence for cytoplasmic-binding proteins and cytoplasmic to nuclear transfer suggests that the initial steps may be similar in anterior pituitary, hypothalamus, and uterus.

It should be emphasized that there is no direct evidence that this binding process is responsible for any of the cellular modifications produced by sex steroids. However, a localization of hormone at chromatin is consistent with the current concept of the earliest change promoted in cellular metabolism. It is thought that sex steroids increase RNA synthesis or the synthesis of selective RNAs in reproductive organs. Specificity could occur by transcribing regions of DNA not utilized or utilized at a slower rate in the absence of the steroid hormone. According to one group, estrogens rapidly increase the synthesis of RNA in the uterus (Hamilton, 1968). Another group cannot find an early over-all increased rate of RNA synthesis but does have the following evidence consistent with the early appearance of RNA responsible for synthesis of a protein fraction. Within one hour after estrogen administration amino acid incorporation is increased in one protein fraction separated by gel electrophoresis. Administration of actinomycin D blocks this stimulation (De Angelo and Gorski, 1970). Synthesis of RNA by endometrial chromatin in the presence of excess RNA polymerase is increased to three times castrate levels 10 minutes after the administration of estradiol (Church and McCarthy, 1970). A qualitative change in the RNA synthesized in the presence of estrogens is suggested by studies of the hybridization of RNA to DNA. In one study radioactive RNA was obtained from the nuclei of rabbit uteri 60 minutes after estradiol administration and 10 minutes after ^{3}H-uridine. Some of this uterine RNA will bind to DNA immobilized on membrane filters. Prior or concomitant addition of an excess of nonradioactive RNA from various tissue sources will reduce the radioactive RNA binding if the nonradioactive and radioactive compete for a limited number of similar binding sites on the DNA. It was found that nonradioactive RNA from the uteri of rabbits treated with estradiol one hour previously competed more effectively than did RNA from castrate uteri. This suggests that new regions of DNA may be involved in synthesizing RNA after estrogen administration (Church and McCarthy, 1970). At four hours after administration of estrogen the nearest neighbor frequency of nucleotides in RNA synthesized by uterine nuclei is changed (Barton and Liao, 1967). (For nearest neighbor frequency analysis, a nucleotide containing radioactive phosphate attached to the 5 position of ribose (α^{32}P ATP, GTP, UTP, and CTP one at a time) is incorporated into RNA utilizing nuclei (or chromatin with an excess of bacterial RNA polymerase). In forming RNA the phosphate group attaches to the 3 position of ribose of the neighboring nucleotide. The RNA is then isolated and hydrolyzed by base which cleaves the phosphodiester bond at the 5 position of ribose. The ^{32}P phosphate remains attached to the neighboring nucleotide. The four nucleotides are separated and the radioactivity in each measured.)

The chick oviduct is a useful model system for progesterone effects in that progesterone induces the synthesis of a specific oviduct protein. The administration of progesterone to estrogen-primed chicks appears to promote the synthesis of RNA from new regions of the DNA. RNA-DNA hybridization and nearest neighbor frequency are changed 6 hours after progesterone in comparison with the estrogen-primed oviduct alone (O'Malley et al., 1969). Progesterone induces the synthesis of a specific protein, avidin (which binds the viatmin biotin) within 10 hours after *in vivo* administration or *in vitro* addition to oviduct monolayer cultures. This protein synthesis appears to be dependent on RNA synthesis since it is inhibited by actinomycin D (O'Malley et al., 1969).

Androgens rapidly increase the synthesis of RNA in seminal vesicles. Following intraperitoneal administration of testosterone, rapidly labelled RNA synthesis is 150 per cent of castrate control level after 20 minutes and 200 per cent castrate control level at 50 minutes (Wicks and Kenney, 1964). It has been suggested that testosterone may be responsible for certain androgen effects, and dihydrotestosterone for others in the prostate. Addition of testosterone to organ cultures of prostate promotes epithelial-cell hyperplasia, and an increase in cell height and secretion. Addition of dihydrotestosterone provokes greater epithelial-cell hyperplasia than does testosterone but does not increase either cell height or secretion (Baulieu, Lasnitzki, and Robel, 1968).

Regulation of Ovulation

In the brain and pituitary the sex steroids influence ovulation by modulation of hypothalamic releasing factors and pituitary gonadotrophins.

The hypothalamus is known to influence anterior pituitary function by a group of releasing factors which are both acid- and heat-stable (McCann and Porter, 1969). The releasing factors, some of which have been shown to be small polypeptides, are discharged into capillaries in the median eminence of the hypothalamus and carried via a portal blood vessel system to the anterior pituitary. These factors have specificity for the pituitary hormones they release. FSH-RF promotes discharge of FSH (follicular stimulating hormones) and LH-RF discharge of LH (luteinizing hormone). Hypothalamic extracts not only regulate the release but also promote the synthesis of pituitary hormones. If the pituitary of a rat is transplanted to a site distant from the hypothalamus only prolactin is produced. The rat hypothalamus also has activity which inhibits the synthesis and discharge of prolactin in the pituitary.

There is some evidence that secretion of releasing factors may be mediated by discharge of various neurotransmitters. Ovulatory discharge of gonadotrophins occurs by 4 p.m. of the day of proestrus in the rat. During a critical period (from 2 to 4 p.m.) ovulation can be inhibited by administration of either a long-acting alpha adrenergic blocking agent (or of other drugs that affect CNS function such as atropine, barbiturates, or morphine) (Everett, 1964). Dopamine discharges both LH and FSH into the medium of organ cultures containing hypothalamus and anterior pituitary. Since dopamine will not discharge either LH or FSH when added to cultures of anterior pituitary without hypothalamus and will not increase pituitary responsiveness to purified releasing factors, the effect of the dopamine appears to be hypothalamic. This effect of dopamine is inhibited by alpha adrenergic blocking agents (Schneider and McCann, 1969). *In vivo* low doses of dopamine injected into the third ventricle adjacent to the hypothalamus increases plasma LH 4-fold 10 minutes later. Perfusion of the anterior pituitary with dopamine via a portal vessel does not increase plasma LH (Kamberi, Mical, and Porter, 1970).

Only a very small portion of intact brain is required to promote ovulation. Rats will ovulate even after the preoptic area has been freed of afferent innervation by cutting all anterior, lateral, and superior connections bilaterally. Ovulation will not occur even if a cut only separates the preoptic region from the medial basal hypothalamus (Halasz, 1969). This indicates that the preoptic region is needed for ovulation. One possible role for the preoptic region may be to provide the neural discharge that initiates the sequence culminating in the discharge of LH-RF; electrolytic stimulation of the preoptic region is known to elicit ovulation (Everett, 1964). Alternatively the preoptic area might influence the synthesis of a pool of LH-RF which must be discharged to promote the release of the ovulatory surge of LH. Lesions of the suprachiasmatic area between the preoptic and anterior hypothalamus reduce the content of LH-RF in the median eminence of male rats (Martini, Fraschini,, and Motta, 1968).

It is generally thought that LH-RF discharge is responsible for the ovulatory surge of LH secretion. In normally cycling rats there are technical difficulties in measuring LH-RF secretion; therefore direct proof of LH-RF discharge preceding LH secretion is not available. Hypothalamic content of LH-RF has been measured. If LH-RF synthesis remains constant, an increase in LH-RF discharge should be reflected by decreased hypothalamic content; however, no such decrease has been found either shortly preceding or during the critical period (Ramirez and Sawyer, 1965; Chowers and McCann, 1965).

Role of Estrogens and Progestational Agents in the Regulation of Ovulation

The role of the estrogens and progestational agents in the regulation of ovulation will be discussed from the vantage point of the sequence of secretion of estrogens, progesterone, and gonadotrophins during the normal menstrual cycle and in association with administration of birth control pills.

Menstrual Cycle

Plasma levels of hormones have recently been accurately measured using radioimmunoassay for FSH and LH and either isotopic derivative formation or competitive protein-binding assays for estrogens and progesterone. In the normal menstrual cycle there is a rise in plasma FSH levels which starts shortly before menstruation. During and after menstruation a slight increase in FSH levels promotes ovarian follicular development. Plasma FSH then declines while plasma estrogens are increasing (Ross et al., 1970). Plasma estrogen levels increase abruptly to maximal levels the day before and day of a peak in plasma LH levels (Baird and Guevara, 1969). This peak in plasma LH (and a peak in plasma FSH found in some cycles) precedes ovulation by approximately one day (Ross et al., 1970; Yussman and Taymor, 1970). Plasma progesterone—which is low throughout the follicular phase—doubles on the day of the LH peak and then continues to rise steadily to 25 times the follicular level by the seventh day after ovulation; subsequently it returns to low levels by a few days before the onset of menses (Ross et al., 1970). Plasma estrogens decline the day after the LH peak, rise slightly during the secretory phase, and decline to low levels before menses start (Baird and Guevara, 1969). Plasma FSH and LH are both low during the secretory phase (Ross et al., 1970).

The marked changes which precede ovulation are elevated plasma estrogens followed by a sharp rise in plasma LH. There is now strong support derived from studies in lower animals for the concept that the elevated plasma estrogen level causes ovulation. In the female rat, plasma estrogens are high shortly before and during the surge in LH secretion (Brown-Grant, Exley, and Naftolin, 1970). Rats injected with antibodies directed against steroidal estrogens do not ovulate. Ovulation can be restored in animals treated with these antibodies by injecting the nonsteroidal estrogen, diethylstilbestrol. By contrast administration of antibodies directed against progesterone does not inhibit ovulation (Ferin et al., 1969).

It is not settled whether estrogens induce ovulation by a hypothalamic or anterior pituitary effect. There is only one report of a positive effect on LH secretion of estrogen implantation in the hypothalamus of an adult animal. Five days after implanting estrogen into the median eminence of adult female rats, plasma LH was markedly elevated; pituitary implantation of estrogen did not increase plasma LH (Palka, Ramirez, and Sawyer, 1966). In adult castrate rats (Ramirez, Abrams, and McCann, 1964) or rabbits (Kanematsu and Sawyer, 1964) the more chronic effect of implanting estrogen into the median eminence is decreased LH secretion. (Actinomycin D administration prevents estrogen reduction in plasma LH in castrates, suggesting that RNA synthesis may be involved in estrogen effects in the brain (Schally et al., 1969).

If estrogens promote ovulation via an hypothalamic effect, estrogens should increase the discharge of LH-RF. Possibly estrogens may exert a positive influence on the dopamine LH-RF system by increasing dopamine discharge; estrogen administration to female castrates increases the turnover of dopamine in arcuate neurons (Fuxe, Hokfert, and Nilson, 1967). However, other studies of the effect of estrogens on LH-RF discharge suggest a negative influence. Chronic treatment of female castrate rats with estrogen decreases the concentration of hypothalamic LH-RF and pituitary LH (Piacsek and Meites, 1966). In hypophysectomized rats, LH-RF is released into plasma by injecting dopamine. Administration of estradiol into the third ventricle two hours before the dopamine prevents the discharge of LH-RF (Scheider and McCann, 1970a). As mentioned previously, dopamine promotes the appearance of LH in the medium in coincubates of hypothalamus and anterior pituitary presumably by increasing LH-RF discharge. Estradiol addition to the hypothalamic-pituitary coincubate inhibits LH release by dopamine. These negative influences may be the mechanisms whereby estrogens decrease the high tonic secretion of LH following castration.

The following information relates to a possible anterior pituitary input of estrogen increasing LH secretion into plasma of adult cycling rats. Estrogen implantation into the anterior pituitary advances ovulation by one day in rats with five-day cycles; hypothalamic implantation of estradiol does not (Weick and Davidson, 1970). However, as previously mentioned, implantation of estrogens into the pituitary of adult cycling rats does not increase plasma LH when measured at five days (Palka, Ramirez, and Sawyer, 1966). Finally, high doses of estradiol added to organ cultures of rat pituitary increase the discharge of LH into the medium (Schneider and McCann, 1970b). (Inhibition by estrogen of both dopamine-mediated LH release from hypothalamic-pituitary coincubates and stimulation of LH release with pituitary alone may require protein synthesis. These estrogen effects are both prevented by either cycloheximide or puromycin) (Schneider and McCann, 1970b).

Oral Contraceptives

Both the sequential and combination oral contraceptives prevent pregnancy predominately by inhibiting ovulation. The inhibition of ovulation has been confirmed by the absence of fresh corpora lutea in ovaries inspected at laparotomy late in the menstrual cycle. Administration of exogenous gonadotrophins (with FSH and LH activity) to women taking combination oral contraceptives produces ovulation (Diszfalusy, 1968). This is consistent with the hypothesis that ovulation is not occurring because the birth control pills are impairing the secretion of gonadotrophins.

Sequential Oral Contraceptives

In sequential oral contraception an estrogen (either mestranol or 17α-ethinyl estradiol) is administered from day 5 to day 20 of the menstrual cycle; a progestin is added during the next five days. (The start of menstruation is designated as day 1.) Thus, the estrogen is the only medication given preceding and during the portion of the cycle when ovulation normally occurs. The amount of estrogen in the pill is thought to be greater than the amount secreted by the ovary, particularly that secreted early in the follicular phase. Plasma FSH levels are low during the follicular phase in women on sequential therapy. By contrast, plasma LH levels may be markedly elevated; in some women there are multiple peaks with levels as high as in the ovulatory surge of the normal cycle (Swerdloff and Odell, 1969). Ovarian follicles are undeveloped in women on sequential oral contraceptives (Diszfalusy, 1968). These findings suggest that the estrogen in the sequential pills inhibits ovulation by decreasing FSH secretion and thereby preventing follicular maturation.

FSH secretion appears to be under the regulation of the medial basal hypothalamic region which includes the median eminence, arcuate, and ventromedial nuclei. The pituitary alone cannot secrete FSH; after stalk section or transplantation to another site in the body it does not secrete FSH. However, FSH secretion (as indicated by follicular development) will occur even if all afferents to the medial basal hypothalamus are transected (Halasz, 1969). Estrogens prevent the rise in plasma FSH following castration even if the connections between the anterior hypothalamus and median eminence are transected (Kalra, Velasco, and Sawyer, 1970).

There is some evidence that negative feedback of estrogen on FSH secretion is a hypothalamic effect. Estradiol implanted in the arcuate nucleus terminates estrous cycling, and the ovaries contain no large follicles (Lisk, 1970). While implantation of estradiol in the rabbit median eminence leads to ovarian atrophy, similar implantation in the adenohypophysis does not (Davidson and Sawyer, 1961). Administration of estradiol to castrate female rats reduces hypothalamic FSH-RF and pituitary FSH content (Martini, Fraschini, and Motta, 1968).

Combined Oral Contraceptives

The combined pill consists of an estrogen (17α-ethinyl estradiol or mestranol) and a progestational agent (either a progesterone derivative or a 19-nortestosterone) administered from day 5 to day 25 of the menstrual cycle. Women on the combined pill have low levels of plasma FSH and LH (Swerdloff and Odell, 1969). The essentials for ovulation that are missing with combined pill therapy are the early increase in plasma FSH and the ovulatory surge of LH. The inhibition of FSH secretion is thought to be due to the negative feedback hypothalamic effect of the estrogen. The absence of the ovulatory surge of LH is most likely an effect of the progestational agent. There is evidence that progestins reduce pituitary responsiveness to median eminence extracts with LH-RF activity (Stevens et al., 1970). However, plasma LH can be increased in women taking combined oral contraceptives by administration of a purified LH-RF (Kastin et al., 1969). Plasma LH is also increased by administration of LH-RF to rats receiving a variety of different combined oral contraceptives (Schally et al., 1970). Consistent with a hypothalamic locus for progesterone inhibition of LH discharge, median eminence implants of progesterone in the median eminence permit follicular development but prevent corpus luteum formation; in contrast corpora lutea are found despite implants of progesterone in the anterior pituitary (Davidson, 1969). Thus, the combined oral contraceptives appear to inhibit ovulation both by estrogen inhibition of FSH secretion and progestational-agent inhibition of the ovulatory surge of LH secretion.

Summary

The hypothalamus and anterior pituitary contain proteins with high specificity and affinity for estrogens. *In vivo* accumulation has been shown in neurons in localized regions of both the hypothalamus and the limbic system and in all cell types of the anterior pituitary. The possibility exists that the attachment of estrogens to cytoplasmic proteins and transfer to the nucleus many be early steps in the regulatory action of estrogens in the brain and pituitary. Neonatally androgen-treated females are less responsive to estrogens, but a defect in estrogen receptor mechanism remains to be established clearly.

After administration of ^{3}H-testosterone, dihydrotestosterone, as well as testosterone, is found in the hypothalamus and pituitary. Possibly dihydrotestosterone may be responsible for some androgen effects.

The metabolic steps of steroid action in the brain are unknown. In peripheral organs concerned with reproduction the sex steroids appear to modulate the synthesis of RNA.

The hypothalamus contains factors that release FSH and LH from the pituitary. Dopamine appears to be a neurotransmitter that promotes the secretion of FSH-RF and LH-RF.

High levels of estrogen in plasma followed by a surge of LH secretion precedes ovulation in women. In the rat, antibodies that react with estrogens prevent ovulation.

Women taking sequential oral contraceptives do not ovulate because the secretion of FSH is inhibited; consequently, the ovarian follicles do not mature. Estrogens appear to inhibit FSH secretion by a hypothalamic effect that results in a reduced secretion of FSH-RF.

Plasma levels of both FSH and LH are low in women receiving combined oral contraceptives. The estrogenic component is thought to be responsible for the decreased FSH secretion, and the progestational agent responsible for the absence of the ovulatory surge of LH secretion.

References

Anand Kumar, T. C., and Knowles, F. 1967. *Nature* 215:54.
Anderson, C. H., and Greenwald, G. S. 1969. *Endocrinology* 85:1160.
Attramadal, A. 1964. In *Proceedings of the Second International Congress of Endocrinology,* Part 1, Excerpta Medica Foundation, Amsterdam, p. 612.
Attramadal, A. 1970a. *Z. Zellforsch.* 104:572.
Attramadal, A. 1970b. *Z. Zellforsch.* 104:597.
Baird, D. T., and Guevara, A. J. 1960. *Clin. Endocr.* 29:149.
Barton, R. W., and Liao, S. 1967. *Endocrinology* 81:409.
Baulieu, E. E., Lasnitzki, I., and Robel, P. 1968. *Biochem. Biophys. Res. Commun.* 32:575.
Brown-Grant, K., Exley, D., and Naftolin, F. J. 1970. *J. Endocr.* 48:295.
Bruschovsky, N., and Wilson, J. D. 1968. *J. Biol. Chem.* 243:2012, 5953.
Chader, G. J., and Villee, C. A. 1970. *Biochem. J.* 118:93.
Chowers, I., and McCann, S. M. 1965. *Endocrinology,* 76:700.
Church, R. B., and McCarthy, B. J. 1970. *Biochim. Biophys. Acta* 199:103.
Davidson, J. M. 1969. *Endocrinology* 87:1365.
Davidson, J. M. 1969. In *Frontiers in Neuroendocrinology,* W. F. Ganong and L. Martini (Eds.), Oxford University Press, New York, p. 343.
De Angelo, A. B., and Gorski, J. 1970. *Proc. Nat. Acad. Sci. U.S.* 66:693.
Diszfalusy, E. 1968. *Amer. J. Obstet. Gynec.* 100:136.
Edwards, D. A. 1968. *Amer. Zool.* 8:749 (abstract).
Eisenfeld, A. J., and Axelrod, J. 1965. *J. Pharmacol. Exp. Ther.* 150:469.
Eisenfeld, A. J., and Axelrod, J. 1966. *Endocrinology* 79:38.
Eisenfeld, A. J. 1967a. *Biochim. Biophys. Acta* 136:498.
Eisenfeld, A. J. 1967b. *Fed. Proc.* 26:365 (abstract).
Eisenfeld, A. J., and Axelrod, J. 1967. *Biochem. Pharmacol.* 16:1781.
Eisenfeld, A. J. 1969. *Nature* 224:1202.
Eisenfeld, A. J. 1970. *Endocrinology* 86:1313.
Eisenfeld, A. J. In *The Regulation of Mammalian Reproduction* (in press).
Everett, J. W. 1964. *Physiol. Rev.* 44:373.
Falk, R. J., and Bardin, C. W. 1970. *Endocrinology* 86:1059.
Fang, S., Anderson, K. M., and Liao, S. 1969. *J. Biol. Chem.* 244:6584.
Ferin, M., Tempone, A., Zimmering, P. E., and Van de Wiele, R. L. 1969. *Endocrinology* 85:1070.

Flerko, B., Mess, B., and Illei-Donhoffer, A. 1969. *Neuroendocrinology* 4:164.

Fuxe, K., Hökfelt, T., and Nilsson, O. 1967. *Life Sci.* 6:2057.

Gerall, A. A., and Kenney, A. M. 1970. *Endocrinology* 87:560.

Glascock, R. F., and Hoekstra, W. G. 1959. *Biochem. J.* 72:673.

Halasz, B. 1969. In *Frontiers in Neuroendocrinology*, W. F. Ganong and L. Martini (Eds.), Oxford University Press, New York, p. 307.

Hamilton, T. H. 1968. *Science* 161:649.

Harris, G. W. 1964. *Endocrinology* 75:527.

Harris, G. W., and Levine, S. 1965. *J. Physiol.* (Lond.) 181:379.

Jensen, E. V., and Jacobson, H. I. 1962. *Recent Prog. Hormone Res.* 18:387.

Jensen, E. V., Jacobson, H. I., Flesher, J. W., Saha, N. N., Gupta, G. N., Smith, S., Colucci, V., Shiplacoff, D., Neumann, H. G., Desombre, E. R., Jungblut, P. W. 1966. In *Steroids Dynamics*, G. Pincus, T. Nakao, and J. F. Tait (Eds.), Academic Press, New York, p. 133.

Jensen, E. V., Hurst, D. J., De Sombre, E. R., Jungblut, P. W. 1967. *Science* 158:385.

Jensen, E. V., Suzuki, T., Kawashima, T., Stumpf, W., Jungblut, P. W., and De Sombre, E. R. 1968. *Proc. Nat. Acad. Sci. U.S.* 59:632.

Jensen, E. V., Suzuki, T., Numata, M., Smith, S., and De Sombre, E. R. 1969. *Steroids* 13:417.

Jensen, E. V., Numata, M., Smith, S., Suzuki, T., and De Sombre, E. R. In *Communication in Development*, A Lang (Ed.), Academic Press, New York (in press).

Kahwanago, I., Heinrichs, W. L., and Herrmann, W. L. 1969. *Nature* 223:313.

Kahwanago, I., Heinrichs, W. L., and Herrmann, W. L. 1970. *Endocrinology* 86:1319.

Kalra, S. P., Velasco, M. E., and Sawyer, C. H. 1970. *Neuroendocrinology* 6:228.

Kamberi, I. A., Mical, R. S., and Porter, J. C. 1970. *Endocrinology* 87:1.

Kamberi, I. A., Schneider, H. P. G., and McCann, S. M. 1970. *Endocrinology* 86:278.

Kanematsu, S., and Sawyer, C. H. 1964. *Endocrinology* 75:579.

Kastin, A. S., Schally, A. V., Gual, C., Midgely, A. R., Jr., Bowers, C. Y., Diaz-Infante, A., Jr. 1969. *J. Clin. Endocr.* 29:1046.

Kato, J., and Villee, C. A. 1967a. *Endocrinology* 80:567.

Kato, J., and Villee, C. A. 1967b. *Endocrinology* 80:1133.

Kato, J., Kobayashi, T., and Villee, C. A. 1968. *Endocrinology* 82:1049.

Korenman, S. G. 1969. *Steroids* 13:163.

Leavitt, W. W., Friend, J. P., and Robinson, J. A. 1969. *Science* 165:496.

Lisk, R. K. 1967. In *Neuroendocrinology*, L. Martini and W. F. Ganong (Eds.), vol. 2, Academic Press, New York, p. 197.

Martini, L., Fraschini, F., and Motta, M. 1968. *Recent Prog. Hormone Res.* 24:439.

Maurer, H. R., and Chalkley, G. R. 1967. *J. Molec. Biol.* 27:431.

McCann, S. M., and Porter, J. C. 1969. *Physiol. Rev.* 49:240.

McEwen, B. S., and Pfaff, D. W. 1970. *Brain Res.* 21:1.

McEwen, B. S., Pfaff, D. W., and Zigmond, R. E. 1970. *Brain Res.* 21:17.

McGuire, J. L., and Lisk, R. D. 1968. *Proc. Nat. Acad. Sci. U.S.* 61:497.

McGuire, J. L., and Lisk, R. D. 1969a. *Neuroendocrinology* 4:289.

McGuire, J. L., and Lisk, R. D. 1969b. *Nature* 221:1068.

Michael, R. P. 1962. *Science* 136:322.

Michael, R. P. 1965a. In *Hormonal Steriods, L. Martini and A. Pecile* (Eds.), vol. 2, Academic Press, New York, p. 469.

Michael, R. P. 1965b. *Brit. Med. Bull.* 21:87.

Mowles, T. F., Ashkanazy, B., and Mix, E., Jr. 1970. *Fed. Proc.* 29:312 (abstract).

Neuman, F., and Elger, W. 1966. *Endokrinologie* 50:209.

O'Malley, B. W., McGuire, W. L., Kohler, P. O., and Korenman, S. G. 1969. *Recent Prog. Hormone Res.* 25:105.

O'Malley, B. W., Sherman, M. R., and Toft, D. O. 1970. *Proc. Nat. Acad. Sci. U.S.* 67:501.

Palka, Y. S., Ramirez, V. D., and Sawyer, C. H. 1966. *Endocrinology* 78:487.

Piacsek, B. E., and Meites, J. 1966. *Endocrinology* 79:432.

Ramirez, V. D., and Sawyer, C. H. 1965. *Endocrinology* 76:282.

Ramirez, V. D., Abrams, R. M., and McCann, S. M. 1969. *Endocrinology* 75:243.

Resko, J. A., Goy, R. W., and Phoenix, C. H. 1967. *Endocrinology* 80:490.

Ross, G. T., Cargille, C. M., Lipsett, M. B., Rayford, P. L., Marshall, J. R., Strott, C. A., and Rodbard, D. 1970. *Recent Prog. Hormone Res.* 26:1.

Roy, S., Mahesh, V. B., and Greenblatt, R. B., 1964. *Acta Endocr.* (Copenhagen) 47:669.

Samparez, S., Thieulant, M. L., and Jouan, P. C. R. 1969. *Acad. Sci. (D)* (Paris) 268:2965.

Schally, A. U., Bowers, C. Y., Carter, W. H., Animura, A., Redding, T. W., and Saito, M. 1969. *Endocrinology* 85:290.

Schally, A. V., Parlow, A. F., Carter, W. H., Saito, M., Bowers, C. Y., and Arimura, A. 1970. *Endocrinology* 86:530.

Schneider, H. P. G., and McCann, S. M. 1969. *Endocrinology* 85:121.

Schneider, H. P. G., and McCann, S. M. 1970a. *Endocrinology* 87:249.

Schneider, H. P. G., and McCann, S. M. 1970b. *Endocrinology* 87:330.

Seiki, K., Higashida, M., Imanishi, Y., Miyamoto, M., Kitagawa, T., and Kotani, M. 1968. *J. Endocr.* 41:109.

Shyamala, G., and Gorski, J. 1969. *J. Biol. Chem.* 244:1097.

Stern, J. M., and Eisenfeld, A. J. 1969. *Science* 166:233.

Stern, J. M., and Eisenfeld, A. J. 1971. *Endocrinology* 88:1117.

Stevens, K. R., Spies, H. G., Hilliard, J., and Sawyer, C. H. 1970. *Endocrinology* 86:970.

Stumpf, W. E. 1968a. *Science* 162:1001.

Stumpf, W. E. 1968b. *Z. Zellforsch.* 92:23.

Swerdloff, R. S., and Odell, W. D. 1969. *J. Clin. Endocr.* 29:157.

Toft, D., and Gorski, J. 1966. *Proc. Nat. Acad. Sci. U.S.* 55:1574

Vertes, M., and King, R. J. B. 1969. *J. Endocr.* 45:xxii (abstract).

Weick, R. F., and Davidson, J. M. 1970. *Endocrinology* 87:693.

Whalen, R. E., Luttge, W. G., and Green, R. 1969. *Endocrinology* 84:217.

Wicks, W. D., and Kenney, F. T. 1964. *Science* 144:1346.

Yussman, M. A., and Taymor, M. L. 1970. *J. Clin. Endocr.* 30:396.

Zigmond, R. E., and McEwen, B. S. 1970. *J. Neurochem.* 17:889.

6

L-Tryptophan, L-Tyrosine, and the Control
of Brain Monoamine Biosynthesis

RICHARD J. WURTMAN
JOHN D. FERNSTROM

It is now well established that the mammalian brain synthesizes serotonin and the catecholamines, dopamine and norepinephrine, from the amino acids L-tryptophan and L-tyrosine. Moreover, a growing body of experimental data supports the hypothesis that these monoamines are released at central synapses to function as neurotransmitters. The initial step in both serotonin and catecholamine biosynthesis is the introduction of a hydroxyl group onto one of the carbon atoms of the aromatic ring. These oxidations are catalyzed by two relatively specific enzymes, tryptophan hydroxylase and tyrosine hydroxylase. The former enzyme catalyzes the hydroxylation of L-tryptophan at the 5-position, to yield the amino acid L-5-hydroxytryptophan (L-5-HTP); tyrosine hydroxylase catalyzes the *meta*-hydroxylation of L-*para*-tyrosine yielding the catechol amino acid L-3, 4-dihydroxyphenylalanine (L-DOPA). Under normal conditions, neither L-5-HTP nor L-DOPA can be detected in the blood or the brain; both are decarboxylated within their neurons of origin soon after they are formed, giving rise to serotonin or dopamine.

On the basis of considerable *in vitro* data and some *in vivo* evidence, it is generally held that the rate at which neurons synthesize dopamine and norepinephrine depends upon the net catalytic activity of the enzyme tyrosine hydroxylase. According to this formulation, processes that increase or decrease tyrosine hydroxylase activity (i.e. by changing the actual amount of enzyme protein within the neuron or by modifying its inhibition by intracellular catecholamines) produce parallel changes in the rate of *in vivo* catecholamine synthesis. Less information is available about the relationship between the formation of brain serotonin and the activity of tryptophan hydroxylase. However, serotonin synthesis is depressed after administration of para-chlorophenylalanine (PCPA), a synthetic amino acid that inhibits tryptophan hydroxylase (Jequier et al., 1967), and this observation has been offered as evidence that tryptophan hydroxylase, like tyrosine hydroxylase, is rate-limiting *in vivo*.

This article explores the possibility that the rates at which a given central neuron synthesizes serotonin or the catecholamines might sometimes be determined not by the amount or activity of a rate-limiting hydroxylase enzyme but by the availability of its amino acid precursor, L-tryptophan or L-tyrosine. The brain cannot make L-tryptophan, nor, in all likelihood, can it synthesize significant amounts of L-tyrosine. Individual neurons can store small quantities of these amino acids in the form of protein, but it is not yet established that L-tryptophan or L-tyrosine released by intraneuronal proteolysis can subsequently be reutilized for amine biosynthesis. Hence the synthesis of biogenic amines by central neurons requires a continuing external source of L-tryptophan and L-tyrosine, probably provided by the blood and the extracellular fluid of the brain. The concentrations of circulating L-tryptophan and L-tyrosine are now recognized to exhibit characteristic diurnal variations and to change in response to disease states, diet, and a number of experimental manipulations and physiological events. Less information is available about the systems that transport these amino acids across the plasma membranes of brain neurons, and almost no data have been offered on the actual concentrations of amino acid within the perikarya or the terminal boutons of "serotoninergic" or "catecholaminergic" neurons. However, there is evidence, described below, that the flux of amino acids into and out of the brain, and the concentrations of these substances within the brain, also are inconstant, varying diurnally and in response to alterations in plasma amino acid composition.

If the concentration of L-tryptophan within serotoninergic neurons should, in response to a particular physiological circumstance, fall to values approaching the K_m of trpytophan hydroxylase, the rate of serotonin biosynthesis might depend on the extent to which the enzyme is saturated with substrate, rather than on the amount of tryptophan hydroxylase in the cell or the physiological activity of the neuron. A similar hypothesis can be proposed for the potential importance of intraneuronal L-tyrosine concentrations as a factor determining the rate at which the brain synthesizes catecholamines.

In addition to L-tyrosine, L-tryptophan, and the enzymes that hydroxylate these amino acids, the availability of cofactors needed for their hydroxylation and decarboxylation (e.g. the reduced pteridine, pyridoxal phosphate) might also influence the rates at which central neurons synthesize monoamines. Experimental data relating to this possibility are also described below.

Biosynthesis of Brain Monoamines

Catecholamines

Enzymatic Synthesis from L-Tyrosine. The biosynthesis of catecholamines in brain neurons, chromaffin cells, and peripheral postganglionic sympathetic neurons (Wurtman, 1966) is initiated by the hydroxylation of free tyrosine at the *meta* position to form the catechol amino acid L-DOPA (Iyer et al., 1963; Levitt et al., 1965; Nagatsu et al., 1964). This reaction is catalyzed by tyrosine hydroxylase, a mixed-function oxidase that requires oxygen, ferrous iron, and, probably, a still undefined reduced pteridine cofactor for optimal activity (Ikeda et al., 1966; Nagatsu et al., 1964). The reduced pteridine combines with the inactive oxidized form of the hydroxylase enzyme, converting it to the active reduced form; the cofactor is, however, oxidized in the process (Ikeda et al., 1966) and must then be regenerated through the activity of a pteridine reductase. This enzyme has been demonstrated in the adrenal medulla (Musacchio and Castellucci, 1969) but apparently has not yet been identified in brain. The levels of reduced pteridine in tissue are probably low, and thus may influence the *in vivo* rate of tyrosine hydroxylation, as described below. The substrate K_m for brain-stem tyrosine hydroxylase has been estimated at $10^{-5}M$ (Nagatsu et al., 1964). The brain of the adult rat contains about 0.1 micromoles of L-tyrosine per gram of tissue (Zigmond and Wurtman, 1970); hence if it is assumed that the amino acid is distributed uniformly throughout brain intracellular and extracellular water, the concentration of tyrosine within the neuron is at least ten times the K_m for tyrosine hydroxylase, and physiological changes in brain tyrosine levels would probably not influence the rate at which the amino acid is hydroxylated *in vivo*. However, no data are available on the actual concentration of free tyrosine within the neurons as a whole or in the regions of the neuron where most of the protein and most of the catecholamine are synthesized (the perikaryon and the terminal boutons respectively). On the basis of anatomical considerations alone, it seems highly unlikely that all of the tyrosine in the neuron comprises a single metabolic pool that is available equally for hydroxylation or incorporation into protein. Hence, estimates of the extent to which tyrosine hydroxylase is saturated *in vivo* must be regarded as purely speculative. L-tryptophan is not a substrate for tyrosine hydroxylase; however, both L-tryptophan and L-phenylalanine are potent inhibitors of brain-stem tyrosine hydroxylase at concentrations of 10^{-4}M (Nagatsu et al., 1964). The inhibition of tyrosine hydroxylase by catecholamines and by synthetic amino acids is described below.

Aromatic L-amino acid decarboxylase (AAAD), a relatively nonspecific enzyme that requires pyridoxal phosphate as a cofactor, catalyzes the decarboxylation of L-DOPA to form dopamine (Lovenberg et al., 1962). AAAD accepts as substrates L-5-HTP, L-tryptophan, L-tyrosine, L-phenylalanine, and the competitive inhibitor α-methyl DOPA. Its K_m for L-DOPA (40×10^{-5}M) is well above the level of L-DOPA present in brain and blood (Anton and Sayre, 1964). Hence, the enzyme functions *in vivo* in a highly unsaturated state. This point supports the hypothesis that the relatively small fraction of intracellular AAAD localized within the same subcellular organelle as tyrosine hydroxylase (Udenfriend, 1966) is of special physiological significance, for it has ready access to newly synthesized molecules of L-DOPA. The relative V_{max} of AAAD for DOPA decarboxylation is very great.

It is generally held that since the activity of AAAD is so much greater in amine-producing tissues than that of tyrosine or tryptophan hydroxylase, AAAD cannot rate-limit catecholamine or serotonin synthesis *in vivo*. This hypothesis is supported by the apparent absence of L-DOPA and L-5-HTP from the brain. Recent observations suggest, however, that AAAD activity might conceivably be rate-limiting under certain conditions: For optimal activity, the *in vitro* assay for the AAAD in human brain requires concentrations of the pyridoxal phosphate cofactor that probably do not exist *in vivo* (Lloyd and Hornykiewicz, 1970); moreover, the administration of endogenous pyridoxine interferes with the therapeutic effects of L-DOPA, possibly by accelerating its catabolism *in vivo* (DuVoisin et al., 1969; R. C. DuVoisin, L. C. Cote, and M. D. Yahr, personal communication). It is therefore possible that the very high AAAD activity demonstrated *in vitro* might not always reflect the ability of cells to decarboxylate amino acids *in vivo;* the activity of the enzyme might be limited by cofactor concentration (which depends upon both the availability of dietary pyridoxine and the activity of enzymes converting pyridoxine to pyridoxal phosphate). Such limited enzyme activity might, for example, exist among people who consume too little pyridoxine or who utilize unusual quantities of the vitamin in metabolizing very large, chronic doses of L-DOPA.

Norepinephrine-synthesizing cells also contain dopamine β-oxidase, an enzyme that catalyzes the side-chain oxidation of dopamine, tyramine, and related substrates. This enzyme, highly localized within synaptic vesicles and chromaffin granules, is discussed elsewhere in this volume.

Tyrosine Hydroxylase and Rate-Limitation of Catecholamine Biosynthesis. In their original report identifying tyrosine hydroxylase in adrenal medulla and brain (Nagatsu et al., 1964), Udenfriend and his collaborators noted that the activity of this enzyme was far lower than that of AAAD or of dopamine β-oxidase; they also observed that the K_m for the over-all conversion of L-tyrosine to L-norepinephrine in the perfused guinea pig heart ($1 \times 10^{-5}M$) was the same as the K_m for tyrosine hydroxylase *in vitro* (Levitt et al., 1965). On the basis of these findings and of the apparent absence of L-DOPA from catecholamine-synthesizing tissues, these authors suggested that tyrosine hydroxylase catalyzed the critical, rate-limiting step in catecholamine biosynthesis. Noting that dopamine, norepinephrine, and epinephrine were all potent inhibitors of tyrosine hydroxylase *in vitro,* they further suggested that end-product inhibition of the enzyme might also occur *in vivo,* and might constitute an important mechanism for maintaining the constancy of tissue catecholamine levels. Studies subsequently performed in many laboratories have further supported the hypothesis that the rate of *tyrosine hydroxylation* usually limits catecholamine biosynthesis *in vivo.* However, when animals have been treated in such a way as to accelerate tyrosine hydroxylation, there has generally been no parallelism between the rate of catecholamine synthesis measured *in vivo* and tyrosine hydroxylase activity assayed *in vitro,* unless the treatment has been applied for a day or longer (Table 6-1). We recognize, therefore, that additional factors besides the amount of tyrosine hydroxylase in a cell must influence the rate at which it forms catecholamines. Such factors probably include the availability of cofactors and of tyrosine itself.

When animals are subjected to experimental manipulations that enhance the release of catecholamines from neurons or chromaffin cells, the rates

Table 6-1   Effects of physiological inputs and drugs on tyrosine hydroxylation an

Reference	Treatment	Duration of treatment	Tissue	Interval after administration of ^{3}H- or ^{14}C-tyrosine
Gordon et al., 1966a	electrical stimulation of stellate ganglia	60 min	rat heart (*in vivo*)	60 min
Alousi et al., 1966	electrical stimulation of isolated hypogastric nerve-vas deferens preparation	60 min	guinea pig vas deferens (*in vitro*)	60 min
Gordon et al., 1966b	exercise	120 min	rat heart, adrenal, brain, spleen (*in vivo*)	60 min
Roth et al., 1967	electrical stimulation of: isolated hypogastric nerve-vas deferens	4 hr	guinea pig (*in vitro*)	4 hr
	isolated splenic nerve	15-60 min	bovine (*in vitro*)	15-60 min
Sedvall et al., 1968	sympathetic decentralization	14 days	rat submaximillary gland (*in vivo*)	20 min (infusion)
	electrical stimulation, cervical sympathetic chain	20 min		
Dairman et al., 1968	phentolamine (5 mg/kg)	60 min	rat heart, adrenals, brain (*in vivo*)	60 min
	phenoxybenzamine (25 mg/kg)	16 hr		
De Quattro et al., 1969	denervation of carotid sinuses and aortic arch (induces hypertension)	2 days or 3 weeks	rabbit heart (left ventricle), adrenal glands (*in vivo*)	30 min
Dairman and Udenfriend, 1970	phenoxybenzamine (20 mg/kg)	2 days	rat heart, adrenals (*in vivo*)	1 hr

rosine hydroxylase activity

Accumulation of isotopically labeled catechol-amines	Tyrosine hydroxylase activity	Remarks
increased	not measured	³H-catecholamine accumulation from ³H-L-DOPA not increased.
increased	not measured	Specific activity of ¹⁴C-L-tyrosine not measured. Norepinephrine in medium inhibited basal and induced ³H-catecholamine synthesis. ³H-L-tyrosine specific activity not measured.
increased	not measured	Specific activity of brain ¹⁴C-L-tyrosine increased; heart and adrenals unchanged. Specific activity of brain ¹⁴C-dopamine unchanged; ¹⁴C-norepinephrine increased.
increased unchanged	not measured	—
decreased	no change (reported in Sedvall and Kopin, 1967)	³H-catecholamine accumulation was corrected for average specific activity of tissue ¹⁴C-L-tyrosine.
increased	no change	³H-catecholamine accumulation from ³H-L-DOPA not increased. ¹⁴C-L-tyrosine content of tissues unchanged.
increased	50 to 100%	³H-catecholamine accumulation was corrected for specific activity of tissue ³H-tyrosine. ³H-norepinephrine turnover also accelerated (20%), but not as much as ³H-norepinephrine accumulation from ³H-tyrosine (120%)
increased	2-fold increase	4- to 6-fold increase in ³H-catecholamine accumulation after 2 days vs 2-fold to 3-fold increase after 16 hr. Specific activity of ¹⁴C-L-tyrosine in heart and adrenals unchanged.

of L-tyrosine hydroxylation and of catecholamine synthesis are accelerated. This acceleration seems to involve at least two mechanisms (Weiner, 1970): one, a rapid effect (within minutes) (Alousi & Weiner, 1966; Gordon et al., 1966a; Sedvall et al., 1968), possibly caused by the depletion of a "small, critical pool" of norepinephrine that inhibits tyrosine hydroxylase activity (Spector et al., 1967; Weiner and Rabadjija, 1968); and the second, a slower effect (within days), associated with increased tyrosine hydroxylase activity (demonstrated *in vitro*) and possibly caused by an acceleration in the biosynthesis of the enzyme protein.

Numerous short-term studies have demonstrated an acceleration in the conversion of isotopically labelled tyrosine to norepinephrine. Noradrenergic neurons have been stimulated by the direct application of electrical impulses postganglionically (Gordon et al., 1966a) or pregangliconically (Sedvall et al., 1968); by physiological activation of reflex mechanisms (placing animals in the cold (Gordon et al., 1966b)); or by treatment with drugs that block the peripheral actions of norepinephrine, thereby causing a reflex increase in the presynaptic input to the noradrenergic neurons (e.g. the α-blocking agent, phenoxybenzamine (Dairman et al., 1968)) (Table 6-1). The stimulated and control animals are then given isotopically labelled tyrosine, and tissues are removed, preferably after a short period, and assayed for labelled and unlabelled tyrosine and catecholamines. The concentration of ^{3}H-catechols (corrected for the average specific activity of the ^{3}H-tyrosine precursor during the study period) is found to be elevated in tissues containing stimulated neurons. The amount of time allowed to lapse between the administration of the labelled amino acid and the removal of tissues is very important to this sort of study: The accumulation of tissue ^{3}H-catechols appears to be linear in the rat for only 3 to 10 minutes after administration of the amino acid (Zigmond and Wurtman, 1970); hence, experiments in which animals are killed at longer intervals after ^{3}H-tyrosine administration tend to underestimate the rate of catecholamine biosynthesis, and may obscure real differences between control and stimulated groups. The increased conversion of isotopically labelled tyrosine to catecholamines that follows the short-term (one day or less) stimulation of noradrenergic neurons is in general unassociated with changes in tyrosine hydroxylase activity (Table 6-1); it may result in part from a mechanism involving the reduced pteridine cofactor needed by the enzyme. Thus, the rate of catecholamine biosynthesis in the isolated hypogastric nerve–vas deferens preparation was found to be increased both during and after a period of electrical stimulation (Weiner and Rabadjija, 1968). The initial enhancement was blocked by addition of norepinephrine to the medium, and may thus have reflected *in vivo* activation of existing enzyme by the dissipation of the hypothetical "small critical pool" of norepinephrine thought to function as an endogenous enzyme inhibitor. The post-stimulation increase was no longer blocked by norepinephrine. Neither during nor after electrical stimulation was there a measurable increase in the tyrosine hydroxylase activity present in tissue homogenates; hence, neither component of the enhancement of catecholamine synthesis seems to have been mediated by an increase in the amount of tyrosine hydroxylase enzyme protein. The post-stimulation rise was blocked by puromycin, suggesting that it resulted from accelerated synthesis of another enzyme necessary for tyrosine hydroxylation, perhaps the hypothetical pteridine reductase. The "small critical pool" of intracellular norepinephrine, thought to be depleted when the neuron is stimulated, may compete with the pteridine cofactor for a site on the oxidized form of the enzyme (Ikeda et al., 1966); alternatively, the "pool" might interact directly with the cofactor to oxidize and thereby inactivate it (Weiner, 1970). In either case, it is apparent that a pteridine reductase enzyme could, by catalyzing the regeneration of the active form of the cofactor, control tyrosine hydroxylation *in vivo,* thereby constituting an important factor in the regulation of catecholamine biosynthesis. As mentioned above, this enzyme has not yet been identified in brain; however, it has been shown that catechols inhibit brain tyrosine hydroxylase (*in vitro*), just as they do the adrenal enzyme (McGeer and McGeer, 1967).

Studies using inhibitors of monoamine oxidase (MAO) have provided additional support for the hypothesis that the *in vivo* hydroxylation of tyrosine is tonically suppressed by intraneuronal norepinephrine. When MAO activity has been inhibited for a sufficient period, tissue norepinephrine levels rise and the conversion of isotopically labelled tyrosine to catechols is suppressed (Ngai et al., 1968). Catechol biosynthesis is *not* suppressed immediately after the MAO inhibitor is administered, even though *in vitro* studies demonstrate that the inhibition of MAO is maximal at this time. We infer, therefore, that the drug affects tyrosine hydroxylation through a secondary mechanism, i.e. by blocking norepinephrine metabolism, thus causing intraneuronal norepinephrine levels to rise.

In the studies demonstrating increased tyrosine hydroxylase activity in tissues receiving a chronically increased presynaptic input, a generalized increase in sympathetic tone has been induced by denervation of the baro-receptor nerves (Chalmers and Wurtman, 1971; De Quattro et al., 1969) or by administration of the drugs 6-hydroxydopamine (Mueller et al., 1969a), phenoxybenzamine (Dairman and Udenfriend, 1970), or reserpine (Mueller et al., 1969b). Reserpine has been shown by direct measurements to increase the electrical activity of preganglionic sympathetic neurons (Iggo and Vogt, 1960); 6-hydroxydopamine and phenoxybenzamine are thought to share this effect by virtue of their respective abilities to destroy postganglionic sympathetic neurons or to block peripheral vascular receptors. The elevations in tyrosine hydroxylase activity observed in sympathetically innervated tissues following treatment with reserpine (Thoenen et al., 1969a) or 6-hydroxydopamine (Thoenen et al., 1969b) are lost if the preganglionic nerves are transected; they are mediated by a "trans-synaptic" effect. Phenoxybenzamine elevates cardiac and adrenal tyrosine hydroxylase activity after two days of treatment (Dairman and Udenfriend, 1970), but not after one day (Dairman et al., 1968). The time-course of this rise in enzyme activity suggests that the rise reflects an increase in the amount of enzyme protein. In support of this hypothesis, it has been shown that the increase caused by reserpine can be blocked by pretreatment with cycloheximide or actinomycin D. However, the hypothesis cannot be confirmed until an assay is developed that allows direct measurement of the tyrosine hydroxylase enzyme protein. The mechanism through which the presynaptic input to catecholamine-producing cells triggers their synthesis of a specific enzyme protein (tyrosine hydroxylase) also awaits discovery. The nature of this mechanism constitutes one of the genuinely important unanswered questions in neurotransmitter research.

Dairman and Udenfriend (1970) have recently presented perhaps the only available data suggesting that an increase in the amount of tyrosine hydroxylase protein within neurons can by itself accelerate catecholamine biosynthesis. Animals pretreated with phenoxybenzamine were given a ganglionic blocking agent one day later (i.e. before tyrosine hydroxylase activity, assayed *in vitro,* became elevated). The anticipated acceleration of ^{14}C-catecholamine biosynthesis from ^{14}C-tyrosine was completely inhibited. However, if the ganglionic blocker was given two days after the phenoxybenzamine (i.e. when *in vitro* tyrosine hydroxylase activity was already elevated), the acceleration of catecholamine biosynthesis was only partially inhibited. If the only difference between animals tested after one and two days was the presence of more intraneuronal tyrosine hydroxylase in the latter group, it can be inferred that an increase in this enzyme does, of itself, cause an acceleration of tyrosine hydroxylation, and that the enzyme is truly rate-limiting in both directions (i.e. that both increases and decreases in enzyme activity cause parallel changes in the rate of *in vivo* tyrosine hydroxylation). However, it is by no means certain that the sole, or even most significant, biochemical difference between the animals receiving the ganglionic blocker one or two days after phenoxybenzamine was a difference in intraneuronal tyrosine hydroxylase levels. Many other factors, such as tyrosine transport, tyrosine concentration in the terminal bouton, or pteridine reductase activity, might have been affected.

There is abundant evidence that tyrosine hydroxylase can be *made* rate-limiting if it is pharmacologically inhibited by a substance like the synthetic L-amino acid, α-methyl para-tyrosine. Its administration brings about a profound reduction in tissue catecholamine stores and in the rate at which isotopically labelled tyrosine is converted to catecholamines (Spector et al., 1965). Of course, this type of experiment can never prove that the enzyme is limiting under physiological conditions. The interpretation of experiments using α-methyl para-tyrosine or related synthetic amino acids are further complicated by the propensity of these agents to produce multiple biochemical effects besides the one for which they are chosen.

In summary, tyrosine hydroxylase activity is probably just one of several factors that can influence the rate at which neurons synthesize catecholamines.

Serotonin

Enzymatic Synthesis from L-*Tryptophan.* The biosynthesis of serotonin from L-tryptophan occurs in certain brain neurons, the pineal organ, mast cells, enterochromaffin cells, and, possibly, platelets (Garattini and Valzelli, 1965; Page, 1968). The initial step in this process is the oxidation of amino acid at the 5-position to form 5-HTP. This step is catalyzed by several different tissue-specific tryptophan hydroxylases (Lovenberg et al., 1968) and by phenylalanine hydroxylase, the enzyme in liver that converts L-phenylalanine to L-tyrosine (Renson et al., 1962). Like tyrosine hydroxylase, tryptophan hydroxylase prepared from rat brain-stem requires oxygen, ferrous iron, and a reduced pteridine cofactor for optimal activity (Lovenberg et al., 1968). Its K_m for tryptophan ($3 \times 10^{-4}M$) is quite high compared with the levels of free tryptophan likely to be present in the brain (approximately 0.05 μmoles/g: Mckean et al., 1968), suggesting that the enzyme normally functions in an unsaturated state, and that changes in brain tryptophan concentration are likely to influence the rate at which tryptophan is hydroxylated. L-phenylalanine is a potent competitive inhibitor of tryptophan hydroxylase; its K_i is equal to the K_m for the natural substrate (Lovenberg et al., 1968). The effects of phenylalanine and other natural and synthetic amino acids on brain serotonin metabolism are discussed below.

As recently as five or six years ago, there was speculation that the circulating amino acid precursor for brain serotonin might be L-5-hydroxytryptophan (L-5-HTP), and not L-tryptophan itself. The liver had been shown to contain an enzyme (phenylalanine hydroxylase) that could convert L-tryptophan to L-5-HTP, and brain serotonin levels were known to increase after the administration of synthetic 5-HTP (Bogdanski et al., 1957). On the other hand, it was difficult to obtain unequivocal evidence that the brain alone could synthesize serotonin from L-tryptophan. Tryptophan hydroxylase activity was finally identified in brain preparations by Gal and his collaborators (1963) and by Grahame-Smith (1964a, b). The technical problems that had afflicted most investigators trying to demonstrate this enzyme were resolved when Lovenberg and his collaborators (1968) established the enzyme's cofactor requirements and described a sensitive and specific radiochemical method for its assay based on the enzymatic conversion of the newly formed labelled 5-HTP to serotonin. Tryptophan hydroxylase has since been localized within synaptosomes (Grahame-Smith, 1967, 1970) and its distribution within the brain has been shown to be similar to that of serotonin (Peters et al., 1968). The hypothesis that circulating L-5-HTP is an important precursor for brain serotonin now seems untenable in view of this additional evidence: (1) under normal circumstances, measurable quantities of 5-HTP cannot be detected in the blood; (2) there is little similarity between the regional distribution of endogenous brain serotonin and the pattern of the increment in serotonin content that follows the administration of 5-HTP (Moir and Eccleston, 1968); (3) brains of eviscerated rats can synthesize serotonin from administered L-tryptophan (Weber and Horita, 1965). The natural history of endogenous 5-HTP is similar to that of L-DOPA; it is synthesized from a circulating aromatic L-amino acid by a small population of cells that do not store or release it, but rapidly decarboxylate it to form a biologically active amine. Administered 5-HTP should be viewed as a drug; it should be anticipated that circulating 5-HTP would have a different fate from that of the amino acid synthesized within the neurons, just as the fate of circulating L-DOPA differs markedly from that of endogenous L-DOPA (Wurtman et al., 1970a).

The decarboxylation of 5-HTP and L-DOPA is probably catalyzed by the same enzyme, aromatic amino acid decarboxylase (AAAD) (Lovenberg et al., 1962). Some of the properties of this enzyme are described above. Its K_m for 5-HTP is less than one-hundredth that for L-tryptophan and its V_{max} is several times greater (Lovenberg et al., 1962). Hence, brain AAAD normally catalyzes the synthesis of little, if any, tryptamine, and tryptamine is not likely to be a physiological precursor for serotonin (Udenfriend et al., 1959).

Tryptophan Hydroxylase and Rate-Limitation of Serotonin Biosynthesis. Insufficient information is available on which to base a judgment about the likelihood that tryptophan hydroxylase activity controls the rate of serotonin synthesis *in vivo*. The capacity of central serotoninergic neurons to hydroxylate a given load of tryptophan appears to increase after electrical stimulation (Eccleston et al., 1970); no evidence, however, has been presented that the activity of tryptophan hydroxylase assayed *in vitro* changes in response to this *in vivo* stimulation. *Para*-chlorophenylalanine, a synthetic amino acid which inhibits tryptophan hydroxylase *in vivo* and *in vitro,* does appear to suppress serotonin biosynthesis; this drug, however, apparently has multiple biochemical actions, which could contribute to this effect. Moreover, as discussed above, the demonstration that an enzyme can be *made* rate-limiting by the administration of inhibitors can never prove that the enzyme is normally limiting.

Norepinephrine also inhibits tryptophan hydroxylase activity *in vitro* (Lovenberg et al., 1968), possibly by interacting with the reduced pteridine cofactor in a manner similar to that described above for tyrosine hydroxylase. This inhibition probably does not occur under physiological conditions, however, since no cells have been shown to contain both norepinephrine and tryptophan hydroxylase. The addition of norepinephrine to cultured pineal organs stimulates serotonin biosynthesis from tryptophan (Shein and Wurtman, 1971).

Apparently, serotonin does not influence its own rate of synthesis by

Table 6-2   Effects of naturally occurring amino acids on brain aromatic amino acid

Reference	Animal	Treatment
Carver, 1965	adult rat (150-175g)	L-phenylalanine, 100 mg i.p.; killed after 15 to 120 min
McKean et al., 1968	adult rat	L-phenylalanine, 1 g/kg i.p.; killed after 15 to 180 min
	adult rat	L-tyrosine, 2 g/kg i.p.; killed after 180 min
	3-week-old rat	diet supplemented with 7% L-phenylalanine for 3 weeks; pair-fed controls
	3-week-old rat	diet supplemented with 7% L-tyrosine for 3 weeks; pair-fed controls
Roberts, 1968	adult rat (fasting)	L-leucine, 130 mg/kg i.v. killed after 10 min
Aoki and Siegel, 1970	7-day-old rat	L-phenylalanine, 1 g/kg i.p.; killed after 60 min
	4-week-old rat	L-phenylalanine, 1 g/kg i.p.; killed after 60 min
Fernstrom and Wurtman (unpublished observations)	adult rat	L-tyrosine, 375 mg/kg i.p.; killed after 60 to 180 min

Levels are given as multiples of control values.

end-product inhibition: concentrations as great as 10^{-4}M have no effect on brain-stem tryptophan hydroxylase activity assayed *in vitro* (Jequier et al., 1969).

Control of Brain Levels of L-Tyrosine and L-Tryptophan

L-tyrosine and L-tryptophan are presumably distributed throughout the water content of the brain. Measurements of these substances in homogenates of whole brain are a composite of their concentrations within intra-

levels

| Plasma | | | Brain | | | |
phenyl-alanine	tyrosine	tryptophan	phenyl-alanine	tyrosine	tryptophan	Remarks
30×	5×	—	14×	3×	—	Most other brain amino acids unchanged.
36×	8×	0.71×	15×	2×	0.75×	Also lowers brain tryptophan, but not brain tyrosine, in infant.
—	—	—	0.93×	44×	—	
—	—	—	10×	1.65×	—	
—	—	—	0.85×	59×	—	
1.03×	0.88×	—	0.43×	0.54×	—	
—	—	—	16×	—	0.56×	Disaggregates brain polyribosomes in 7-day-old, but not 4-week-old rats.
—	—	—	6×	—	0.50×	
—	4× (1 hr)	0.65× (1 hr)	—	2× (1 hr)	0.80× (1 hr)	Brain serotonin unchanged.

cellular fluid, the extracellular space, and, to a lesser extent, the plasma trapped within brain capillaries (0.4 to 1.2 per cent of brain volume (Sokoloff, 1961)) and the cerebrospinal fluid trapped within the ventricular system. Plasma L-tyrosine and L-tryptophan concentrations tend to be higher than those of brain (Guroff and Udenfriend, 1962; McKean et al., 1968), and cerebrospinal fluid concentrations tend to be lower (Bito et al., 1966; van Sande et al., 1970); however, these ratios vary from species to species, and fluctuate diurnally. At present, it is not known whether the concentrations of L-tyrosine and L-tryptophan within the extracellular fluid of the brain are the same as those within cells, whether these concentrations are similar within different populations of brain cells, or even whether the concentrations within the perikaryon and the terminal boutons of a given brain neuron are the same.

Under normal circumstances, the level of L-tyrosine or L-tryptophan in the brain depends upon two sets of rates. "Source rates" are rates at which additional molecules of the free amino acids are entering the brain pool (by uptake from the blood via the brain extracellular fluid, or by intracellular proteolysis); "sink rates" are those at which molecules are leaving this pool (by secretion into the blood, incorporation into protein, conversion to hydroxylated derivatives and then to amines, or, in the case of L-tyrosine, by transamination). From minute to minute, brain amino acid levels reflect a steady state. However, these levels do change over long periods, presumably because one or more source or sink rates have been modified. This section considers the sources and sinks thought to influence free L-tyrosine and L-tryptophan levels in the brain.

Sources and Sinks of Brain L-Tyrosine

SOURCES: (A) *Uptake from the Plasma*. The rate at which the brain takes up L-tyrosine from the blood apparently depends on its concentration in the plasma and the activity of a transport system which L-tyrosine shares with such other large, neutral L-amino acids as L-tryptophan, L-leucine, and L-methionine (Blasberg and Lajtha, 1965; Guroff and Udenfriend, 1962). If large amounts of L-tyrosine are administered (300 to 500 mg/kg, i.p. (Chirigos et al., 1960) Table 6-2), brain and plasma L-tyrosine levels both increase to about the same extent (fivefold after one hour). One hour after rats receive a tracer dose of isotopically labelled L-tyrosine, the specific activity of the amino acid in whole brain is about 25 per cent greater than in plasma (Chirigos et al., 1960; Zigmond and Wurtman, 1970) (Table 6-3). This implies that, under normal conditions, variations in the rate at which tyrosine is taken up from the circulation are an important factor in determining brain tyrosine levels. It is not known whether catecholamine-producing neurons, which must utilize especially large quantities of tyrosine, have a special additional transport mechanism for this amino acid, in addition to the "large, neutral amino acid" system (Blasberg and Lajtha, 1965, 1966).

Table 6-3   Accumulation of ^{3}H-tyrosine and ^{3}H-catecholamine in brain after the administration of ^{3}H-tyrosine at different times of day

		Time			
		9 a.m.	3 p.m.	9 p.m.	3 a.m.
Tissue	Compound Measured	(D12)	(L6)	(L12)	(D6)
	TYROSINE				
blood	^{3}H-tyrosine (mμc/ml)	290	278	269	253
blood	tyrosine (μg/ml)	31.7*	29.5	24.3	25.9
blood	specific activity (mμc/μg)	9.15*	9.43	11.07	9.77
brain	^{3}H-tyrosine (mμc/g)	267	266	243	233
brain	tyrosine (μg/g)	16.8*	18.1	15.3	14.4
brain	specific activity (mμc/μg)	15.9*	14.7	15.9	16.2
	$\dfrac{\text{specific activity}_{\text{brain}}}{\text{specific activity}_{\text{blood}}}$	1.74*	1.56	1.44	1.66
	CATECHOLAMINES				
brain	^{3}H-catecholamine (mμc/g)	0.43*	0.47	0.34	0.26
brain	norepinephrine (μg/g)	0.41	0.40	0.40	0.43
brain	specific activity (mμc/μg)	1.05*	1.18	0.85	0.60
	$\dfrac{^3\text{H-catecholamine}_{\text{brain}}}{\text{specific activity}_{\text{brain tyrosine}}}$ (μg/g)	0.027*	0.032	0.021	0.016

Animals were killed one hour after receiving ^{3}H-tyrosine (50 μc/100 g) i.p. Lights were on between 9 a.m. and 9 p.m. daily.
* variance due to time significant at $P < 0.01$.
D = hour of darkness; L = hour of light.

PLASMA L-TYROSINE LEVELS. The plasma receives molecules of free L-tyrosine from three sources (Fig. 6-1) (Wurtman, 1970):

(1) Dietary protein. (Table 6-4) A fraction of the L-tyrosine ingested manages to pass unchanged from the portal to the systemic circulation (Elwyn, 1970). Most amino acid entering the liver from the gut is probably transaminated, retained as free L-tyrosine, or incorporated into hepatic proteins which are then stored (e.g. enzymes) or secreted (e.g. albumin).

(2) De novo synthesis in the liver, by the hydroxylation of phenylalanine.

(3) Secretion from the free L-tyrosine pools present in various tissues. The flux of L-tyrosine and other amino acids between the blood and specific tissues is influenced by a variety of hormones. For example, glucagon enhances the uptake by the liver of the nonutilizable amino acids α-aminoisobutyric acid (AIBA) and cycloleucine (Chambers et al., 1968; Tews et al., 1970), and growth hormone accelerates amino acid

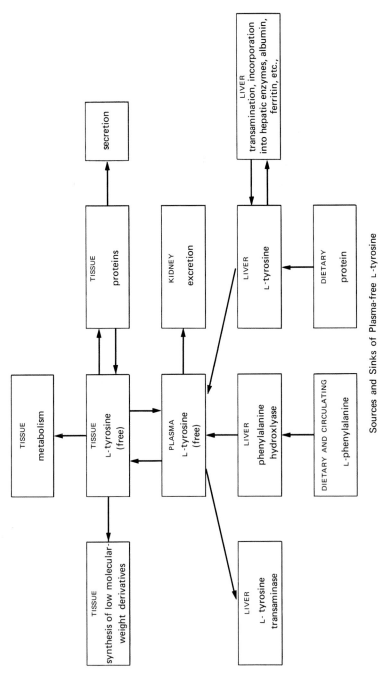

Sources and Sinks of Plasma-free L-tyrosine

uptake in skeletal muscle (Kostyo and Knobil, 1959). Insulin decreases the net outward flux of tyrosine from skeletal muscle into blood, but has no effect on the flux of tryptophan (Pozefsky et al., 1969). Insulin administration or the administration of a glucose load (which stimulates the secretion of endogenous insulin) lowers the concentrations of L-tyrosine and most other amino acids in the blood (Munro, 1964); paradoxically, intraperitoneal insulin elevates plasma tryptophan levels in the rat (Fernstrom and Wurtman, 1971) (Table 6-5). Theoretically, an increase in the rate of protein catabolism should enhance the secretion of free amino acids from the tissues into the blood. However, it appears that most of the additional L-tyrosine or L-tryptophan molecules liberated when the lysis of skeletal muscle protein is accelerated (e.g. in starvation) are not secreted as such but are transaminated and oxidized (Marliss et al., 1971). Most of the alpha-amino nitrogen leaves the muscle as alanine or glutamate.

The plasma loses L-tyrosine into the following major sinks (Fig. 6-1):

(1) Uptake by the tissues, whereupon it enters the tissue free-tyrosine pool and can be incorporated into proteins, converted by specialized tissues into biologically active low-molecular-weight compounds (e.g. catecholamines, thyroxine, melanin), transaminated, and metabolized, or secreted back into the circulation.

(2) Excretion into the urine. Small but significant quantities of L-tyrosine are lost into the urine of normal males (Tewksbury and Lohrenz, 1970).

(3) Transamination in the liver. Transamination is catalyzed by tyrosine transaminase, forming the product para-hydroxyphenylpyruvic acid. The activity of tyrosine transaminase in the rat liver undergoes marked diurnal changes. In animals receiving light for 12 hours per day, enzyme activity rises more than fourfold during the eight hours surrounding the end of the daily light period (Wurtman and Axelrod, 1967). This rhythm persists despite removal of the pituitary, adrenals (Wurtman and Axelrod, 1967), or pancreas (Fuller et al., 1969), and probably results from the cyclic ingestion of dietary protein (Wurtman, 1969, 1970; Wurtman

Figure 6-1. The amino acid enters the plasma from: dietary L-tyrosine that is not destroyed or utilized in passing from the portal to the systemic circulation; synthesis in the liver from L-phenylalanine; or secretion from the tissue-free L-tyrosine pool. L-tyrosine leaves the plasma by: uptake into the tissues (after which it can be metabolized, incorporated into proteins, or converted to low-molecular-weight derivatives such as thyroxine or catecholamines); excretion into the urine; or, destruction in the liver, catalyzed by tyrosine transaminase.

Table 6-4   The tyrosine, phenylalanine, and tryptophan contents of various foods

Food Source	Amino Acid (mg/100 g food)		
	Tyrosine	Phenylalanine	Tryptophan
whole cow's milk	196	182	49
beef meat	850	1000	275
whole egg	475	626	151
white, raw potatoes	50	72	20
whole corn	226	167	30
Charles River Rat and Mouse Formula	930	1160	—*
Big Red Laboratory Animal Food†	890	1180	290

* Information not available.
† If normal daily food intake per adult rat is 12 to 15 grams, the animal consumes daily: 34 to 43 mg tryptophan
          142 to 177 mg phenylalanine
          107 to 134 mg tyrosine

Chart compiled from data taken from R. J. Block and K. W. Weiss, *Amino Acid Handbook*, Charles C Thomas, Springfield, Ill., 1956, p. 249, and from B. T. Burton, ed., *The Heinz Handbook of Nutrition*, 2nd edition, McGraw-Hill, 1965, p. 424.

et al., 1968b). Towards the end of the daily light period, the rat becomes active and begins to consume food more rapidly. If its food contains L-tryptophan, as most proteins do (Table 6-4), its portal circulation begins to deliver relatively high concentrations of this amino acid to the liver. The availability of these high tryptophan concentrations causes some of the unbound messenger RNA in hepatic cells to become aggregated to ribosomes, forming polysomes (Fishman et al., 1969). Apparently some of these newly formed polysomes are coded for the synthesis of tyrosine transaminase enzyme protein; the synthesis of the enzyme is accelerated, and the levels of tyrosine transaminase protein in the liver rise in parallel with enzyme activity (D. Granner and M. Civen, unpublished observation). If animals are forced to consume their daily protein intake in 24 separate hourly meals instead of being allowed to eat cyclically, the hepatic tyrosine transaminase rhythm is extinguished, even though other daily rhythms not generated by cyclic food intake (such as the rhythm in adrenal corticosterone content) persist (Cohn et al., 1970). If animals are allowed to eat according to their usual schedule but are given a diet containing no protein or no tryptophan, the enzyme rhythm is also extinguished (Wurtman et al., 1968b). Shifting by 12 hours the daily lighting schedule under which the animals are maintained causes a corresponding shift in both the daily eating cycle and the enzyme rhythm (Zigmond et al., 1969). It is perhaps surprising that dietary tryptophan produces major changes in the activity of tyrosine transaminase, an enzyme that metabolizes tyrosine rather than tryptophan itself. The physiological significance of the tyrosine transaminase rhythm appears to lie in the ability of this enzyme to serve as a "gate" that limits the amount of tyrosine allowed to enter the body (Wurtman, 1970). Tyrosine transaminase activity is low when the animal starts to eat protein; hence most of the amino acid is not destroyed when it passes through the liver. However, enzyme activity rapidly rises during the feeding, so that L-tyrosine molecules entering the portal blood five or six hours after the animal starts to eat confront much higher transaminase activities, and have a correspondingly greater chance of being destroyed before they can enter the general circulation. Such a "gating system" might be useful if L-tyrosine were toxic in large amounts, or if a sudden elevation in plasma tyrosine after a high-protein meal could cause the overproduction of a tyrosine derivative (such as catecholamines) in the tissues. While it has not yet been demonstrated that the parenteral administration of large amounts of tyrosine causes the overproduction of brain norepinephrine, it is known that L-tyrosine is toxic in doses not much larger than the amount normally consumed daily (Alam, 1965). It is also well established that induced elevations in plasma tyrosine concentration are followed by parallel elevations in brain tyrosine (Table 6-2 (Chirigos et al., 1960)).

Small quantities of L-tyrosine might also be decarboxylated in the liver or elsewhere to form tyramine. However, para-tyrosine is a poor substrate for aromatic L-amino acid decarboxylase (Lovenberg et al., 1962).

The concentrations of L-tyrosine in the plasma of humans (Feigen et al., 1968; Wurtman et al., 1967, 1968c) and rats (Coburn et al., 1968) undergo characteristic diurnal changes: In humans tyrosine levels are lowest between 2:00 and 4:00 a.m., and rise by 60 to 100 per cent to a peak by midmorning; in rats the rhythm is shifted by about eight hours, in keeping with their eating schedule. The tyrosine rhythm persists for two weeks in humans consuming little or no protein (Wurtman et al., 1968c), although the shape of the daily tyrosine curve is shifted somewhat. Since a no-protein diet would be expected to extinguish the rhythms in the amount of tyrosine entering the blood from dietary protein and in hepatic tyrosine transaminase activity, it seems likely that additional mechanisms must be involved in producing the tyrosine rhythm. One such mechanism is the regulation, by hormones such as insulin, of the flux of free amino acids into and out of the tissues. The secretion of insulin after a carbohydrate meal would be expected to decrease the rate at which skeletal muscle secretes tyrosine into the blood (Pozefsky et al., 1969; Zinneman et al., 1966); it is not surprising, therefore, that among subjects given the no-protein diet, plasma tyrosine levels fall sharply after 8:00 a.m., or soon after their largely carbohydrate breakfast (Wurtman et al., 1968c). It can be concluded that, among humans consuming a balanced diet, the plasma tyrosine rhythm probably results from several factors. At least two of these factors depend on dietary protein (i.e. the postprandial overflow of amino acids into the systemic circulation, and the rhythms in hepatic tyrosine transaminase activity); and one depends on dietary carbohydrate (i.e. changes in the flux of amino acids between the blood and the tissues resulting from the secretion of insulin and, probably, glucagon and growth hormone).

Brain tyrosine levels in the rat also exhibit a diurnal rhythm (Zigmond and Wurtman, 1970) (Table 6-3) which lags several hours behind the plasma rhythm. In both tissues, tyrosine concentrations are low at the end of the light period and during the first six hours of the dark period, that is, when hepatic tyrosine transaminase activities are highest (Wurtman and Axelrod, 1967). Blood levels reach a peak at the end of the dark peroid and decline slightly during the next six hours, whereas brain levels do not peak until the middle of the light period.

TRANSPORT OF L-TYROSINE INTO THE BRAIN. The brain concentrates L-tyrosine from the circulation (Chirigos et al., 1960) by a stereospecific transport system. The uptake of exogenous L-tyrosine can be inhibited by the concurrent administration of all large, neutral amino acids (phenylalanine, tryptophan, histidine, the branch-chain amino acids, and the sulfur-containing amino acids). The same transport system apparently operates *in vivo* to take up phenylalanine and tryptophan; however, the maximal brain-to-plasma ratio attainable after tryptophan administration (0.25) is considerably less than that observed after tyrosine (1.25) (Chirigos et al., 1960; Guroff and Udenfriend, 1962; Zigmond and Wurtman, 1970). The ratio of the specific activities of tyrosine in brain and blood one hour after administration of the labelled amino acid varies with the time of day that label is injected (Zigmond and Wurtman, 1970) (Table 6-3); this variation suggests that tyrosine transport into the brain may be influenced by diurnal rhythms in the physiological activity of brain neurons. This hypothesis is supported by the demonstration that transection of the sciatic nerve reduces the uptake of the nonutilizable amino acid AIBA by rat soleus and plantaris muscle (Goldberg and Goodman, 1969), and that the addition of norepinephrine to cultured rat pineal organs enhances their steady-state concentrations of ^{14}C-tryptophan (Wurtman et al., 1969a). No information, however, is available concerning the effects of increasing or decreasing the presynaptic inputs to brain neurons on the neurons' ability to take up amino acids.

Lajtha and his colleagues have identified five physiologically distinct transport systems that mediate the uptake of amino acids by brain slices, plus one for the putative neurotransmitter γ-aminobutyric acid (GABA) (Blasberg, 1968; Blasberg and Lajtha, 1965; Blasberg and Lajtha, 1966; Lajtha and Mela, 1961; Lajtha and Toth, 1961). These systems handle small neutral amino acids, large neutral amino acids (e.g. tyrosine and tryptophan), small basic amino acids, large basic amino acids, and acidic amino acids. The kinetics of transport for any amino acid can be described phenomenologically using the K_m and V_{max} of classical Michaelis-Menten kinetics (Blasberg, 1968). The transport constants must be determined from initial uptake experiments (i.e. of unidirectional flux) and *not* from steady-state systems, since brain cells also secrete the amino acids back into the medium. Amino acids in a given transport class competitively inhibit the uptake of other compounds in their class (Blasberg, 1968).

It is assumed that amino acids pass without difficulty from the blood into the extracellular fluid of the brain, and that the transport systems operate at the interface of the extracellular fluid and the neuronal plasma membrane. This assumption cannot yet be confirmed, since there is no generally accepted method for measuring the amino acid concentrations of brain extracellular fluid. Bito and his colleagues (1966) have attempted to estimate these concentrations by placing dialysis sacs within the substance of dog brain for several weeks, and then measuring amino acid concentrations in the dialysate, the plasma, and the cerebrospinal fluid. In general, amino acid levels in the dialysate were close to those observed in plasma, and considerably higher than those in the cerebrospinal fluid. These data and the observation that the choroid plexus contains an active transport system for concentrating amino acids (Lorenzo and Cutler, 1969) support the notion that the cerebrospinal fluid is a sink, not a source, for brain amino acids.

(B) *Liberation from Intracellular Proteins and Synthesis from Phenylala-*

nine. Almost no information is available about the possible reutilization of amino acids liberated by the intracellular lysis of brain proteins. The brain is known to contain specific proteinases (Lajtha and Marks, 1966) that turn over with an average half-life of 14 days in the rat (Lajtha and Toth, 1966). However, no studies have been done to determine whether the L-tyrosine (or L-tryptophan) released by proteolysis within catecholaminergic (or serotoninergic) neurons is available for reincorporation into proteins, or for conversion to monoamines.

The brain apparently lacks a true phenylalanine hydroxylase, but tryptophan hydroxylase in the pineal organ can catalyze the synthesis of tyrosine from phenylalanine, and phenylalanine can competitively inhibit the 5-hydroxylation of tryptophan by brain tryptophan hydroxylase (Lovenberg et al., 1968). It is therefore conceivable that the brain might synthesize small amounts of tyrosine.

SINKS. Besides serving as the precursor for brain catecholamines, brain tyrosine can also be incorporated into proteins, transaminated by a mitochondrial tyrosine transaminase, or, probably, secreted into the blood.

A particle-bound tyrosine transaminase has been identified in rat brain by at least three groups of investigators (Gibb and Webb, 1969; Mark et al., 1970; Miller and Litwack, 1969). Unlike the hepatic enzyme, brain tyrosine transaminase activity is not enhanced by the addition of pyridoxal phosphate to the incubation medium. Its K_m for substrate is about $3 \times 10^{-3}M$, or about the same as that of the hepatic enzyme (Wurtman and Larin, 1968). The activity of brain homogenates is increased tenfold by treatment with the detergent Triton X-100. This activity, expressed per unit of weight of DNA, is almost 30 per cent greater than that of unstimulated liver (i.e. liver preparations to which no pyridoxal phosphate has been added) (Mark et al., 1970). No information is available as to whether the activity of the particulate brain tyrosine transaminase exhibits characteristic diurnal variations similar to those observed in rat liver. Since the daily variations in the concentration of tryptophan perfusing the brain via the systemic blood are much smaller than the changes in portal venous tryptophan following protein ingestion (Wurtman, 1970), we anticipate that the brain enzyme would show less propensity to vary diurnally than hepatic tyrosine transaminase.

Gibb and Webb (1969) have suggested that brain tyrosine transaminase might function to limit the amounts of brain tyrosine available for hydroxylation and conversion to catecholamines. It is not known whether the hydroxylating and transaminating enzymes are present in the same cells, or whether significant quantities of tyrosine are actually metabolized by transamination in the brain. However, the K_m of brain tyrosine transaminase is more than one hundred times that of tyrosine hydroxylase (Mark et al., 1970; Nagatsu et al., 1964).

No information appears to be available about the flux of tyrosine, or of any other amino acid, across the intact brain.

Sources and Sinks of Brain L-Tryptophan

Like its uptake of L-tyrosine, the rate at which the brain takes up circulating L-tryptophan appears to depend upon both the concentration of the amino acid in the plasma and the activity of a transport system shared with other large, neutral L-amino acids. The administration of large doses of exogenous L-tryptophan (800 mg/kg, i.p. (Ashcroft et al., 1965)) causes a 40-fold rise in brain tryptophan concentrations after two hours; small doses of the amino acid are also effective in elevating brain tryptophan (Table 6-6). Brain L-tryptophan levels do not rise as high after a large dose as plasma concentrations (Guroff and Udenfriend, 1962); in this sense, the response of the brain to exogenous L-tryptophan differs from its response to L-tyrosine. The uptake of L-tryptophan by brain *in vivo* apparently can be inhibited by a variety of natural (Table 6-2) and synthetic amino acids. These are discussed below.

The tryptophan content of rat brains undergoes characteristic diurnal variations (Fig. 6-2).

PLASMA L-TRYPTOPHAN. The plasma receives L-tryptophan molecules from two sources only: dietary tryptophan and secretion from the free amino acid pools of various tissues. Since tryptophan tends to be the limiting amino acid in many dietary proteins (Table 6-4) as well as in human protein, tryptophan levels in the plasma are lower than those of most other amino acids, and the net flux of tryptophan between brain and blood per unit time is probably also lower. A sensitive and simple assay for free tryptophan has been developed only within the past few years (Denckla and Dewey, 1967), and therefore relatively little information is available about the effects of hormones and other physiological inputs on tryptophan flux. Plasma tryptophan concentrations are raised by doses of insulin that lower tyrosine and ^{14}C-cycloleucine levels (Fernstrom and

Table 6-5   Effect of insulin on levels of L-tryptophan and amino acid in plasma

Amino Acid	Tryptophan Level ($\mu g/ml$)		% Change
	Control	Insulin-Treated	
L-tryptophan	11.06 ± 0.60	16.59 ± 0.86*	+50
L-tyrosine	16.05 ± 0.61	13.16 ± 0.59*	−18
L-phenylalanine	11.78 ± 0.30	10.76 ± 0.86	−9
L-serine	24.62 ± 1.16	16.95 ± 1.25*	−31
L-glycine	29.63 ± 1.37	18.25 ± 2.00*	−38
L-alanine	25.30 ± 0.93	11.67 ± 0.52*	−54
L-valine	21.46 ± 1.30	17.25 ± 1.80	−20
L-isoleucine	13.74 ± 0.82	7.13 ± 0.40*	−48
L-leucine	21.34 ± 1.17	16.58 ± 2.05	−22
^{14}C-cycloleucine (DPM × 10^{-3})	164.2 ± 10.63	124.0 ± 6.06*	−24

Fasting rats (150 to 200 g) were killed two hours after receiving insulin (2U/kg, i.p.).
* $P < 0.01$ differs from control group.

Wurtman, 1971) (Table 6-5); we must infer, therefore, that the *in vivo* behavior of tryptophan cannot necessarily be predicted from the behavior of structurally related amino acids.

The main sinks for plasma tryptophan are probably uptake by the tissues (followed by incorporation into proteins, conversion to serotonin, secretion back into the circulation, or, possibly, transamination), and destruction in the liver, catalyzed by tryptophan pyrrolase. Hepatic tryptophan pyrrolase activity also undergoes characteristic diurnal fluctuations in the mouse (Rapoport et al., 1966) and rat (Fuller, 1970). Enzyme activity is lowest at the start of the daily dark period and rises about twofold during the next eight hours. Bilateral adrenalectomy lowers the basal enzyme level but does not extinguish the enzyme rhythm. The similar diurnal patterns of tyrosine transaminase and tryptophan pyrrolase suggest that the rhythms in these enzymes are generated by a common mechanism; but the response of the pyrrolase rhythm to no-protein or tryptophan-free diets has not been studied. The daily rhythm in tryptophan pyrrolase activity apparently influences the fate of dietary tryptophan; the proportion of a dietary tryptophan load (3 g) appearing in the urine as kynurenine derivatives varies according to the hour of its administration (Rapoport and Beisel, 1968). It is not known whether this variability reflects rhythms in the proportion of dietary tryptophan metabolized during its initial passage through the liver, or in the rate at which circulating tryptophan is destroyed.

Small amounts of L-tryptophan are present in the urine (Denckla and Dewey, 1967). It is possible that some tryptophan is decarboxylated by AAAD to form tryptamine (Lovenberg et al., 1962).

Plasma L-tryptophan concentrations undergo characteristic diurnal fluctuations which are similar to those of L-tyrosine (Wurtman et al., 1968c) and which persist in subjects given a very low protein diet for two weeks. The L-tryptophan rhythm can be extinguished by feeding subjects at four-hour intervals (Young et al., 1969).

Experimental Evidence Relating the Availability of L-Tyrosine and L-Tryptophan to Brain Monoamine Synthesis

Problems in Interpreting Experimental Observations

To demonstrate that the rate of catecholamine synthesis within brain neurons varies with the availability of L-tyrosine (or the rate of serotonin synthesis with L-tryptophan), one would, ideally, monitor the concentration of the amino acid and the rate of monoamine synthesis at the terminal bouton, *in vivo,* and then demonstrate that within the physiologic range of L-tyrosine concentrations, a dose-response relationship existed between these concentrations and the rates of catecholamine biosynthesis. This ideal experiment has not been performed, nor does it seem likely that it will be during the period in which anyone might be inclined to read this chapter. No technique is available which permits reliable measurements of amino acid concentrations within brain neurons, uncontaminated by glia or extracellular water, *in vitro,* let alone *in vivo.* Furthermore, the possibility of assaying the L-tyrosine or L-tryptophan within a small subset of brain neurons (i.e. catecholaminergic or serotoninergic neurons), let alone within a single region of those neurons (the terminal boutons), seems distant indeed. All of the methods proposed for estimating monoamine synthesis rates *in vivo* are flawed, some more than others. Isotopic methods, which measure the accumulation of brain monoamines after administration of labelled L-tyrosine or L-tryptophan, require that the animal be killed at a very short interval after injection of the amino acid (Zigmond and Wurtman, 1970), lest significant amounts of the newly formed amine be released or metabolized prior to assay. It seems less than likely that during this short interval ^{3}H-tyrosine injected into the peritoneal cavity can become a true tracer for the brain tyrosine pool that serves as catecholamine precursor. Experiments in which monoamine synthesis rates are estimated by measuring changes in brain monoamine *lev-*

els (i.e. after the administration of enzyme inhibitors, or large doses of precursor or other amino acids) are perhaps most flawed (Anton-Tay and Wurtman, 1971; Wurtman et al., 1969b), since such changes reflect alterations in *both* the synthesis and the turnover of the amine, and turnover rates are almost certain to be modified when the levels of the amine change in its cell of origin. The direction of change may be hard to predict: Increases in brain serotonin *levels* that follow the administration of monoamine oxidase (MAO) inhibitors (Aghajanian et al., 1970) or of L-tryptophan (Aghajanian and Asher, unpublished observations) may be associated with a *decrease* in the physiological activity of the serotonin-containing neurons, and thus with decreases in the synthesis and turnover of neurotransmitter in brain.

As discussed below, there is a wealth of evidence that experimental manipulations which increase or decrease the availability of L-tryptophan to the brain can cause corresponding changes in brain serotonin content, probably because such manipulations modify the rate at which the amine is synthesized. Unfortunately, most of these experimental manipulations produce animals in which L-tryptophan metabolism is so unphysiological that they provide no basis for deciding whether the availability of this amino acid controls serotonin synthesis in normal subjects. (These manipulations do, however, provide potentially useful insights into the abnormalities of brain and behavior associated with diseases of amino acid metabolism.) Even if the doses of L-tryptophan used to induce a rise in brain serotonin content are not terribly large in themselves, it should be recognized that in nature, the animal or human rarely if ever consumes tryptophan without also consuming all of the other twenty-odd L-amino acids found in mammalian proteins. The fate of any amino acid when administered alone is very different from its fate as part of a complete amino acid mixture. For example, the likelihood that a given dose of an amino acid will be incorporated into protein *in vivo* is reduced to almost nil when it is administered alone (Harper, 1964). The ability of brain homogenates to incorporate individual amino acids into protein also depends upon the total amino acid pattern in the incubation medium (Peterson and McKean, 1969). Hence, the ability of L-tryptophan, administered by itself, to change brain serotonin metabolism tells little or nothing about the changes that might occur when L-tryptophan enters the body naturally as a constituent of dietary proteins.

Interpretation of such data is further complicated by the very large number of possible mechanisms by which large doses of natural or synthetic amino acids might influence the conversion of L-tyrosine to catecholamines, or of L-tryptophan to serotonin. For example, it might be expected that α-methyl DOPA, a known inhibitor of AAAD (Sharman and Smith, 1962; Sourkes, 1954) would inhibit brain serotonin synthesis by blocking the decarboxylation of 5-HTP; however, 5-HTP does not accumulate in the brains of dogs treated with α-methyl DOPA. This paradox caused Eccleston et al. (1968) to conjecture that, *in vivo,* α-methyl DOPA also acts as a tryptophan hydroxylase inhibitor. As a catechol, α-methyl DOPA could suppress the hydroxylation of tryptophan by oxidizing the reduced pteridine cofactor; it does not appear to inhibit the hepatic hydroxylase (probably phenylalanine hydroxylase) in this manner (Fuller, 1965). As a large, neutral amino acid, it might be expected to compete with L-tryptophan for uptake into serotonin-producing neurons (Blasberg, 1968). Pretreatment with α-methyl DOPA, however, causes an increase in the peak brain L-tryptophan levels observed in animals given a tryptophan load (Eccleston et al., 1968). This increase could reflect inhibition of tryptophan hydroxylase, but it could also result from competition between α-methyl DOPA and L-tryptophan for a transport system that normally *extrudes* L-tryptophan from the brain. If a large dose of α-methyl DOPA blocked the uptake of L-tryptophan into the brain, it might, like phenylalanine (Aoki and Siegel, 1970), disaggregate brain polysomes and suppress brain protein synthesis. The resulting deceleration of a process that utilized tryptophan might cause brain L-tryptophan levels to rise, further saturating tryptophan hydroxylase and *accelerating* serotonin biosynthesis. Some amino acids (e.g. L-leucine) can modify the fates of others by intermediate hormonal mechanisms (e.g. by releasing insulin from the pancreatic β-cells) (Fajans et al., 1967). The list of possible interactions between the amino acids could be extended *ad infinitum.* Its length underscores the necessity for caution in assigning mechanisms to the effects of amino acid administration. L-DOPA, administered to Parkinsonian patients with the intent of restoring dopamine concentrations in the corpus striatum, produces profound effects on the metabolism of a different neurotransmitter (norepinephrine) in different regions of the brain (the cerebral cortex and hypothalamus) (Chalmers et al., 1971), in part by depleting the brain of a derivative of another amino acid (S-adenosylmethionine (Wurtman et al., 1970b)) and thereby interfering with methylation reactions. It appears likely that

L-DOPA exerts a variety of effects on brain monoaminergic neurons, just as might any of the amino acids administered to animals to study the relationships between brain L-tyrosine or L-tryptophan and monoamine biosynthesis.

L-Tyrosine and Catecholamines

Relatively few data have been published concerning possible effects that major changes in brain L-tyrosine would have on catecholamine biosynthesis. Several laboratories have reported changes in brain catecholamine levels among animals receiving treatments that ought to have affected the concentration of L-tyrosine; brain tyrosine, however, usually was not measured or was found to be unchanged.

Green et al. (1962) gave weanling rats a diet containing nine times the control concentration of DL-phenylalanine (9 per cent vs 1 per cent) for 15 to 17 days, and observed a 339 per cent increase in brain dopamine concentration at the end of this period. Brain norepinephrine was unchanged in these animals, but brain serotonin was decreased by 33 per cent (Table 6-2). Brain L-tyrosine and L-tryptophan concentrations were not measured.

Shoemaker and Wurtman (1970, 1971) and Serini et al. (1966) examined the effects of two types of protein malnutrition on the rate at which brain monoamine levels increased postnatally in rats. In the former study, pregnant female rats were given diets containing 8 per cent or 24 per cent protein *ad libitum*. Throughout the weaning period, the mothers continued to receive the same diets, but their litters were divided and redistributed so that four groups of animals were generated according to whether they received nourishment from "control" or "deprived" mothers, before or after birth. Weanling rats nourished by "deprived" mothers had 12 per cent less norepinephrine in their brains at 12 days of age, and 30 per cent less by 24 days of age. Brain dopamine was also significantly depressed at day 24. The initial uptake by brain of ^{3}H-norepinephrine placed in the cisterna magna was not decreased in the "deprived" animals (unpublished observations), suggesting that the failure of brain norepinephrine to attain normal levels reflected not a decrease in the number of noradrenergic cells but a decrease in the norepinephrine content per cell. Brain tyrosine hydroxylase activity was significantly *elevated* in the "deprived" animals, a change that may reflect an increase in the reflex presynaptic input to these cells. (Similar increases have been observed in guinea pig brain (Chalmers and Wurtman, 1971) and heart (DeQuattro et al., 1969) following transection of the baroreceptor nerves.) The combination of decreased norepinephrine levels and elevated tyrosine hydroxylase activity suggests that a factor other than enzyme activity might be limiting norepinephrine biosynthesis. This factor could be the precursor amino acid, L-tyrosine, although brain tyrosine levels were not depressed in crude homogenates prepared from the "deprived" animals.

Serini and his associates (1966) produced experimental protein malnutrition by placing 16 or more newborn rats with each lactating female; control litters contained four newborn animals. The concentrations of norepinephrine and serotonin in the brain were significantly lower than normal until the eighth day of life; norepinephrine levels were probably depressed until the 21st day, at which time all rats were placed on a diet containing adequate amounts of protein. Brain L-tyrosine and L-tryptophan concentrations were not measured.

The concentration of L-tyrosine in the rat brain, the uptake of ^{3}H-tyrosine from the blood into the brain, and the rate at which brain ^{3}H-tyrosine is converted to ^{3}H-catecholamines all show parallel diurnal rhythms (Table 6-3); all of these functions attain their nadir in the middle of the daily dark period, and reach a peak 6 to 12 hours later (Zigmond and Wurtman, 1970). These data are compatible with the hypothesis that within the normal (or "dynamic") range, the level of tyrosine in the brain influences the rate at which the brain synthesizes catecholamines. Of course, a temporal correlation does not prove a causal relationship.

L-Tryptophan and Serotonin

There is abundant experimental evidence that procedures which cause major changes in brain L-tryptophan content can produce parallel alterations in brain serotonin. Techniques that have been utilized to manipulate brain L-tryptophan levels include:

(1) the induction of tryptophan deficiency by synthetic diets (Table 6-6);

(2) the increase in the size of the total tryptophan pool in the body by use of high-tryptophan diets or parenteral administration of the amino acid (Table 6-6);

Table 6-6   Effect of dietary or injected L-tryptophan on brain serotonin levels

Reference	Animal	Treatment
Zbinden et al., 1958	rabbit, guinea pig, rat, mouse	tryptophan-deficient synthetic diet, 1. 31 days
Gal et al., 1961	rat	tryptophan-deficient diet, 6 weeks
Gal and Drewes, 1962	adult rat	tryptophan-deficient diet (casein ac' hydrolysate with added niacin), 5 wee‖
Wang et al., 1962	18 day-old rat	diet containing 1-5% L-tryptophan, 1‹ weeks
Green et al., 1962	rats weighing 35-45 g	diet containing 0.09% tryptopha‹ 0.22% tryptophan (control), or 1.1‹ tryptophan, 15-17 days
Culley et al., 1963	adult rat	tryptophan-deficient diet (casein ac‹ hydrolysate); 0.5% L-tryptophan adde for controls; 2-32 days
Boullin, 1963	weanling rat	tryptophan-free synthetic diet; contro‹ received 0.4% L-tryptophan; 14-35 day‹ pair-fed
Ashcroft et al., 1965	adult rat	L-tryptophan, 800 mg/kg i.p.; kill‹ after 0.5-8 hr
Eccleston et al., 1965	adult rat	L-tryptophan, 400-1600 mg/kg i.‹ killed after 1-4 hr
Weber and Horita, 1965	adult rat	L-tryptophan, 50-300 mg/kg i.p., to ra‹ pretreated with MAO inhibitor; kill‹ after 2 hr
Thomas and Wyson, 1967	weanling rat	tryptophan-poor diet (0.056%) or co‹ trol diet (0.23%); 3-4 weeks
Weber, 1966	adult rat	L-tryptophan, 204 mg/kg i.p.; kill‹ after 2 hr
Moir and Eccleston, 1968	adult rat	L-tryptophan, 50-1600 mg/kg i.p.; kill‹ after 0.5-4 hr
	adult dog	L-tryptophan, 50 mg/kg i.v.; killed aft‹ 1-4 hr (D,L-5-HTP or L-5-HTP, 10 m‹ kg i.v.; killed after 1-4 hr)
Eccleston et al., 1968	adult dog	L-tryptophan, 50 mg/kg i.v.; killed aft‹ 1-4 hr
Horita and Carino, 1970	adult rat	L-tryptophan, 2500 mg/kg, i.p.; su‹ vivors killed after 24 hr
Meek et al., 1970	adult spinal rat	L-tryptophan, 100-750 mg/kg i.p.; kill‹ after 2 hr

Change in Brain Serotonin	Remarks
.48 vs 0.76 µg/g (rat)	—
.47 vs 0.99 µg/g (mouse)	—
ecreased by 70%	No change in brain norepinephrine.
.16 vs 0.47 µg/g	Similar findings if sulfasuxidine added to diet.
78 (1%, 2 weeks)	High phenylalanine diet (7%,. 1 week)
s. 0.58 mg/g (controls)	depressed serotonin.
icreased 32% with high tryptophan, naffected by low tryptophan	High phenylalanine diet (9%) depressed serotonin, raised dopamine.
.35 vs 0.54 µg/g after 4 days; 0.18 vs .51 µg/g after 32 days	Plasma tryptophan 0.6 vs 1.7 mg/100 ml after 4 days; 0.35 vs 2.1 mg/100 ml after 32 days.
12 vs 0.60 µg/g	No serotonin detectable in 11 of 19 animals; convulsions in 16, ataxia in 13 of 19.
62 vs 0.32 µg/g after 1 hr; 0.32 after hr	Brain tryptophan increased 40-fold after 2 hr, 5-HIAA increased 4-fold after 4 hr.
62 vs 0.32 µg/g 1 hr after 400 mg/kg; gger dose prolongs effect, but doesn't nhance peak	No 5-HTP detectable in brain, indicating that hydroxylation is rate-limiting; MAO inhibition causes brain serotonin to reach 1.27 µg/g with 400 mg/kg.
gnificant rise with 75 mg/kg	Viscera not needed for rise in brain serotonin; hence hydroxylation occurs in brain.
24 vs 0.39 µg/g (if niacin added to yptophan-poor diet)	If no niacin added to tryptophan-poor diet, animals develop signs of pellagra, and brain serotonin is not depressed (0.36 µg/g)
73 vs 0.56 µg/g	—
53 (0.5 hr) or 0.63 (1.0 hr) vs 0.38 ;/g, after 50 mg/kg dose	Peak brain serotonin level and rate of rise of brain serotonin plus 5-HIAA as great after 50 mg/kg tryptophan as after 1600 mg/kg; hence, hydroxylation is rate-limiting.
crement in each brain region related its concentration in control dogs	Increment in regional serotonin contents after 5-HTP not related to concentrations in control animals; hence, plasma 5-HTP is not normal precursor for brain serotonin.
proximate doubling after 1 hr in mid-ain, hypothalamus, thalamus, caudate, ppocampus, hindbrain	Approximate 5-fold increase in tryptophan concentrations of all regions, including those without detectable serotonin (cortex, cerebellum).
78 vs 0.48 µg/g	Enormous dose no more effective than 50 mg/kg in elevating brain serotonin.
iorescence intensity of serotonin-con-ining neurons increased with 500-750 g/kg doses	Increase in extensor reflex with 500 to 750 mg/kg doses.

(3) administration of hormones (e.g. hydrocortisone) or drugs (e.g. α-methyl tryptophan) which might be expected to accelerate the destruction of tryptophan by inducing or stabilizing hepatic tryptophan pyrrolase;

(4) administration of other natural L-amino acids (e.g. L-phenylalanine, L-leucine) which might be expected to lower brain tryptophan levels by competing with it for transport into neurons (Table 6-2).

In addition, several experimental manipulations [such as administration of para-chlorophenylalanine (PCPA)] previously thought to influence brain serotonin levels by mechanisms unrelated to tryptophan availability, have recently been shown to cause changes in brain tryptophan concentration that parallel those in serotonin concentration (Tagliamonte et al., 1970).

It is not certain that any of these experimental manipulations change brain serotonin levels by raising or lowering the plasma tryptophan to levels that remain within the dynamic range observed in normal animals. The possibility that physiological variations in plasma tryptophan could drive changes in brain serotonin synthesis is, however, suggested by the observation that the levels of tryptophan and serotonin in rat brains oscillate with similar diurnal rhythms (Fig. 6-2). It is also relevant that the lowest doses of tryptophan thus far reported to raise brain serotonin levels (50 mg/kg) provide amounts of the amino acid within the range that the laboratory rat normally consumes in its daily diet (200 to 300 mg/kg). The changes in brain tryptophan and serotonin produced by administering large doses of L-phenylalanine or L-leucine may mimic pathologic alterations that occur in phenylketonuria and "maple syrup disease," two inborn errors of amino acid metabolism described below.

Effects of L-Tryptophan Deprivation or Administration. The first investigators to describe changes in brain serotonin content in animals deprived of dietary tryptophan were probably Zbinden et al. (1958) (Table 6-6), who fed rats, mice, and other animals a synthetic tryptophan-deficient diet for 15 to 31 days and observed decreases of 35 to 50 per cent in brain serotonin concentrations. Similar observations were made by Gal et al. (1961), Gal and Drewes (1962), Culley et al. (1963), and Thomas and Wysor (1967), who used casein acid hydrolysates as the source of tryptophan-poor protein, and by Boullin (1963), who used synthetic diets. The decrease in brain serotonin was unaccompanied by changes in brain norepinephrine (Gal et al., 1961), but was associated with depressed

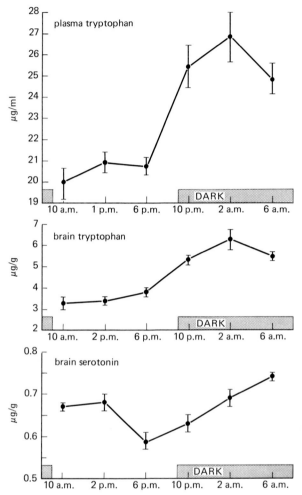

Figure 6-2.   Daily rhythms in the concentrations of L-tryptophan in rat plasma, and of L-tryptophan and serotonin in brain. Groups of 15 animals, given access *ad libitum* to a 24 per cent protein diet and exposed to light between 9:00 a.m. and 9:00 p.m. daily, were killed at the times indicated.

changes, convulsions, and ataxia (Boullin, 1963). The decrease in brain serotonin did not occur unless animals were given extra niacin to block the development of pellagra (Thomas and Wysor, 1967); it was not affected by addition of dietary sulfasuccidine (Gal and Drewes, 1962) and thus was not dependent on the metabolism of tryptophan by intestinal flora. A decline in brain serotonin did occur among weanling rats given a diet containing 0.056 per cent tryptophan for three to four weeks (Thomas and Wysor, 1967), but not among similar animals given a diet containing 0.09 per cent tryptophan (Green et al., 1962). (Control diets contained about 0.2 to 0.3 per cent tryptophan.)

Wang et al. (1962) and Green et al. (1962) independently discovered that brain serotonin concentration could be increased by feeding rats diets rich in tryptophan (1.1 per cent). Brain tryptophan concentrations apparently have not been measured by any of the above groups reporting diet-induced changes in brain serotonin.

The administration of as little as 50 mg/kg (the lowest dose tested) of L-tryptophan i.p. to rats causes, after one hour, a 66 per cent increase in brain serotonin concentration (Moir and Eccleston, 1968). Much larger doses of L-tryptophan cause only a slightly greater increase in brain serotonin concentration or in the rate at which brain 5-hydroxyindoleacetic acid (5-HIAA) levels rise; the increase in brain 5-HIAA after administration of 5-HTP, however, continues to be dose-related to considerably larger doses of amino acid (Moir and Eccleston, 1968). These findings, plus the absence of 5-HTP from brains of rats given very large doses of L-tryptophan (Eccleston et al., 1965) have been taken as evidence that tryptophan hydroxylation is rate-limiting in brain serotonin biosynthesis. Attempts to identify this rate-limiting step by administering 5-HTP are complicated by the fact that the exogenous amino acid is delivered by the circulation to the entire brain, and that large amounts of it are probably converted to serotonin by cells that do not normally produce this amine but happen to contain AAAD (i.e. dopaminergic or noradrenergic neurons). Thus, although brain 5-HIAA levels continue to increase even after very large doses of 5-HTP, it is still possible that decarboxylation is rate-limiting in serotonin-containing neurons.

Two studies have recently provided evidence that the increase in brain serotonin after L-tryptophan administration reflects changes in cells that normally contain this monoamine. Using a specific histochemical fluorescence method, Meek et al. (1970) have found that doses of L-tryptophan (500 to 750 mg/kg, i.p.) which potentiate the extensor reflex in spinal rats also cause an increase in the fluorescence of serotoninergic neurons in the brain stem. Aghajanian and Asher (personal communication) have observed that doses of L-tryptophan which cause brain serotonin levels to increase (100 mg/kg) also depress the spontaneous activity of neurons

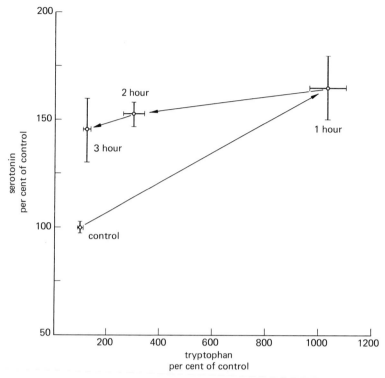

Figure 6-3. Changes in brain tryptophan and serotonin concentrations at various times after administration of L-tryptophan (125 mg/kg, i.p.) to rats. Concentrations in control animals were: tryptophan, 6.72 ± 0.34 μg/g brain; serotonin, 0.39 ± 0.01 μg/g brain.

in the raphe nucleus. This depression was also observed among animals in which brain serotonin levels had been increased by treatment with monoamine oxide inhibitors, but not those in which the effect of the inhibitor had been blocked by concurrent treatment with para-chlorophenylalanine (Aghajanian et al., 1970).

The sequence of changes in brain L-tryptophan and serotonin after a single injection (125 mg/kg, i.p.) of the amino acid are illustrated in Fig. 6-3.

Adrenocortical Hormones, Tryptophan Pyrrolase, and Tryptophan Hydroxylase. If adult rats are treated simultaneously with cortisone (7.5

mg/kg) and tryptophan (80 mg/kg), the increase in brain serotonin levels produced by injecting tryptophan alone is blocked. Brains of animals receiving tryptophan for five days contained 0.96 μg/g of serotonin, compared with 0.63 μg/g in control brains and 0.66 μg/g in brains from cortisone-treated animals. Brains of animals receiving both cortisol and tryptophan contained only 0.69 μg/g of serotonin (Shah et al., 1968). Since livers of cortisol-treated rats exhibited a sizable increase in tryptophan pyrrolase activity, Shah and his associates postulated that the failure of brain serotonin levels to rise in animals receiving both L-tryptophan and cortisol resulted from increased hepatic destruction of the amino acid, and a consequent decrease in the amount available for conversion to brain serotonin. (Brain L-tryptophan levels were not measured in this study.) Studies on human subjects have shown that hydrocortisone treatment does indeed accelerate the metabolism of tryptophan in the liver, increasing the excretion of kynurenine and of related products of tryptophan pyrrolase (Altman and Greengard, 1966). The ability of tryptophan pyrrolase induction to block the increase in brain serotonin that follows the feeding or i.p. administration of tryptophan would imply that the tryptophan pyrrolase exerts a major influence on the fate of tryptophan in the *portal* circulation. It does not necessarily follow, however, that changes in hepatic tryptophan pyrrolase activity significantly modify the size of the free tryptophan pool in the *systemic* circulation or in the brain. That tryptophan pyrrolase induction need not modify systemic tryptophan levels is suggested by the finding that cortisone treatment *per se* had no effect on brain serotonin content.

Curzon and Green (1968) observed that cortisol injections (5 mg/kg, i.p.) caused rapid, short-lived declines in the concentrations of serotonin and 5-HIAA within rat brain; the levels of both indoles fell by one-third between six and eight hours after cortisol administration, returning to normal by the eleventh hour. Daily injections of cortisol were found to lower brain serotonin content for two days, but not thereafter. Since cortisol administration was known to increase hepatic tryptophan pyrrolase activity, and since allopurinol, an agent which decreases pyrrolase activity, blocked the cortisone-induced fall in brain serotonin content (Green and Curzon, 1968), the authors postulated that the effect of cortisol on brain serotonin resulted from a critical shortage in the supply of tryptophan available to the brain for conversion to serotonin. This hypothesis seemed supported by the observation that immobilization, an experimental model of stress, simultaneously increased hepatic tryptophan pyrrolase activity and lowered the levels of serotonin and 5-HIAA in the brain (Curzon and Green, 1969a). It failed, however, to explain the subsequent observation that the fall in brain serotonin after hydrocortisone treatment had an entirely different time-course from the fall in plasma tryptophan concentration (Curzon and Green, 1969b). More recently, Green and Curzon have observed that kynurenine, 3-hydroxykynurenine, and 3-hydroxyanthranilic acid inhibit the uptake of ^{14}C-tryptophan into brain slices (Green and Curzon, 1970) and have postulated that these three *products* of the action of tryptophan pyrrolase inhibit the synthesis of serotonin by decreasing the amount of tryptophan available to the brain. In none of the above studies were data provided on the actual levels of tryptophan in the brain; hence it is not possible to draw any conclusions as to whether cortisol treatment actually produces a physiologically significant decrease in brain tryptophan content. There is little direct evidence that the amount of tryptophan in the brain bears any simple relationship to the activity of tryptophan pyrrolase in the liver.

Azmitia and McEwen (1969) observed a 75 per cent fall in the activity of tryptophan hydroxylase within the rat midbrain one to two weeks after bilateral adrenalectomy; enzyme activity could be partially restored by treatment with corticosterone. The rate at which the brain stem converted intravenously administered ^{3}H-tryptophan to ^{3}H-serotonin (corrected for the specific activity of the precursor amino acid) was also decreased in rats adrenalectomized ten days previously (Azmitia et al., 1970). The level of serotonin in the brain stem was not altered in adrenalectomized rats, nor was the concentration or uptake of tryptophan. Hence, if brain-stem serotonin synthesis is depressed after adrenalectomy, this depression is presumably a consequence of decreased tryptophan hydroxylase activity, and not of inadequate amounts of precursor amino acid. The literature on possible effects of adrenocortical hormones on brain serotonin content is contradictory. Adrenalectomy has been reported to increase, decrease, and leave unchanged brain serotonin levels; similar claims have been made for the effects of exogenous glucocorticoids. This literature is discussed by Shah et al. (1968), and by Azmitia et al. (1970).

Alpha-Methyl Tryptophan. Alpha-methyl tryptophan, a synthetic derivative of the amino acid, causes profound changes in the metabolism of

L-tryptophan. Its administration causes a great and prolonged increase in the activity of hepatic tryptophan pyrrolase, resulting partly from the induction of new enzyme protein (Civen and Knox, 1960) and partly from the stabilization of existing enzyme (Schimke et al., 1965; Sourkes and Townsend, 1955). Probably as a result of this increase, the metabolism of ^{14}C-tryptophan to ^{14}CO$_2$ is accelerated (Sourkes et al., 1970), the excretion of kynurenic and anthurenic acids in the urine is increased (Madras and Sourkes, 1965), and the concentrations of tryptophan in blood, liver, and brain decline (Sourkes et al., 1970). The concentrations of serotonin (Curzon and Green, 1969a) and of 5-HIAA (Sourkes et al., 1970) in rat brain decline markedly within hours after rats are treated with α-methyl tryptophan (25 mg/kg, i.p.). Only the L-form of the synthetic amino acid produces this effect (Sourkes et al., 1970), and, like its ability to induce tryptophan pyrrolase (Civen and Knox, 1960), this action of α-methyl tryptophan is not impaired by adrenalectomy (Curzon and Green, 1969a).

Alpha-methyl tryptophan is converted *in vivo* to a compound with fluorescence properties similar to those of authentic serotonin and which may be α-methyl serotonin (Sourkes, in press). This compound could act as a "false neurotransmitter" (Wurtman, 1966), and might contribute significantly to what is measured as "brain serotonin." Hence, the actual effect of α-methyl tryptophan on brain serotonin content may be even greater than the 35 per cent reduction observed by Sourkes et al. (1970).

Since brain tryptophan levels are severely depressed in animals treated with α-methyl tryptophan (0.12 mg/100 g vs 0.31 mg/100 g in control animals), it seems likely that the reduction in brain serotonin content and synthesis does indeed reflect the inadequacy of amino acid precursor. In support of this interpretation, it has been shown that α-methyl tryptophan is only a weak inhibitor of brain tryptophan hydroxylase (McGeer and Peters, 1969) or of aromatic L-amino acid decarboxylase (Lovenberg et al., 1962; Murphy and Sourkes, 1961). Alpha-methyl 5-HTP, however, which could be formed *in vivo* from the synthetic amino acid by the action of brain tryptophan hydroxylase or liver phenylalanine hydroxylase, is a potent inhibitor of aromatic L-amino acid decarboxylase (Moran and Sourkes, 1963; Murphy and Sourkes, 1961). Hence, it is still theoretically possible that α-methyl tryptophan might suppress serotonin synthesis by a mechanism unrelated to its effect on brain tryptophan content.

It is not yet certain that the decrease in brain tryptophan comes about solely because more of the amino acid is destroyed by hepatic tryptophan pyrrolase. For example, α-methyl tryptophan treatment causes hepatic polyribosomes to become disaggregated (Oravec, 1969; Sourkes, in press); probably because brain tryptophan levels become limiting, as in Munro's experimental system: Baliga et al., 1968), and suppresses the incorporation of ^{14}C-leucine into new proteins (Oravec, 1969). Hence, the synthetic amino acid might be suppressing serotonin biosynthesis by interfering with the formation of proteins necessary for the transport or metabolism of tryptophan, or of any of the cofactors needed for serotonin synthesis. Similarly, α-methyl tryptophan lowers brain norepinephrine levels (Sourkes et al., 1961), possibly by inhibiting tyrosine hydroxylase (Zhalyaskov et al., 1968) or by substituting for the catecholamine as a "false neurotransmitter." It is possible that this decrease could, via transsynaptic mechanisms, modify the physiological activity of serotonin-containing neurons, causing them to synthesize less of their neurotransmitter. Alpha-methyl tryptophan might also be expected to compete with tryptophan for transport into brain cells; in this regard, it might be interesting to determine whether the synthetic amino acid also lowers brain levels of other amino acids (such as tyrosine or methionine) which share a common transport system with tryptophan but which are not substrates for tryptophan pyrrolase.

L-*Phenylalanine and* L-*Leucine.* The mental deficits associated with two inborn errors of amino acid metabolism, phenylketonuria and maple syrup disease (branched-chain amino aciduria), probably generated the initial interest in examining effects of elevated plasma phenylalanine or leucine concentrations on brain serotonin metabolism. Both amino acids have now been shown to decrease brain serotonin levels when administered in large doses to experimental animals; both probably produce this effect by lowering the levels of tryptophan in the brain (Table 6-2). In 1957, Pare et al. reported that phenylketonuric patients had subnormal concentrations of serum serotonin and urinary 5-HIAA. In a subsequent publication (Pare et al., 1958) these authors showed that serum serotonin levels could be increased if plasma phenylalanine was lowered by giving subjects a low-phenylalanine diet. The relationship between phenylketonuria and serotonin production was quickly confirmed in other laboratories (Baldridge et al., 1959; Berendes et al., 1958) and the biosynthetic defect was localized to the step of tryptophan hydroxylation by demonstration that although phenylketonurics could synthesize large amounts of serotonin from exogenous 5-HTP, they failed to exhibit a normal increase in urinary 5-HIAA when given an oral load of L-tryptophan (100 mg/kg) (Perry et al., 1964). This defect could have reflected decreased activity of the hydroxylating enzyme or an inability of the substrate to reach the enzyme (because of impaired tryptophan transport into serotonin-producing neurons). Both mechanisms appear to operate: phenylalanine is a good inhibitor of tryptophan hydroxylase in rat brain (Lovenberg et al., 1968) and phenylalanine administration markedly reduces brain tryptophan levels (Aoki and Siegel, 1970; McKean et al., 1968) (Table 6-2). The excretion of catecholamines has also been reported to be abnormally low in phenylketonuric children (Nadler and Hsia, 1961). Decreased catecholamine synthesis in this disease state could also reflect inhibition of a rate-limiting enzyme (i.e. tyrosine hydroxylase) or inadequate concentrations of the precursor amino acid (i.e. L-tyrosine).

In 1961, Waisman's and Yuwiler's laboratories simultaneously demonstrated that "experimental phenylketonuria" induced by feeding high-phenylalanine diets to weanling rats also was associated with low brain serotonin levels. Yuwiler and Louttit (1961) provided rats with a phenylalanine-fortified diet containing an additional 5 g/kg body weight of the amino acid each day; after eight weeks of treatment, brain serotonin levels were approximately 20 per cent lower than those of control animals (0.47 μg/g vs 0.58 μg/g). Using a similar experimental preparation, Wang et al. (1962) showed that the fall in brain serotonin could be blocked by providing extra dietary tryptophan. Boggs et al. (1963) reported that serotonin synthesis (as reflected in urinary 5-HIAA excretion) could also be suppressed by feeding primates high-phenylalanine diets, and Boggs and Waisman (1964) demonstrated that the extent to which brain serotonin was depressed in rats fed phenylalanine was related to the amount of the amino acid in the diet. Using the initial rate at which brain serotonin increases after MAO inhibition as an index of serotonin biosynthesis, Yuwiler and Geller (1969) have obtained additional evidence that the low brain serotonin levels of rats fed phenylalanine result from impaired synthesis of the amine and not from accelerated turnover. At present, insufficient information is available to sustain conclusions as to whether the impairment in brain serotonin synthesis in animals fed phenylalanine results primarily from the decrease in brain tryptophan content or the inhibition of tryptophan hydroxylase activity. It is also not certain that the abnormalities in serotonin metabolism observed in phenyl-ketonuric patients arise solely from the effects of hyperphenylalaninemia on tryptophan hydroxylation.

If weanling rats are fed a diet supplemented with L-leucine for 30 to 40 days, the amount of serotonin in the brain is reduced in proportion to the leucine intake. In the study by Yuwiler and Geller (1965) total brain serotonin was decreased from 1.08 μg in control animals to 0.97 μg and 0.86 μg respectively in animals given 5 per cent and 8 per cent L-leucine-supplemented diets. The larger leucine dose was also associated with a significant reduction in brain weight; but even with this reduction, brain serotonin concentration was significantly lower than in control rats (0.47 μg/g vs 0.60 μg/g). A single large intravenous dose of L-leucine lowers the concentrations of tyrosine and phenylalanine in the brain (Roberts, 1968) (Table 6-2); however, no data are available on the effects of acute or chronic leucine administration on brain tryptophan content. Since the transport of L-tryptophan into brain neurons is apparently mediated by the same system that transports L-tyrosine, L-phenylalanine, and L-leucine, and since the decline in brain amino acid levels that follows L-leucine administration results from both impaired transport and accelerated utilization (i.e. for protein synthesis), it seems likely, if unproved, that the fall in brain serotonin observed in leucine-fed rats is associated with a parallel decrease in brain tryptophan levels. As discussed above, leucine could also lower brain serotonin levels by inhibiting enzymes involved in serotonin biosynthesis (e.g. aromatic L-amino acid decarboxylase (Tashian, 1961)), or by modifying the turnover of serotonin and the physiological activity of serotonin-containing neurons (Ramanamurthy and Srikantia, 1970). L-leucine is a potent stimulator of insulin secretion (Fajans et al., 1967) and could thus influence brain serotonin secondarily, by direct effects of insulin or indirect effects of the resulting hypoglycemia.

Natives of the Hyderabad region of India suffer from an endemic form of pellagra which is associated with the use of jowar (*Sorghum vulgare*) as the staple protein source (Belavady et al., 1963). Jowar differs from maize, the more common etiologic agent in pellagra, in that it contains adequate amounts of tryptophan and of utilizable nicotinic acid; however, like maize, jowar has a high leucine content. Gopalan and his associates have performed extensive studies on tryptophan metabolism in patients suffering from jowar-induced pellagra, as well as on humans and experimental animals given excessive amounts of L-leucine. The urinary excre-

tion of 5-HIAA is low in pellagrins (12 mg/day vs 28 mg/day in normal
male control subjects), and is depressed in both normal and sick subjects
by supplemental dietary leucine (10 g/day for 5 days: normal subjects
then excrete 18 mg of 5-HIAA per day; pellagrins excrete 6.8 mg/day)
(Belvady et al., 1963). Weanling rats fed high-leucine diets for four
weeks had low brain serotonin levels. Animals consuming a 10 per cent
casein diet fortified with 3 per cent L-leucine had about 20 per cent less
brain serotonin than pair-fed control animals consuming the unfortified
diet (Ramanamurthy and Srikantia, 1970); brain weight was not affected
by this treatment, and supplementation with 8 per cent L-leucine was no
more effective in reducing brain serotonin than 3 per cent L-leucine. Rats
allowed to consume *ad libitum* a diet containing 10 per cent jowar protein
had considerably less brain serotonin than littermates given 10 per cent
casein *ad libitum,* but the body weight of animals given jowar protein was
markedly reduced, probably as a consequence of low food intake. The observation that consumption of a *naturally occurring* foodstuff is associated
with a major alteration in the metabolism of a brain neurotransmitter is
of considerable potential clinical significance.

Para-chlorophenylalanine. The administration of the synthetic amino acid
para-chlorophenylalanine (PCPA) to rats results in *selective* depletion of
brain serotonin in mice, rats, and dogs (Koe and Weissman, 1966). Since
PCPA is a potent competitive inhibitor of tryptophan hydroxylase *in vitro*
and an irreversible inactivator of this enzyme *in vivo* (Jequier et al.,
1967), it has generally been assumed that the fall in brain serotonin levels
that it induces reflects an impairment in serotonin biosynthesis resulting
from inhibition of tryptophan hydroxylase. More recent studies suggest
that the deceleration in serotonin biosynthesis might also result from a
decrease in the availability of L-tryptophan to serotoninergic neurons.
Brains of animals pretreated for three days with PCPA take up a smaller
fraction of a dose of injected ^{14}C-tryptophan than brains of control animals (Gal et al., 1970); PCPA, phenylalanine, and tyrosine all inhibit
the uptake of ^{14}C-tryptophan by synaptosomes prepared from rat brain
(Grahame-Smith and Parfitt, 1970); PCPA administration causes a 50
per cent fall in brain tryptophan levels (Tagliamonte et al., 1970). PCPA
is a potent inhibitor of heptatic phenylalanine hydroxylase (Koe and
Weissman, 1966), and its administration causes a marked rise in brain
phenylalanine levels (Jequier et al., 1967). Hence its apparent ability to

inhibit the transport of L-tryptophan into brain might result from increased phenylalanine levels in plasma or brain. PCPA might also interfere with tryptophan transport by substituting for phenylalanine in newly
synthesized proteins utilized in the transport process (Gal et al., 1970)
or by acting through its brain metabolite, para-chlorophenylacetaldehyde
(Gal et al., 1970), to form a Schiff base with such a theoretical protein.
PCPA treatment has also been shown to produce a transient decline in
brain norepinephrine levels (Welch and Welch, 1967) even though the
synthetic amino acid is apparently not an effective inhibitor of tyrosine
hydroxylase. It might be useful to determine whether PCPA treatment
lowers brain tyrosine levels, presumably by interfering with tyrosine synthesis in the liver or its transport into the brain.

A variety of drugs that enhance serotonin biosynthesis have been shown
to elevate brain tryptophan levels; these include d-amphetamine, reserpine, and lithium. L-DOPA lowers brain serotonin levels (Everett and
Borcherding, 1970), and like phenylalanine (Aoki and Siegel, 1970) it
disaggregates the polyribosomes in infant rat brains (Weiss et al., 1971).
Its effect on brain tryptophan, however, is opposite to that of phenylalanine; single doses elevate tryptophan concentrations, and therefore do not
lower brain serotonin by limiting the tryptophan supply (Weiss et al.,
1971). It is possible that the fall in brain serotonin that follows L-DOPA
administration results from a "false neurotransmitter" mechanism, in
which catecholamine molecules formed by the decarboxylation of L-DOPA
within serotonin-containing neurons compete with the natural transmitter
for storage sites (Ng et al., 1970).

Summary

The rates at which the brain synthesizes the catecholamines and serotonin
are influenced by several factors in addition to the levels of tyrosine hydroxylase or tryptophan hydroxylase within "aminergic" neurons. These
factors include the availability of the precursor amino acids, L-tyrosine
and L-tryptophan, and, probably, of such cofactors as reduced pteridines
and pyridoxal phosphate. There is considerable experimental evidence
that the content of serotonin in the brain can be varied by manipulating
the amount of L-tryptophan available to the experimental animal; temporal correlations seem to exist between the diurnal peaks in brain norepi-

nephrine and L-tyrosine concentrations, as well as between peaks in serotonin and L-tryptophan.

Addendum

The task of compiling this review (which was completed in December
1970) generated in the authors considerable enthusiasm about exploring
the possibility that physiological changes in plasma tryptophan concentrations actually do influence brain serotonin. Accordingly, a series of experiments was initiated, which, so far, have shown the following:

1. The administration of a very low dose of tryptophan (12.5 mg/kg,
or less than 6 per cent the amount of the amino acid normally consumed
each day) to rats at the time of day when plasma and brain tryptophan
concentrations are normally lowest (Fig. 6-2) causes a 20 to 25 per cent
($P<0.01$) increase in brain serotonin content, without driving plasma or
brain tryptophan concentrations above their normal daily ranges (Fernstrom and Wurtman, 1971b).

2. The administration of doses of insulin (1-2U/kg, by any parenteral
route of administration) which elevate plasma tryptophan levels in rats
(Fernstrom and Wurtman, 1971a, 1971c) also cause significant increases
in brain tryptophan and brain serotonin (Fernstrom and Wurtman, 1971d).

3. The voluntary consumption of a carbohydrate meal causes, in rats,
sequential rises in plasma tryptophan, brain tryptophan, and brain serotonin (Fernstrom and Wurtman, 1971d). This effect is probably mediated
at least in part by the secretion of insulin. The rapid response of brain
serotonin levels to food-induced changes in plasma tryptophan suggests
that "serotoninergic" neurons may serve as sensors for food consumption,
and for peripheral amino acid metabolism. It also suggests that the daily
rhythm in brain serotonin content results at least in part from diet-induced
rhythmic changes in plasma tryptophan.

4. The effect of a particular foodstuff on brain serotonin levels in rats
also depends upon its protein content. Preliminary data suggest that foods
containing large amounts of amino acids which compete with tryptophan
for uptake into central neurons cause less of an increment in brain tryptophan and serotonin, per unit increase in plasma tryptophan, than pure
carbohydrate diets.

5. The chronic consumption of a diet in which the only protein source

is a tryptophan-poor protein (i.e. corn) causes marked reductions in brain serotonin content and concentration; this reduction can be blocked by fortifying the corn diet with tryptophan (Fernstrom and Wurtman, 1971e).

References

Aghajanian, G. K., Graham, A. W., and Sheard, M. H. 1970. *Science* 169:1100.

Alam, S. Q. 1965. Ph.D. Thesis, Department of Nutrition and Food Science, Massachusetts Institute of Technology, Cambridge, Massachusetts.

Alousi, A., and Weiner, N. 1966. *Proc. Nat. Acad. Sci. U.S.* 56:1491.

Altman, K., and Greengard, O. 1966. *J. Clin. Invest.* 45:1527.

Anton, A. H., and Sayre, D. F. 1964. *J. Pharmacol. Exptl. Therap.* 145:326.

Anton-Tay, F., and Wurtman, R. J. 1971. In *Frontiers in Neuroendocrinology*, W. F. Ganong and L. Martini (Eds.), Oxford University Press, New York.

Aoki, K., and Siegel, F. L. 1970. *Science* 168:129.

Ashcroft, G. W., Eccleston, D., and Crawford, T. B. B. 1965. *J. Neurochem.* 12:483.

Axelrod, J., Shein, H. M., and Wurtman, R. J. 1969. *Proc. Nat. Acad. Sci. U.S.* 62:544.

Azmitia, E. C., Jr., and McEwen, B. S. 1969. *Science* 166:1274.

Azmitia, E. C., Jr., Algeri, S., and Costa, E. 1970. *Science* 169:201.

Baldridge, R. C., Borofsky, L., Baird, H., Reickle, F., and Bullock, D. 1959. *Proc. Soc. Exptl. Biol. Med.* 100:529.

Baliga, B. S., Pronczuk, A. W., and Munro, H. N. 1968. *J. Mol. Biol.* 34:199.

Belavady, B., Srikentia, S. G., and Gopalan, C. 1963. *Biochem. J.* 87:652.

Berendes, H., Anderson, J. A., Ziegler, M. R., and Ruttenberg, D. 1958. *Am. J. Dis. Children* 96:430.

Bito, L., Davson, H., Levin, E., Murray, M., and Snider, N. 1966. *J. Neurochem.* 13:1057.

Blasberg, R. G. 1968. *Recent Prog. Brain Res.* 29:245.

Blasberg, R., and Lajtha, A. 1965. *Arch. Biochem. Biophys.* 112:361.

Blasberg, R., and Lajtha, A. 1966. *Brain Res.* 1:86.

Bogdanski, D. F., Weissbach, H., and Udenfriend, S. 1957. *J. Neurochem.* 1:272.

Boggs, D. E., and Waisman, H. A. 1964. *Arch. Biochem. Biophys.* 106:307.

Boggs, D. E., McLay, D., Kappy, M., and Waisman, H. A. 1963. *Nature* 200:76.

Boullin, D. J. 1963. *Psychopharmacologia* 5:28.

Carver, M. J. 1965. *J. Neurochem.* 12:45.

Chalmers, J. P., and Wurtman, R. J. 1971. *Circulation Research* 28:480.

Chalmers, J. P., Baldessarini, R. J., and Wurtman, R. J. 1971. *Proc. Nat. Acad. Sci. U.S.* 68:662.

Chambers, J. W., George, R. H., and Bass, A. D. 1968. *Endocrinology* 83:1185.

Chirigos, M. A., Greengard, P., and Udenfriend, S. 1960. *J. Biol. Chem.* 235:2075.

Civen, M., and Knox, W. E. 1960. *J. Biol. Chem.* 235:1716.

Coburn, S. P., Seidenberg, M., and Fuller, R. W. 1968. *Proc. Soc. Exptl. Biol. Med.* 129:338.

Cohn, C., Joseph, D., Larin, F., Shoemaker, W. J., and Wurtman, R. J. 1970. *Proc. Soc. Exptl. Biol. Med.* 133:460.

Culley, W. J., Saunders, R. N., Mertz, E. T., and Jolly, D. H. 1963. *Proc. Soc. Exptl. Biol. Med.* 113:645.

Curzon, G., and Green, A. R. 1968. *Life Sci.* 7:657.

Curzon, G., and Green, A. R. 1969a. *Brit. J. Pharmacol.* 37:689.

Curzon, G., and Green, A. R. 1969b. *Biochem. J.* 111:15P.

Dairman, W., and Udenfriend, S. 1970. *Mol. Pharmacol.* 6:350.

Dairman, W., Gordon, R., Spector, S., Sjoerdsma, A., and Udenfriend, S. 1968. *Mol. Pharmacol.* 4:457.

Denckla, W. D., and Dewey, R. H. 1967. *J. Lab. Clin. Med.* 69:160.

DeQuattro, V., Nagatsu, T., Maronde, R., and Alexander, N. 1969. *Circulation Res.* 24:545.

Dixit, B. N., and Buckley, J. P. 1967. *Life Sci.* 6:755.

DuVoisin, R. C., Yahr, M. D., and Cote, L. D. 1969. *Trans. Amer. Neurol. Assn.* 94:81.

Eccleston, D., Ashcroft, G. W., and Crawford, T. B. B. 1965. *J. Neurochem.* 12:493.

Eccleston, D., Ashcroft, G. W., Moir, A. T. B., Parker-Rhodes, A., Lutz, W., and O'Mahoney, D. 1968. *J. Neurochem.* 15:947.

Eccleston, D., Ritchie, I. M., Roberts, M. H. T. 1970. *Nature* 226:84.

Elwyn, D. H. 1970. In *Mammalian Protein Metabolism,* H. N. Munro (Ed.), vol. 4, Academic Press, New York, pp. 523-58.

Everett, G., and Borcherding, J. W. 1970. *Science* 168:849.

Fajans, S., Floyd, J. C., Jr., Knopf, R. F., and Conn, J. W. 1967. *Recent Prog. Hormone Res.* 23:717.

Feigen, R. D., Klainer, A. S., and Beisel, W. R. 1968. *Metabolism* 17:764.

Fernstrom, J. D., and Wurtman, R. J. 1971a. *Federation Proc.* 30:250.

Fernstrom, J. D., and Wurtman, R. J. 1971b. *Science* 173:149.

Fernstrom, J. D., and Wurtman, R. J. 1971c. *Metabolism* (in press).

Fernstrom, J. D., and Wurtman, R. J. 1971d. *Science* 174:1023.

Fernstrom, J. D., and Wurtman, R. J. 1971e. *Nature, New Biology* 234:62.

Fishman, B., Wurtman, R. J., and Munro, H. N. 1969. *Proc. Nat. Acad. Sci. U.S.* 64:677.

Fuller, R. W. 1965. *Life Sci.* 4:1.

Fuller, R. W. 1970. *Proc. Soc. Exptl. Biol. Med.* 133:620.

Fuller, R. W., Jones, G. T., Snoddy, H. D., and Salter, I. H. 1969. *Life Sci.* 8:685.

Gal, E. M., and Drewes, P. A. 1962. *Proc. Soc. Exptl. Biol. Med.* 110:368.

Gal, E. M., Drewes, P. A., and Barraclough, C. A. 1961. *Biochem. Pharmacol.* 8:23.

Gal, E. M., Poczick, M., and Marshall, F. D., Jr. 1963. *Biochem. Biophys. Res. Commun.* 12:29.

Gal, E. M., Roggeveen, A. E., and Millard, S. A. 1970. *J. Neurochem.* 17:1221.

Garattini, S., and Valzelli, L. 1965. *Serotonin,* Elsevier Publishing Co., Amsterdam.

Gibb, J. W., and Webb, J. G. 1969. *Proc. Nat. Acad. Sci. U.S.* 63:364.

Goldberg, A. L., and Goodman, H. M. 1969. *Am. J. Physiol.* 216:1116.

Gordon, R., Reid, J. V. D., Sjoerdsma, A., and Udenfriend, S. 1966a. *Mol. Pharmacol.* 2:610.

Gordon, R., Spector, S., Sjoerdsma, A., and Udenfriend, S. 1966b. *J. Pharmacol. Exptl. Therap.* 153:440.

Grahame-Smith, D. G. 1964a. *Biochem. J.* 92:52.

Grahame-Smith, D. G. 1964b. *Biochem. Biophys. Res. Commun.* 16:586.

Grahame-Smith, D. G. 1967. *Biochem. J.* 105:351.

Grahame-Smith, D. G., and Parfitt, A. G. 1970. *J. Neurochem.* 17:1339.

Green, A. R., and Curzon, G. 1968. *Nature* 220:1095.

Green, A. R., and Curzon, G. 1970. *Biochem. Pharmacol.* 19:2061.

Green, H., Greenberg, S. M., Erickson, R. W., Sawyer, J. L., and Ellizon, T. 1962. *J. Pharmacol. Exptl. Therap.* 136:174.

Guroff, G., and Udenfriend, S. 1962. *J. Biol. Chem.* 237:803.

Harper, A. E. 1964. In *Mammalian Protein Metabolism,* H. N. Munro and J. B. Allison (Eds.), vol. 2, Academic Press, New York, pp. 87-130.

Horita, A., and Carino, M. A. 1970. *Biochem. Pharmacol.* 19:1521.

Iggo, A., and Vogt, M. 1960. *J. Physiol.* 150:114.

Ikeda, M., Fahien, L. A., and Udenfriend, S. 1966. *J. Biol. Chem.* 241:4452.

Iyer, N. T., McGeer, P. L., and McGeer, E. G. 1963. *Can. J. Biochem. Physiol.* 41: 1565.

Jequier, E., Lovenberg, W., and Sjoerdsma, A. 1967. *Mol. Pharmacol.* 3:274.

Jequier, E., Robinson, D. S., Lovenberg, W., and Sjoerdsma, A. 1969. *Biochem. Pharmacol.* 18:1071.

Koe, B. K., and Weissman, A. 1966. *J. Pharmacol. Exptl. Therap.* 154:499.

Kostyo, J. L., and Knobil, E. 1959. *Endocrinology* 65:395.

Lajtha, A., and Marks, N. 1966. *Protides of the Biological Fluids,* Elsevier Publishing Co., Amsterdam, pp. 103-14.

Lajtha, A., and Mela, P. 1961. *J. Neurochem.* 7:210.

Lajtha, A., and Toth, J. 1961. *J. Neurochem.* 8:216.

Lajtha, A., and Toth, J. 1966. *Biochem. Biophys. Res. Commun.* 23:294.

Levitt, M., Spector, S., Sjoerdsma, A., and Udenfriend, S. 1965. *J. Pharmacol. Exptl. Therap.* 148:1.

Lloyd, K., Hornykiewicz, O. 1970. *Brain Res.* 22:426.

Lorenzo, A. V., and Cutler, R. W. P. 1969. *J. Neurochem.* 16:577.

Lovenberg, W., Weissbach, H., and Udenfriend, S. 1962. *J. Biol. Chem.* 237:89.

Lovenberg, W., Jequier, E., and Sjoerdsma, A. 1968. *Advan. Pharmacol.* 6A:21.

Madras, B. K., and Sourkes, T. L. 1965. *Biochem. Pharmacol.* 14:1499.

Mark, J., Pugge, H., and Mandel, P. 1970. *J. Neurochem.* 17:1393.

Marliss, E. B., Aoki, T. T., Pozefsky, T., Most, A., and Cahill, G. F., Jr. 1971. *J. Clin. Invest.* 50:814.

McGeer, E. G., and McGeer, P. L. 1967. *Can. J. Biochem.* 45:115.

McGeer, E. G., and Peters, D. A. V. 1969. *Can. J. Biochem.* 47:501.

McKean, C. M., Boggs, D. E., and Peterson, N. A. 1968. *J. Neurochem.* 15:235.

Meek, J., Fuxe, K., and Anden, N. E. 1970. *European J. Pharmacol.* 9:325.

Miller, J. E., and Litwack, G. 1969. *Arch. Biochem. Biophys.* 135:149.

Moir, A. T. B., and Eccleston, D. 1968. *J. Neurochem.* 15:1093.

Moran, J. F., and Sourkes, T. L. 1963. *J. Biol. Chem.* 238:3006.

Mueller, R. A., Thoenen, H., and Axelrod, J. 1969a. *Science* 163:468.

Mueller, R. A., Thoenen, H., and Axelrod, J. 1969b. *J. Pharmacol. Exptl. Therap.* 169:74.

Munro, H. N. 1964. In *Mammalian Protein Metabolism,* H. N. Munro and J. B. Allison (Eds.), vol. 1, Academic Press, New York, p. 442.

Murphy, G. F., and Sourkes, T. L. 1961. *Arch. Biochem. Biophys.* 93:338.

Musacchio, J. M., and Castellucci, L. B. 1969. *Pharmacologist* 11(2):274.

Nadler, H. L., and Hsia, D. Y. 1961. *Proc. Soc. Exptl. Biol. Med.* 107:721.

Nagatsu, T., Levitt, M., and Udenfriend, S. 1964. *J. Biol. Chem.* 239:2910.

Ng, K. Y., Chase, T.-N., Colburn, R. W., and Kopin, I. J. 1970. *Science* 170:76.

Ngai, S. H., Neff, N. H., and Costa, E. 1968. *Life Sci.* 7:847.

Oravec, M. 1969. Ph.D. Thesis, McGill University, Montreal, Canada; cited in T. L. Sourkes. 1971. *Federation Proc.* 30:897.

Page, I. H. 1968. *Serotonin,* Yearbook Medical Publishers, Inc., Chicago.

Pare, C. M. B., Sandler, M., and Stacey, R. S. 1957. *Lancet* i:551.

Pare, C. M. B., Sandler, M., and Stacey, R. S. 1958. *Lancet* ii:1099.

Perry, T. L., Hansen, S., Tischler, B., and Hestrim, M. 1964. *Proc. Soc. Exptl. Biol. Med.* 115:118.

Peters, D. A. V., McGeer, P. L., and McGeer, E. G. 1968. *J. Neurochem.* 15:1431.

Peterson, N. A., and McKean, C. M. 1969. *J. Neurochem.* 16:1211.

Pozefsky, T., Felig, P., Tobin, J. D., Soeldner, J. S., and Cahill, G. F., Jr. 1969. *J. Clin. Invest.* 48:2273.

Ramanamurthy, P. S. V., and Srikantia, S. G. 1970. *J. Neurochem.* 71:27.

Rapoport, M. I., and Beisel, W. R. 1968. *J. Clin. Invest.* 47:934.

Rapoport, M. I., Feigen, R. D., Bruton, J., and Beisel, W. R. 1966. *Science* 153:1642.

Renson, J., Weissbach, H., and Udenfriend, S. 1962. *J. Biol. Chem.* 237:2261.

Roberts, S. 1968. *Progr. Brain. Res.* 29:235.

Roth, R. H., Stjärne, L., von Euler, U. S. 1967. *J. Pharmacol. Exptl. Therap.* 158:373.

Schimke, R. T., Sweeney, E. W., and Berlin, C. M. 1965. *J. Biol. Chem.* 240:4609.

Sedvall, G., and Kopin, I. J. 1967. *Biochem. Pharmacol.* 16:39.

Sedvall, G., Weise, V. K., and Kopin, I. J. 1968. *J. Pharmacol. Exptl. Therap.* 159:274.

Serini, F., Principi, N., Perletti, L., and Sereni, L. P. 1966. *Biol. Neonatorum* 10:254.

Shah, N. S., Stevens, S., and Himwich, H. E. 1968. *Arch. Intern. Pharmacodyn.* 171:285.

Sharman, D., and Smith, S. E. 1962. *J. Neurochem.* 9:403.

Shein, H. M., and Wurtman, R. J. 1971. *Life Sci.* 10:935.

Shoemaker, W. J., and Wurtman, R. J. 1970. *Federation Proc.* 29:496.

Shoemaker, W. J., and Wurtman, R. J. 1971. *Science.* 171:1017.

Sokoloff, L. 1961. In *Regional Neurochemistry,* S. S. Kety and J. Elkes (Eds.), Pergamon Press, Oxford, p. 107.

Sourkes, T. L. 1954. *Arch. Biochem.* 51:444.

Sourkes, T. L. 1971. *Federation Proc.* 30:897.

Sourkes, T. L., and Townsend, E. 1955. *Can. J. Biochem. Physiol.* 33:735.

Sourkes, T. L., Murphy, G. F., Chavez, B., and Zielinska, M. J. 1961. *J. Neurochem.* 8:109.

Sourkes, T. L., Missala, K., and Oravec, M. 1970. *J. Neurochem.* 17:111.

Spector, S., Sjoerdsma, A., and Udenfriend, S. 1965. *J. Pharmacol. Exptl. Therap.* 147:86.

Spector, S., Gordon, R., Sjoerdsma, A., and Udenfriend, S. 1967. *Mol. Pharmacol.* 3:549.

Tagliamonte, A., Tagliamonte, P., Perez-Cruet, J., and Gessa, G. 1970. *Pharmacologist* 12(2):236.

Tashian, R. E. 1961. *Metab. Clin. Exptl.* 10:393.

Tewksbury, D. A., and Lohrenz, F. N. 1970. *Metabolism* 19:363.

Tews, J. K., Woodcock, N. A., and Harper, A. E. 1970. *J. Biol. Chem.* 245:3026.

Thoenen, H., Mueller, R. A., and Axelrod, J. 1969a. *Nature* 221:1264.
Thoenen, H., Mueller, R. A., and Axelrod, J. 1969b. *J. Pharmacol. Exptl. Therap.* 169:249.
Thomas, R. G., and Wysor, W. G. 1967. *Proc. Soc. Exptl. Biol. Med.* 126:374.
Udenfriend, S. 1966. In *Mechanisms of Release of Biogenic Amines,* U. S. von Euler, S. Rosell, and B. Uvnas (Eds.), Pergamon Press, Oxford, pp. 103-8.
Udenfriend, S., Creveling, C. R., Posner, H., Redfield, B. G., Daly, J., and Witkop, B. 1959. *Arch. Biochem.* 83:501.
van Sande, M., Mardens, Y., Ariaenssesns, K., and Lowenthal, A. 1970. *J. Neurochem.* 17:125.
Wang, H. L., Harwalker, V. H., and Waisman, H. A. 1962. *Arch. Biochem. Biophys.* 96:181.
Weber, L. J. 1966. *Proc. Soc. Exptl. Biol. Med.* 123:35.
Weber, L. J., and Horita, A. 1965. *Biochem. Pharmacol.* 14:1141.
Weiner, N. 1970. *Ann. Rev. Pharmacol.* 10:273.
Weiner, N., and Rabadjija, M. 1968. *J. Pharmacol. Exptl. Therap.* 164:103.
Weiss, B., Wurtman, R. J., and Munro, H. N. *Federation Proc.* (in press).
Welch, B., and Welch, A. 1967. *J. Pharm. Pharmacol.* 19:632.
Wurtman, R. J. 1966. *Catecholamines,* Little, Brown, Boston.
Wurtman, R. J. 1969. *Advan. Enzyme Regulation* 7:57.
Wurtman, R. J. 1970. In *Mammalian Protein Metabolism,* H. N. Munro (Ed.), vol. 4, Academic Press, New York, pp. 445-70.
Wurtman, R. J., and Axelrod, J. 1967. *Proc. Nat. Acad. Sci. U.S.* 6:1594.
Wurtman, R. J., and Larin, F. 1968. *Biochem. Pharmacol.* 17:817.
Wurtman, R. J., Chou, C., and Rose, C. 1967. *Science* 158:660.
Wurtman, R. J., Axelrod, J., and Kelly, D. E. 1968a. *The Pineal,* Academic Press, New York.
Wurtman, R. J., Shoemaker, W. J., and Larin, F. 1968b. *Proc. Nat. Acad. Sci. U.S.* 59:800.
Wurtman, R. J., Rose, C. M., Chou, C., and Larin, F. 1968c. *New Engl. J. Med.* 279:171.
Wurtman, R. J., Shein, H. M., Axelrod, J., and Larin, F. 1969a. *Proc. Nat. Acad. Sci. U.S.* 62:749.
Wurtman, R. J., Anton-Tay, F., and Anton, S. 1969b. *Life Sci.* 8:1015.
Wurtman, R. J., Chou, C., and Rose, C. 1970a. *J. Pharmacol. Exptl. Therap.* 174:351.
Wurtman, R. J., Rose, C. M., Matthysse, S., Stephenson, J., and Baldessarini, R. J. 1970b. *Science* 169:395.
Young, V., Hussein, M. A., Murray, E., and Scrimshaw, N. S. 1969. *Am. J. Clin. Nutr.* 22:1563.
Yuwiler, A., and Geller, E. 1965. *Nature* 208:83.
Yuwiler, A., and Geller, E. 1969. *J. Neurochem.* 16:999.
Yuwiler, A., and Louttit, R. 1961. *Science* 134:831.
Zbinden, G., Pletscher, A., and Studer, A. 1958. *Z. Ges. Exptl. Med.* 129:615.
Zhelyaskov, D. K., Levitt, M., and Udenfriend, S. 1968. *Mol. Pharmacol.* 4:445.
Zigmond, M. J., and Wurtman, R. J. 1970. *J. Pharmacol. Exptl. Therap.* 172:416.
Zigmond, M. J., Shoemaker, W. J., Larin, F., and Wurtman, R. J. 1969. *J. Nutr.* 98:71.
Zinneman, H. H., Nuttall, F. Q., Goetz, F. C. 1966. *Diabetes* 15:5.

7

The Sympathetic Neuro-Humoral System and White Adipose Tissue

SUNE ROSELL

A multitude of biogenic substances are known to stimulate the hormone-sensitive lipase system in adipose tissue (Rudman et al., 1965). Such stimulation leads to lipolysis, i.e. hydrolysis of triglycerides into free fatty acids (FFA) and glycerol. Our knowledge concerning the lipolytic actions of different substances is to a large extent based on *in vitro* experiments on the rat epididymal fat pad. However, there are large species variations in the actions of lipolytic substances as well as regional differences in the same species. This review will be mainly confined to canine white adipose tissue *in vivo*. One reason for choosing this species is that catecholamines play a significant role as lipolytic agents in the dog. Furthermore, the influence of the adrenergic neuro-humoral system on the vascular reactions in adipose tissue has been most extensively studied in dogs and therefore it is possible to relate metabolic and vascular reactions to each other in that species.

Cholinergic Innervation of Adipose Tissue

On the basis of the presence of cholinesterase, it has been suggested that adipose tissue contains cholinergic receptors (Salvador and Kuntzman, 1965) and thus may be innervated by cholinergic fibers of sympathetic or parasympathetic origin. It has also been shown that a cholinesterase inhibitor, neostigmine, lowers the fasting concentrations of plasma FFA in the conscious dog. This finding might indicate that stimulation of cholinergic receptors inhibits the release of FFA (Colville et al., 1964), but another possible explanation is that neostigmine inhibits the lipase activity (Dixon and Webb, 1964). Similarly, Weiss and Maickel (1968) observed that atropine can enhance the lipolytic response to nerve stimulation in isolated tissue, using histochemical techniques. Ballantyne (1968) demonstrated the presence of at least two cholinesterase enzymes in white adipose tissue from different species. The adipocytes appeared to contain both an acetyl- and a buturylcholinesterase, whereas the nerve fibers to the vessels seemed to contain only buturylcholinesterase. No direct nerve supply to the individual adipocytes was found. The fact that the nerves did not contain acetylcholinesterase led Ballantyne to propose that there are no cholinergic fibers to adipose tissue. This opinion is supported by the finding that the vascular responses to electrical stimulation of the nervous supply to the canine subcutaneous adipose tissue is not influenced by atropine (Ngai, Rosell, and Wallenberg, 1966) and that acetylcholine has very weak vasoactive effects in that tissue. Thus acetylcholine is roughly 1000 times less potent as a vasodilator than prostaglandin E_1, and 100 times less potent than histamine (Fredholm, Öberg, and Rosell, 1970). Naturally, these findings raise some questions as to the physiological significance of cholinergic fibers to white adipose tissue.

Adrenergic Innervation of Adipose Tissue

With the use of the histochemical fluorescence method of Falck and Hillarp (Falck et al., 1962) monoaminergic fluorescent nerve fibers could be found only around arteries and arterioles and occasionally around veins (Wirsén, 1965a). In contrast, the adipocytes did not seem to have any contacts with adrenergic nerve terminals. Later Wirsén (1965b) incubated adipose tissue in α-methylnorepinephrine to increase the amine content of nerve fibers but still failed to reveal any adrenergic nerve terminals around adipocytes in white adipose tissue. These histochemical findings have been confirmed by Ballantyne and Raftery (1969). There is thus strong morphological evidence that the adipocytes in white adipose tissue, in contrast to those in brown adipose tissue (see Cottle, 1970), are not in synaptic contact with adrenergic nerve fibers. This is true for adipose tissue in species which respond with increased lipolysis following administration of catecholamines. Consequently, it has been suggested that the lipolysis which has been noted following stimulation of adrenergic nerves to white adipose tissue is secondary to blood flow changes (Ballantyne and Raftery, 1969) or that circulating catecholamines are of greater quantitative importance for lipolysis than the sympathetic innervation (Wirsén, 1965b). As will be discussed later the stimulation of sympathetic nerves to adipose tissue elevates the lipolytic rate even if blood is kept constant (Rosell, 1966). Furthermore, by comparing the lipolytic effect of circulating catecholamines with that of sympathetic nerve activation it was found that the sympathetic innervation of subcutaneous adipose tissue, at least to the inguinal region of the dog, plays a greater role than circulating epinephrine or norepinephrine (Ballard and Rosell, 1971a). There is thus a divergence of opinion regarding the relative importance of the sympathetic innervation of adipose tissue for the regulation of lipolysis, the opinion depending on whether the problem has been studied from the morphological or physiological standpoint.

Responses to Sympathetic Nerve Activity

Lipolysis

Lipolysis elevates the venous outflow of FFA and glycerol from adipose tissue. Of these two products, glycerol is generally used as a measure of the rate of lipolysis since it is utilized in the white adipose tissue to only a minor extent or not at all (Steinberg and Vaughan, 1965) since this tissue has little capacity to phosphorylate glycerol (Margolis and Vaughan, 1965; Robinson and Newsholme, 1967). FFA, on the other hand, is partially re-esterified as indicated by the finding that often less than three moles of FFA per mole of glycerol are released *in vitro* (Steinberg and Vaughan, 1965) or appear in the venous outflow from adipose tissue *in vivo* (Fredholm and Rosell, 1968).

Electrical stimulation of nerves to canine *subcutaneous adipose tissue* produces increased outflow of FFA and glycerol as well as vascular responses (Rosell, 1966; Ngai, Rosell, and Wallenberg, 1966; Rosell, 1969; Fredholm, 1970). These effects are seen with stimulation frequencies which are supposed to be within the physiological range. Folkow (1952) concluded that the impulse activity in postganglionic sympathetic nerves to skeletal muscle is in the order of 1 to 2 imp/sec and rarely exceeds 6 to 8 imp/sec under physiological conditions. It is reasonable to assume that

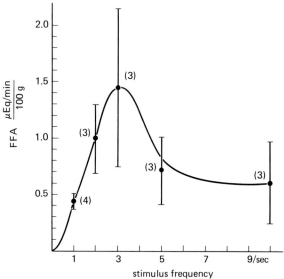

FFA=free fatty acids

Figure 7-1   Relation between stimulation frequency and the rate of release of FFA in canine subcutaneous adipose tissue. The figures within brackets indicate the number of stimulations. The vertical lines represent $\pm$ S.E.M. (From Rosell, *Acta Physiol. Scand.* 67:343, 1966)

this is also the case in sympathetic nerves to adipose tissue. As is evident from Fig. 7-1, the maximum FFA release in canine subcutaneous adipose tissue is obtained with about 3 imp/sec.

Release of FFA has also been found following supramaximal stimulation of nerves to isolated rat and rabbit adipose tissue *in vitro* (Correll, 1963). However, it is questionable whether lipolysis in rabbits is influenced by adrenergic sympathetic nervous activity under physiological conditions, since catecholamines have a weak adipokinetic action when added to adipose tissue from that species *in vitro* (Rudman et al., 1963). Moreover, Braun and Hechter (1970) found that in ghost preparations from rabbit epididymal fat cells epinephrine had little or no stimulatory effect on the adenyl cyclase which forms increasing amounts of adenosine-3', 5' monophosphate. They suggested therefore that in the rabbit fat cell membrane, in contrast to the rat adipocyte membrane, adenyl cyclase is not coupled to an epinephrine receptor.

Electrical stimulation of the appropriate sympathetic nerves also causes an elevated venous outflow of FFA and glycerol in canine *omental adipose tissue* (Fig. 7-2) (Ballard and Rosell, 1971a). This is in agreement with the results of Nash et al. (1961) and Paoletti et al. (1961). In the same type of tissue they also found an elevated venous outflow of FFA following nerve stimulation, but their experiments did not yield consistent results and no quantitative data were reported. One explanation may be that a high stimulation frequency was applied (16 imp/sec) and the vasoconstriction may have been strong enough to trap the released FFA within the tissue.

In contrast, stimulation of the superior mesenteric nerves had no observable effects on the outflow of glycerol or FFA from the *canine mesentery* (Ballard and Rosell, 1969). To induce lipolysis, norepinephrine had to be injected in approximately ten times higher doses than those required to produce similar effects in subcutaneous adipose tissue. It therefore seems as if receptors for catecholamines are less abundant in the mesenteric adipose tissue than in subcutaneous and omental tissue in the same species. Consequently, the sympathetic neuro-humoral system seems to be of little physiological importance for lipolysis in the mesentery. Aronovsky et al. (1963) suggested that in some regions the adipose tissue

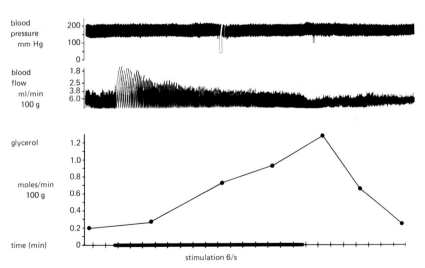

Figure 7-2   Systemic blood pressure, blood flow, and release of glycerol in canine omental adipose tissue. Tissue weight: 39 g. The mixed nerves to the tissue were stimulated electrically for 15 minutes (6 v, 2 msec, 6/s). (From Ballard and Rosell, *Circulation Res.*, 1971, in press)

may have a supportive function rather than serving as an energy depot. They found that catecholamines did not exert any adipokinetic effects when added to adipose tissue from the orbital socket and the paw of the cat. Whether the fat in the mesentery has only a supportive function remains to be evaluated.

The differences demonstrated for the effects of sympathetic nerve activity show that there are regional differences in the sympathetic neurohumoral control of lipolysis. Perhaps circulating hormones, rather than this system, play a greater physiological role in some regions. This possibility has not yet been evaluated experimentally.

Pharmacologic Characterization. Beta-receptor blocking agents (propranolol, pronethalol, D(-)-INPEA) inhibit the lipolysis caused by sympathetic nerve activity in subcutaneous (Fredholm and Rosell, 1968) as well as omental adipose tissue (Ballard and Rosell, 1971a). This is in agreement with the action of β-receptor blocking agents in *in vitro* systems (see Wenke 1966; Sutherland et al., 1968) and with the finding by Bär and Hechter (1969) that β-receptor blocking agents antagonize the increase in adenyl cyclase activity induced by catecholamines in fat cell ghosts.

Interestingly enough, low concentrations of adrenergic α-receptor blocking agents potentiate venous outflow of FFA and glycerol following stimulation of sympathetic nerves with "physiological" frequencies (Fredholm and Rosell, 1968) (Fig. 7-3). The finding that phentolamine, unlike β-receptor blocking agents, does not inhibit the activation of adenyl cyclase by epinephrine in fat cell ghosts (Birnbaumer and Rodbell, 1969) is in agreement with our results even if this does not explain the potentiation. One factor of importance for the potentiation seems to be the vascular reactions to sympathetic nerve activity in canine subcutaneous adipose tissue. As will be discussed, the vasoconstriction following sympathetic nerve stimulation is converted into vasodilatation following stimulation after administration of α-receptor blocking agents. It is conceivable that this promotes a more rapid and effective venous outflow of the products of lipolysis and may thus partly explain the shortened latency as well as the potentiation.

In contrast, high concentrations of α-adrenolytics *in vitro* inhibit the lipolytic action of catecholamines in a noncompetitive way (Wenke, 1966). Westermann and Stock (1970) found that phentolamine and thy-

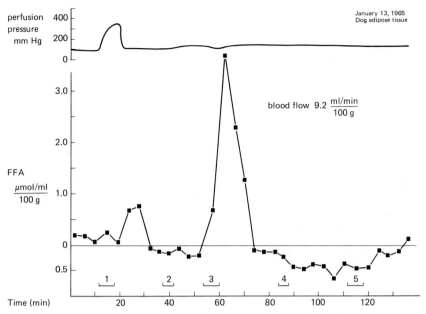

Figure 7-3   Canine subcutaneous adipose tissue perfused with constant flow of 9.2 ml/min/100 g. Electrical stimulation of the nerve to the tissue. Samples for FFA determinations collected during 3-minute intervals. At (1), stimulation, 6 imp/sec; (2), 60 μg of dihydroergotamine; (3), stimulation, 6 imp/sec; (4), 100 μg of propranolol i.a.; (5), stimulation, 6 imp/sec. (From Fredholm and Rosell, *J. Pharm. Exp. Therap.* 159:1, 1968)

moxamine also inhibit the lipolytic action of ACTH and theophylline and suggested therefore that α-receptor blocking agents do not interfere with the adenyl cyclase receptor site but prevent the activation of triglyceride lipase. The effects of high concentrations of adrenergic α-receptor antagonists may explain the confusion concerning the type of receptor responsible for adrenergic stimulation of lipolysis (see Havel, 1965). Thus, Correll (1963) and Nash et al. (1961) could inhibit the lipolytic effect of nerve stimulation by high concentrations of dibenamine.

Inhibition of Lipolysis. Whether vascular changes are the sole explanation for the potentiation and shortened latency of the venous outflow of glycerol and FFA after α-receptor blockade remains to be elucidated, especially since it has been suggested that prostaglandins may act as feedback inhibitors. Prostaglandins of the E type counteract the lipolysis (Bergström, Carlson, and Weeks, 1968), and it has been shown that prostaglandin E_1 blocks the lipolysis following sympathetic nerve activity both *in vitro* (Berti and Usardi, 1964) and *in vivo* (Fredholm and Rosell, 1970b). Shaw and Ramwell (1968) found that stimulation of nerves to the rat epididymal adipose tissue *in vitro* released prostaglandins. This finding was confirmed in canine subcutaneous adipose tissue (Fredholm, Rosell, and Strandberg, 1970). On the basis of such experiments it has been proposed that prostaglandins may act as feedback inhibitors of lipolysis (Bergström, Carlson, and Weeks, 1968; Shaw and Ramwell, 1968; Horton, 1969). Moreover, Davies, Horton, and Withrington (1968) noted an outflow of prostaglandin-like material from the dog's spleen when the appropriate nerve was stimulated and that the release was inhibited by α-receptor blockade. A release of prostaglandins, via activation of α-receptors, which modify the lipolysis caused by β-receptor stimulation is a very attractive hypothesis indeed and would partly explain the potentiation of FFA and glycerol release on sympathetic nerve stimulation after α-receptor blockade. From experiments using human adipose tissue *in vitro* Burns and Langley (1968) and Efendić (1970) have also suggested that α-receptor activity inhibits lipolysis. Accordingly, Burns, Langley, and Robison (1970) found that epinephrine induced a higher concentration of cyclic AMP in the presence of phentolamine than in the absence of that α-receptor blocking drug. Whether this response is confined to human adipocytes remains to be investigated. Fredholm (1970) found no evidence for the presence of an inhibitory α-receptor mechanism in canine subcutaneous adipose tissue. Furthermore, Laity (1969) noted that the release of prostaglandins from the rat diaphragm was actually potentiated by α-receptor blockade. In view of their pronounced inhibitory effect on lipolysis and potent vasodilator properties it is very likely that some of the prostaglandins have a physiological function in adipose tissue, but at present it is difficult to define such a function.

Vascular Reactions

Blood Flow. Resting blood in canine adipose tissue is usually between 7 to 12 ml/min/100 g, regardless of whether it is located in the mesentery, subcutis or the omentum (Ngai, Rosell, and Wallenberg, 1966; Öberg and Rosell, 1967; Ballard and Rosell, 1969; 1971a). Fredholm, Öberg, and Rosell (1970) noted that the highest resting blood flow, calculated per 100 g tissue, was found in the smallest tissue preparations, which indicates that the degree of adiposity may play a role. This is supported by the recent finding that the resting blood flow is significantly lower, per unit weight, in canine subcutaneous adipose tissue containing larger adipocytes than in adipose tissue with smaller ones (Di Girolamo et al., 1970). In humans, Larsen, Lassen, and Quaade (1966) also noted a smaller blood flow per unit weight the thicker the subcutaneous fat layer. Irrespective of the large variation between individuals, the data both from man and experimental animals (see also Mayerle and Havel, 1969; Lewis and Mathews, 1968) show that the adipose tissue blood flow is of the same order of magnitude as in resting skeletal muscle.

Activation of the sympathetic nerves to subcutaneous and omental adipose tissue induces changes in all the consecutive vascular sections, i.e. the resistance, exchange, and capacitance section. However, the mesenteric blood flow does not seem to be markedly influenced by sympathetic nerve activity (Ballard and Rosell, 1969), and therefore data referring to that tissue have not been presented here.

In the omentum and the subcutaneous adipose tissue the total blood flow decreases in proportion to the frequency of stimulation (Ngai, Rosell, and Wallenberg, 1966). With continued stimulation for several minutes there is a gradual return of blood flow to prestimulatory levels. This is especially pronounced in the omentum where the constriction may even be converted to a vasodilatation, despite continued stimulation (Fig. 7-2) (Ballard and Rosell, 1971). This reversal is especially pronounced at higher stimulation frequencies (6 to 9 imp/sec). The reversal of the total blood flow is very similar to the autoregulatory escape in the cat intestine (Folkow et al., 1964a) but the mechanisms for these vascular effects may not be the same since the capillary and capacitance reactions are different. In the intestine the escape is confined to the resistance section (Folkow et al., 1964b; Wallentin, 1966), whereas this is not the case in the omentum.

The vasoconstriction is characterized as an α-receptor effect. After α-blockade, sympathetic nerve stimulation induces a pronounced vasodilatation which in turn is blocked by β-receptor blocking agents (Ngai, Rosell, and Wallenberg, 1966; Ballard and Rosell, 1971).

Exchange Function. To evaluate the exchange function of the vascular bed the capillary filtration coefficient (CFC) has been determined in subcutaneous and omental adipose tissues by means of the plethysmographic method of Folkow and Mellander (see Cobbold et al., 1963). The vascular beds in these two tissues seem to be particularly well suited for exchange, as evidenced by the resting CFC values. In the subcutaneous adipose tissue the CFC averaged 0.027 ml/min $\times$ 100 g $\times$ mm Hg (Öberg and Rosell, 1967), which is approximately 1.5 to 2 times the value found in resting skeletal muscle (Cobbold et al., 1963). In the omentum even higher resting CFC values were obtained (mean value = 0.05 ml/min $\times$ 100 g $\times$ mm Hg) (Ballard and Rosell, 1971). These results indicate that the total surface area over which filtration occurs is larger in the vascular beds of adipose tissue than of skeletal muscle. This indicates that the number of patent capillaries per unit weight is larger and/or that the porosity of the capillary endothelium is higher in adipose tissue than in skeletal muscle.

Sympathetic nerve stimulation induced a further increase in CFC both in the subcutaneous and omental adipose tissue, despite a concomitant decrease in total blood flow (Fig. 7-4). This is surprising since in other vascular beds, including skeletal muscle, skin, and intestine, there is a decreased CFC under similar conditions (Folkow and Mellander, 1960; Öberg, 1964; Folkow et al., 1964b). This has been taken as support for the hypothesis that sympathetic nerve activity increases the tone of the precapillary sphincter vessels, thus diminishing the number of capillaries open to flow and consequently the surface area over which filtration occurs. By the same token, an elevated CFC as seen in the adipose tissue would indicate a relaxation of the precapillary sphincter tone and thus an increased capillary surface area. To investigate this possibility, the disappearance of ^{133}Xe and ^{125}I from a depot in subcutaneous adipose tissue (Linde and Rosell, unpublished) and in the omentum (Ballard and Rosell, 1971) was determined under constant flow conditions. The blood flow was kept constant to eliminate the influence of changes in total blood flow on the disappearance rate. Under these conditions sympathetic nerve activity caused a decrease in disappearance rate, indicating a diminished diffusion of the tracer from tissue to blood, presumably due to a decrease in the number of open capillaries. There is thus an apparent discrepancy between the results from the filtration and diffusion measurements. To explain this difference the hypothesis was advanced that sympathetic nerve activity not only affects the precapillary sphincter tone but also the permeability of the exchange vessels (Rosell, 1969, Fredholm, Öberg,

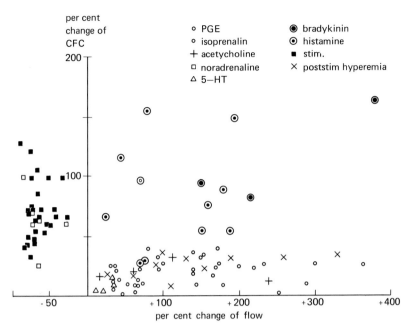

Figure 7-4   Relation between per cent change in blood flow and in CFC in sub-cutaneous adipose tissue, produced by administration of various vasoactive drugs and by regional vasomotor fiber stimulation. (From Fredholm, Öberg, and Rosell, *Acta Physiol. Scand.* 79:564, 1970)

and Rosell, 1970; Fredholm, 1970). The hydrodynamic conductivity, as measured by CFC, is dependent not only on the total capillary surface area available for exchange processes but also on the permeability (the number and dimensions of the pores), and alterations of the CFC do not provide information regarding which of these two factors has changed. Therefore the pronounced increase in CFC may be due to an increase in pore size which is, however, to some extent offset by an increased precapillary sphincter tone. This results in a diminished number of patent capillaries which may impair diffusion as indicated by the slowed disappearance rate of ^{133}Xe or ^{125}I. Indirect support for the idea that sympathetic nerve activity may actually increase the pore size is the fact that the high CFC values found in subcutaneous adipose tissue following sympathetic nerve stimulation could only be initiated by infusion of vasodilator substances that are known to increase permeability in other tissues e.g. histamine and bradykinin (Fredholm, Öberg, and Rosell, 1970) (Fig. 7-4).

Infusion of prostaglandin E_1, acetylcholine, and isoprenaline in concentrations high enough to produce maximal vasodilatation caused only a moderate increase in CFC. It is reasonable to assume that the smooth muscles of the vascular bed are maximally relaxed during infusion of vasodilator substances in high concentrations, and consequently a maximal capillary surface area is obtained. However, to induce very pronounced increments of the CFC, like those found on sympathetic nerve stimulation, another factor or factors have to be operating and increased permeability may be such a factor. This hypothesis is also supported by the finding that when nerve stimulation was superimposed during infusion of prostaglandin E_1, acetylcholine, or isoprenaline, a further increase of CFC was obtained. This was not the case when sympathetic nerve activity was induced during infusion of histamine or bradykinin (Fredholm, Öberg, and Rosell, 1970). So far, only indirect experimental evidence has been obtained for an increased permeability in the vascular bed of subcutaneous adipose tissue during sympathetic nerve stimulation.

There is also an increased CFC in the omentum during sympathetic nerve activity, but it gradually returns to prestimulatory values, despite continued stimulation, as does the total blood flow (Ballard and Rosell, 1971a). As in subcutaneous tissue, CFC does not decrease below resting values during stimulation, which indicates that principally the same mechanisms are involved in the two tissues.

It is reasonable to assume that the effects of sympathetic nerve activity on the exchange functions of the vascular bed are intimately connected with the metabolic events in the tissue. However, the changes in the hydrodynamic conductivity just described do not seem to be secondary to the lipolytic processes since these effects can be clearly separated by pharmacological means. The pronounced elevation of CFC following sympathetic nerve activity is blocked by adrenergic α-blocking agents, whereas lipolysis is inhibited by adrenergic β-blocking drugs. Consequently, it is at present difficult to ascribe changes in the exchange section of the vascular bed to certain metabolic processes in the canine subcutaneous adipose tissue.

Capacitance Function. It is possible to follow changes in the capacitance of the vascular bed with plethysmographic methods. These changes are supposed to be confined to the venous part. There are decreases in regional blood volume both in the omentum and the subcutaneous tissue, the degree of decrease being related to the stimulation frequency. This effect can be blocked with α-receptor blocking agents (Öberg and Rosell, 1967; Ballard and Rosell, 1971). The results indicate an adrenergic innervation also of the venous sections of these vascular beds, which is in agreement with the morphological findings.

Responses to Circulating Catecholamines

From a large number of studies in man and animals it is evident that epinephrine and norepinephrine in the plasma have lipolytic effects (see Havel, 1965). However, from the physiological point of view it is questionable if the concentrations of catecholamines normally found in plasma are high enough to induce lipolysis. If such concentrations are found the question remains how important the circulating catecholamines are in comparison to the direct sympathetic innervation of adipose tissue. In order to determine this a series of experiments was performed in which epinephrine and norepinephrine were infused intra-arterially to canine subcutaneous adipose tissue (Ballard, Cobb, and Rosell, 1971). It was found that the concentration of added norepinephrine or epinephrine required to elicit a significant venous outflow of glycerol exceeded the plasma level reported to be present in dogs under normal conditions. However, during severe stress, like bleeding or exercise at intensities around or above maximal capacity, circulating catecholamines may reach such high concentrations that they may influence vascular and metabolic events in adipose tissue (Kovách et al., 1970; Ballard and Rosell, 1971b).

Quantitative comparisons thus indicate that the innervation of adipose tissue is the most important link in the sympathetic control of the circulation and lipolysis.

Fate of the Adrenergic Transmitter Substance in Subcutaneous Adipose Tissue

The finding that stimulation of adrenergic nerves to adipose tissue in certain regions induces enhanced lipolysis is in apparent contradiction to the histological evidence indicating a lack of adrenergic innervation of adipocytes in white adipose tissue. This is especially remarkable in view of the fact that the lipolytic rate is increased with stimulation frequencies well within the physiological range (1 to 4 imp/sec). These findings may indi-cate that the transmission process at the adrenergic nerve terminals is dif-ferent from that in other organs, e.g. brown adipose tissue, salivary glands (Cottle, 1970; Norberg and Hamberger, 1964). Generally the nerve terminals are arranged in a ground plexus in intimate contact with the effector cell (Hillarp, 1946).

In order to study the transmission process ³H-norepinephrine was in-fused intra-arterially into canine subcutaneous adipose tissue and after a wash-out period the venous outflow of ³H-radioactivity was followed (Fredholm and Rosell, 1970a). As in other tissues the venous radioactiv-ity could be separated into ³H-norepinephrine and deaminated and O-methylated metabolites, which indicates that the enzymatic handling did not differ from that known to occur in other tissues (Axelrod, 1959). The venous outflow of ³H-norepinephrine was elevated during sympa-thetic nerve activity but, interestingly enough, there was the same latency as for glycerol and FFA. Similarly, α-receptor blockade potentiated the ³H-norepinephrine outflow, and the latency was shortened. These experi-ments indicated to us that not only FFA and glycerol but also the adren-ergic transmitter substance itself may be trapped in the tissue by the vasoconstriction. Depending on the arrangement of the adrenergic nerve terminal system in white adipose tissue, the delayed increase in the rate of outflow of glycerol and FFA may be due to two factors (Fredholm, 1970). First, the adrenergic transmitter substance which is released in close contact with the smooth muscles in the vascular bed causes vaso-constriction which impairs its own transport to the adipocytes. Conse-quently, there is a delay in the stimulation of lipolysis. Second, the prod-ucts of lipolysis, glycerol and FFA, are also trapped in the tissue. During nerve activity after α-receptor blockade, on the other hand, the transmit-ter induces relaxation of the smooth muscles and the transport from the nerve terminal to the adipocytes may be facilitated. Thus, lipolysis is in-duced with shorter latency and the products of lipolysis can diffuse into the blood more easily. Furthermore, if less of the released transmitter substance stays around the nerve terminal system the inactivation proc-esses, including re-uptake into the nerve terminal, may be less efficient, and therefore more norepinephrine may be available for stimulation of the adipocytes. Such a mechanism may explain the potentiation of the outflow of glycerol and FFA during nerve stimulation after α-receptor blockade and also the increased outflow of ³H-norepinephrine.

Adipose Tissue and Hemorrhagic Shock

From the preceding chapters it may be evident that the sympathetic neuro-humoral control of lipolysis and blood circulation in adipose tissue has been studied in some detail. However, most of the information stems from studies in which the sympathetic nerves have been stimulated peripherally. Such studies do not provide information about the central nervous influence on the adipose tissue and furthermore they do not show under what circumstances the sympathetic system to adipose tissue is activated.

Hemorrhagic shock is a situation characterized by intense sympathetic activity and it would therefore be of interest to see how adipose tissue reacts under such circumstances, especially since fat metabolism during shock is a largely neglected field of research (see, for example, Mills and Mayer, 1965). Kovách et al. (1970) measured blood flow and some metabolic changes in canine subcutaneous adipose tissue during standardized hemorrhagic shock. The vascular bed of this tissue was found to be very sensitive to hypotension. During bleeding to 55 mm Hg for 90 minutes the blood flow was reduced to about 10 per cent of the resting blood flow (Fig. 7-5). This decrease is much more pronounced than that which occurs in most other organs under similar experimental conditions. Thus, in skeletal muscle, liver, myocardium, and hypothalamus the blood flow fell to about 60 per cent of the resting flow and the renal cortical blood flow to about 40 per cent (Kovách, personal communication). Moreover, after 180 minutes of hypotension (90 minutes at 55 mm Hg and 90 minutes at 35 mm Hg) reinfusion of the shed blood failed to restore a normal blood flow in the subcutaneous adipose tissue, indicating vascular damage. This suggests that subcutaneous adipose tissue may be one of the organs where irreversible shock is manifested at an early stage of shock which the dogs develop with the above procedure (Kovách, 1967). In contrast, dogs pretreated with phenoxybenzamine, an α-receptor blocking drug, did not develop signs of vascular damage during the bleeding periods and the blood flow remained at about 70 per cent of the resting blood flow, which was enough to keep the oxygen consumption at a normal level (Fig. 7-5). In addition, reinfusion restored blood flow to normal. It is conceivable that the protective effect of phenoxybenzamine was a consequence of the comparatively high blood flow during the hypotensive period, which resulted in a more or less normal tissue metabolism. The reason why phen-

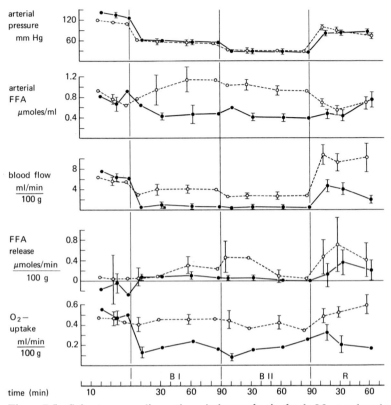

Figure 7-5   Subcutaneous adipose tissue in hemorrhagic shock. Mean values (± S.E.) during control period, bleeding to 55 mm Hg for 90 minutes (B I), to 35 mm Hg for 90 minutes. (B II) and after reinfusion of the shed blood (R). Solid circles show experiments without phenoxybenzamine and open circles show experiments with phenoxybenzamine. (From Kovách et al., *Circulation Res.* 26:733, 1970)

oxybenzamine provided the tissue with blood was presumably due to at least two factors: protection from vasoconstriction caused by α-receptor blockade and vasodilatation due to β-receptor stimulation (Fredholm and Rosell, 1968).

The severe blood flow reduction found in subcutaneous tissue during hypotension may not occur in adipose tissue at other localities, since, as has been discussed already, Ballard and Rosell (1971) found that in the omentum both sympathetic nerve stimulation and infusion of catecholamines induced vasoconstriction only initially. This constriction was followed by a vasodilatation which was more pronounced the more intense the stimulus. Therefore in the omentum during severe hypotension the diminution of blood flow may not be as deleterious as in the subcutaneous tissue.

The impairment of blood flow in the subcutaneous adipose tissue had metabolic consequences as well. Thus, despite a presumably high sympatho-adrenal activity during bleeding, the release rate of FFA did not rise. Another factor which may also have played a role in this connection is that lactate inhibits the outflow of FFA (Issekutz et al., 1965), presumably due to an enhanced re-esterification (Fredholm, 1971). During hemorrhagic shock there is a pronounced elevation of the blood lactate concentration as well as acidosis, and these factors may have contributed to the absence of FFA release (Nahas and Poyart, 1967; Triner and Nahas, 1965).

The vascular and metabolic reactions in adipose tissue during hypotension and shock need further study to evaluate the pathophysiological changes. To do this may be of clinical importance since the studies referred to indicate that adipose tissue, at least localized subcutaneously, seems to be one of the shock organs.

References

Aronovsky, E., Levari, R., Kornblueth, W., and Wertheimer, E. 1963. *Invest. Ophthal.* 2:259.

Axelrod, J. 1959. *Physiol. Rev.* 39:751.

Ballantyne, B. 1968. *Arch. Int. Pharmacodyn.* 173:343.

Ballantyne, B., and Raftery, A. T. 1969. *J. Physiol.* 205:31P.

Ballard, K., and Rosell, S. 1969. *Acta Physiol. Scand.* 77:442.

Ballard, K., and Rosell, S. 1971a. *Circ. Res.* 28:389.

Ballard, K., and Rosell, S. 1971b. *Metabolism in Skeletal Muscle During Exercise,* Pergamon Press, New York.

Ballard, K., Cobb, C. A., and Rosell, S. 1971. *Acta Physiol. Scand.* 81:246.

Bär, H. P., and Hechter, O. 1969. *Proc. Nat. Acad. Sci. U.S.* 63:350.

Bergström, S., Carlson, L. A., and Weeks, J. R. 1968. *Pharmacol. Rev.* 20:1.

Berti, F., and Usardi, M. M. 1964. *G. Arterioscler.* 2:261.

Birnbaumer, L., and Rodbell, M. 1970. *Adipose Tissue. Regulation and Metabolic Function,* Georg Thieme, Stuttart.

Braun, T., and Hechter, O. 1970. *Adipose Tissue. Regulation and Metabolic Function,* Georg Thieme, Stuttgart.

Burns, T. W., and Langley, P. 1968. *J. Lab. Clin. Med.* 72:813.

Burns, T. W., Langley, P. E., and Robison, G. A. 1970. *Clin. Res.* 18:86.

Cobbold, A., Folkow, B., Kjellmer, I., and Mellander, S. 1963. *Acta Physiol. Scand.* 57:180.

Colville, K. I., Salvador, R. A., Lindsay, L. A., and Burns, J. J. 1964. *Nature* 204:888.

Correll, J. W. 1963. *Science* 140:387.

Cottle, W. H. 1970. *Brown Adipose Tissue,* American Elsevier Publishing Co. Inc., New York.

Davies, B. N., Horton, E. W., and Withrington, P. G. 1968. *Brit. J. Parmacol.* 32:127.

Di Girolamo, M., Skinner, N. S., Jr., Hanley, H. G., and Sachs, R. G. 1970. *Circulation* 42. suppl. III: abstr. 553.

Dixon, M., and Webb, E. C. 1964. *Enzymes,* Academic Press, New York, p. 365.

Efendic, S. 1970. Thesis, Stockholm.

Falck, B., Hillarp, N. Å., Thieme, G., and Torp, A. 1962. *J. Histochem. Cytochem.* 10:348.

Folkow, B., Lewis, D. H., Lundgren, O., Mellander, S., and Wallentin, I. 1964a. *Acta Physiol. Scand.* 61:445.

Folkow, B., Lewis, D. H., Lundgren, O., Mellander, S., and Wallentin, I. 1964b. *Acta Physiol. Scand.* 61:458.

Folkow, B. 1952. *Acta Physiol. Scand.* 25:49.

Fredholm, B. B. 1970. *Acta Physiol. Scand.* suppl. 354.

Fredholm, B. B. 1971. *Acta Physiol. Scand.* 81:110.

Fredholm, B., and Rosell, S. 1968. *J. Pharmacol. Exp. Therap.* 159:1.

Fredholm, B. B., and Rosell, S. 1970a. *Acta Physiol. Scand.* 80:404.

Fredholm, B. B., and Rosell, S. 1970b. *Acta Physiol. Scand.* 80:450.

Fredholm, B. B., Linde, B., Öberg, B., and Rosell, S. 1968. *Bibliotheca Anatomica* No. 19:241.

Fredholm, B. B., Öberg, B., and Rosell, S. 1970. *Acta Physiol. Scand.* 79:564.

Fredholm, B. B., Rosell, S., and Strandberg, K. 1970. *Acta Physiol. Scand.* 79:18A.

Havel, R. J. 1965. *Handbook of Physiology,* Section 5, "Adipose Tissue," American Physiological Society, Washington, D.C.

Hillarp, N.-Å. 1946. *Acta Anat.* suppl. 4.

Horton, E. W. 1969. *Physiol. Rev.* 49:122.

Issekutz, Jr., B., Miller, H. I., Paul, P., and Rodahl, K. 1965. *Amer. J. Physiol.* 209:1137.

Kovách, A. G. B. 1967. *Fed. Proc.* 20:122.

Kovách, A. G. B., Rosell, S., Sándor, P., Koltay, E., Kovách, E., and Tomka, N. 1970. *Circ. Res.* 26:733.

Laity, J. L. H. 1969. *Brit. J. Pharmacol.* 37:698.

Larsen, O. A., Lassen, N. A., and Quaade, F. 1966. *Acta Physiol. Scand.* 66:337.

Lewis, G. P., and Matthews, J. 1968. *Br. J. Pharmacol.* 34:564.

Margolis, S., and Vaughan, M. 1962. *J. Biol. Chem.* 237:44.

Mayerle, J. A., and Havel, R. J. 1969. *J. Appl. Physiol.* 26:513.

Mills, L. C., Mayer, J. H. 1965. *Shock and Hypotension,* Grune and Stratton, New York.

Nahas, G. G., and Poyart, C. 1967. *Amer. J. Physiol.* 212:765.

Nash, C. W., Smith, R. L., Maickel, R. P., and Paoletti, R. 1961. *Pharmacologist* 3:55.

Ngai, S. H., Rosell, S., and Wallenberg, L. R. *Acta Physiol. Scand.* 1966. 68:397.

Öberg, B. 1964. *Acta Physiol. Scand.* 62 suppl. 62:1.

Öberg, B., and Rosell, S. 1967. *Acta Physiol. Scand.* 71:47.

Paoletti, R., Maickel, R. P., Smith, R. L., and Brodie, B. B. 1961. *Proc. First Int. Pharm. Meet.* 2:29.

Robinson, J., and Newsholme, E. A. 1967. *Biochem. J.* 104:2C.

Rosell, S. 1966. *Acta Physiol. Scand.* 67:343.

Rosell, S. 1969. *Drugs Affecting Lipid Metabolism,* Plenum Press, New York.

Rudman, D., Borwn, S. J., and Malkin, M. F. 1963. *Endocrinology* 72:527.

Rudman, D., Di Girolamo, M., Malkin, M. F., and Garcia, L. A. 1965. *Handbook of Physiology,* Section 5, "Adipose Tissue," American Physiological Society, Washington, D.C.

Salvador, R. A., and Kuntzman, R. 1965. *J. Pharmacol. Exp. Therap.* 150:84.

Shaw, J. E., and Eamwell, P. W. 1968. *J. Biol. Chem.* 243:1498.

Steinberg, D., and Vaughan, M. 1965. *Handbook of Physiology,* Section 5, "Adipose Tissue," American Physiological Society, Washington, D.C.

Sutherland, E. W., Robinson, G. A., and Butcher, R. W. 1968. *Circulation* 37:279.

Triner, L., and Nahas, G. G. 1965. *Science* 150:1725.

Wallentin, I. 1966. *Acta Physiol. Scand.* 69 suppl. 279.

Weiss, B., and Maickel, R. P. 1968. *Intern. J. Neuropharmacol.* 7:395.

Wenke, M. 1966. *Adv. Lipid. Res.* 4:69.

Westermann, E., and Stock, K. 1970. *Adipose Tissue. Regulation and Metabolic Function,* Georg Thieme, Stuttgart.

Wirsén, C. 1965a. *Handbook of Physiology,* Section 5, "Adipose Tissue," American Physiological Society, Washington, D.C.

Wirsén, C. 1965b. *Acta Physiol. Scand.* 65 suppl. 252:1.

8

Hypertension and the Sympathetic Nervous System

JACQUES DE CHAMPLAIN

The regulation of blood pressure involves the interaction of various systems and factors (Guyton et al., 1969). Hypertensive diseases could result from a variety of dysfunctions occurring at various levels of this complex regulatory mechanism (Page, 1963). Among systems and factors which have been most often studied and proposed as a triggering mechanism in various forms of hypertensive diseases are the pressor renal system, the endocrine system—especially in regard to the adrenal cortex and medulla—the sympathetic nervous system, the ionic balance—mainly involving sodium and/or potassium—and finally genetic factors predisposing to hypertension. In relatively few cases of clinical hypertension, however, has it been possible to recognize a specific etiological cause for an elevated blood pressure with the exception of hypertension associated with tumors of the adrenal cortex or medulla, with renal artery stenosis, or with a coarctation of the aorta. In the majority of cases the etiology has remained unknown or at best controversial.

The increased sensitivity to catecholamine in most cases of hypertension (Mendlowitz, 1967) and the observation that most hypotensive drugs also alter the disposition of catecholamine or the activity of the sympathetic nervous system (Axelrod, 1968; Carlsson, 1966; Abrams, 1969) constitute strong indirect evidence that the sympathetic nervous system may play an important role in the pathogenesis and maintenance of elevated blood pressure. Initial studies on urinary catecholamines, however, have failed to detect any significant abnormality (with the exception of pheochromocytoma) in the catecholamine metabolism in most hypertensive patients. These negative findings have restrained for many years further research on the role of the sympathetic nervous system in the pathogenesis of hypertension.

More recently, however, studies making use of more sophisticated means of investigation have provided much evidence of a dysfunction of the sympathetic nervous system in various forms of experimental and human hypertensive diseases. This new incursion of the sympathetic system in the field of hypertension was stimulated by the fundamental studies of von Euler (1956), Axelrod (1965), and many others who have contributed to the refinement of our concepts of adrenergic mechanisms and drug actions. Moreover, improvement in the sensitivity and specificity of techniques, the use of labelled amines of high specific activities, and the availability of drugs with highly specific effects on the adrenergic functions have permitted investigators to design better experimental approaches and to reach a higher degree of sophistication in the interpretation of findings.

The Autonomic Nervous System and the Control of Blood Pressure

The observation by Claude Bernard (1851) that the section of the cervical sympathetic chain caused a vasodilatation of the blood vessels of the face, followed by Charles Brown-Séquard's (1854) demonstration that the stimulation of the cervical sympathetic chain produced a vasoconstriction of the same vessels, first established that blood vessels are indeed controlled by tonically active nerve fibers.

The remarkable constancy of blood pressure in normal man, preserving at all times adequate perfusion of vital organs according to their metabolic needs, is now known to be largely dependent on the autonomic control of the cardiovascular system. Although there was for a long time a strong traditional belief that the autonomic nervous system was characterized by gross undiscriminating responses, recent studies have shown the fallacy of that view in demonstrating that the autonomic nervous system is also capable of finely differentiated and discriminating vascular or glandular responses (Miller, 1969).

The autonomic mechanisms responsible for the regulation of blood pressure within a narrow range of variations are activated through a complex vasoregulatory reflex arc, functioning by means of a negative feedback mechanism (Edis and Shepherd, 1970). Classically, the carotid sinuses, the aortic arch, and other large vessels are identified as the major barosensory areas in the vascular system. These sensitive structures are activated by local vascular distension induced by an increase in intra-arterial pressure. Through a system of afferent fibers, the information generated by such stimulus is relayed to the central nervous system to inhibit the tonic activity of the vasomotor and cardiomodulator centers localized in the reticular formation of the medulla oblongata. These centers are also influenced or modulated by higher integrative centers localized in the hypothalamus, the limbic system, and the cortex. The integration of these various influences brings about a continuous readjustment of the activity of the vasomotor and cardiomodulator centers which is transmitted to the peripheral cardiovascular system by means of an efferent fibers network.

The efferent parasympathetic component of the autonomic nervous system is constituted by a network of inhibitory fibers distributed to the heart and by a relatively minor outflow of cholinergic vasodilator fibers generally distributed to a few hemodynamically insignificant areas. In contrast, the efferent sympathetic component is more closely and dynamically related to the peripheral cardiovascular system by a dense plexus of excitatory fibers distributed to the heart and to all vascular beds with the exception of the intracerebral vessels. With a specific and sensitive fluorescent histochemical technique (Falck et al., 1962), it has been possible to visualize the distribution of these fibers in a variety of vascular segments (Norberg, 1967; Burnstock et al., 1970). Small arterioles which are crucial to the homeostasis of arterial blood pressure (Mellander and Johansson, 1968) were found to be the most densely innervated segments of the vascular tree (see Fig. 8-1) (Norberg, 1967; Burnstock et al., 1970). Although the majority of these fibers terminate at the adventitial-medial border and rarely penetrate the muscle coat, the contraction of the smooth muscle fibers of the vessel upon nerve stimulation is believed to occur by electronic coupling of the smooth muscle cell (Burnstock et al., 1970). In addition to this network of fibers, the sympathetic system is also responsible for the control of the catecholamine secretion by the adrenal medulla (Malmejac, 1964). Since the heart and blood vessels contain specific receptors to catecholamines (Ahlquist, 1948), these structures can therefore be influenced either by the norepinephrine liberated from the sympathetic nerve endings or by the catecholamines liberated from the adrenal medulla.

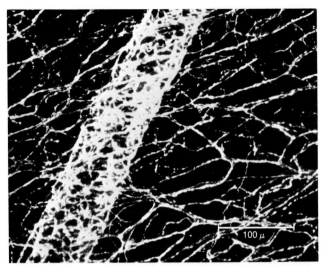

Figure 8-1   Normal adrenergic innervation of the dilator muscle and small artery in stretched preparation of the rat iris. The sympathetic innervation of the dilator muscle is constituted by a dense network of adrenergic terminal fibers characterized by the presence of varicosities. Although the rat iris is considered to be one of the most densely innervated tissues, the innervation of the small artery crossing the preparation is considerably denser than that of the dilator muscle. The preparation was treated by the technique of Falck, Hillarp, and coworkers (1962). The microphotograph is reproduced at a magnification of 275X.

Vascular Reactivity in Hypertension

The observations by Goldenberg and his coworkers (1948) that the injection of norepinephrine could mimic the hemodynamic changes encountered in essential hypertension and that hypertensive patients were hypersensitive to norepinephrine, first drew attention to the possible participation of the sympathetic nervous system in the pathogenesis of hypertension. The pressor hypersensitivity to catecholamines as well as to other pressor agents in various forms of experimental and human hypertension was confirmed by numerous other studies (Mendlowitz, 1967). Moreover, Kato and Komata (1969) have recently found that the reactivity of α-receptors is greater whereas the reactivity of β-receptors is smaller in hypertensive patients. The vascular reactivity to norepinephrine was also found increased in various vascular beds of hypertensive patients (Table 8-1). In various forms of experimental hypertension, similar observations were made on hind limb preparations and on isolated femoral, carotid, mesentery, and tail arteries. However, this phenomenon was not as marked on all vascular segments, and the reactivity of the aorta of these animals was either normal or decreased (Table 8-1).

Table 8-1 Vascular responsiveness to pressor agents in human and experimental hypertension

Authors	Region	Catecholamine (NE and/or E)	Angiotensin
Human hypertension			
Lee and Holze (1951)	conjunctiva	increased	
Greisman (1952)	nailfold	increased	
Jackson (1958)	conjunctiva	increased	
Mendlowitz and Nafchi (1958)	nailfold	increased	
Moulton et al. (1958)	skeletal muscle	increased	
Doyle et al. (1959)	forearm	increased	normal
Daly and Duff (1960)	hand	increased	increased
Desoxycorticosterone and Sodium hypertension			
Redleaf and Tobian (1958)	aorta	decreased	
Mallov (1959)	aorta	decreased	
Hinke (1965)	caudal artery	increased	
Demura et al. (1965)	hindlimb	increased	increased
Oono (1966)	hindlimb	normal	normal
Bohr and Sitrin (1970)	femoral artery	increased	
Chronic renal hypertension			
Zweifach et al. (1948)	mesentery	increased	
McQueen (1956)	hindlimb	increased	
Redleaf and Tobian (1958)	aorta	decreased	
Mallov (1959)	aorta	decreased	
Gordon and Magueira (1962)	aorta	increased	
Nolla-Panades (1963)	hindlimb	increased	
Demura et al. (1965)	hindlimb	increased	increased
Page et al (1966)	hindlimb*	normal	decreased
Oono (1966)	hindlimb	increased	increased
Baum and Shropshire (1967)	hindlimb	increased	increased
McGregor and Smirk (1968)	mesentery	increased	increased
Moerman et al. (1969)	carotid*	increased	
Zimmerman et al. (1969)	cutaneous bed*	increased	
Bandick and Sparks (1970)	femoral artery	increased	
Genetic spontaneous hypertension			
Laverty (1961)	hindlimb	increased	
McGregor and Smirk (1968)	mesentery	increased	increased
Spector et al. (1969)	aorta	decreased	
Clineschmidt et al. (1970)	aorta	normal	

* Experiments were carried on in dogs. In all others, rats were used.

These findings indicated that there is either a decreased inactivation of norepinephrine or else an increased sensitivity of the effector cells in the vessels of hypertensive patients or animals. Decreased inactivation of norepinephrine by denervation or by blockade of re-uptake mechanism can cause an hypersensitivity to norepinephrine (Trendelenburg, 1965). However, recent studies have shown that the spontaneous rhythmicity of vascular smooth muscle cells was increased in rats with renal and DOCA hypertension, thus suggesting that the increased receptor sensitivity may be due to changes in the vascular smooth muscle contraction mechanism (Bohr and Sitrin, 1970; Bandick and Sparks, 1970). Whether the contraction mechanism is affected at the level of the contractile proteins or at the level of cyclic AMP and energy metabolism or else at the level of excitation-contraction coupling has not been determined. Moreover, since the hypersensitivity is not limited to norepinephrine but has also been observed with other pressor agents, this would indicate that the mechanism involved is not related exclusively to the adrenergic nerve function but is rather associated with the state of contraction of the smooth muscle cell.

Sivertsson (1970) has proposed that the increase in vascular reactivity to norepinephrine in hypertensive patients may be due to an increased wall to lumen ratio due to the thickening of the vessel wall in this condition. Although this explanation may be acceptable for the studies made on the systemic pressor response, it is less applicable to studies made on isolated arterial strips in hypertensive animals. The changes in vascular responsiveness have also been attributed to disturbances in the ionic balance (Raab, 1959), but the mode of evaluation of intracellular ion distribution is not accurate enough to permit any conclusion on whether the sympathetic fibers or the smooth muscle cells are affected by the changes in electrolyte concentrations.

Whatever the mechanism involved, the conclusion remains the same: in hypertensive patients or animals, even normal circulating catecholamine levels could contribute to the maintenance of an elevated blood pressure because of an increased vascular responsiveness. It would theoretically be possible to detect signs of sympathetic hyperfunction in presence of a normal sympathetic activity in these subjects. The exact role played by this phenomenon in the pathogenesis of hypertension is not known, but it could certainly contribute, in association with a dysfunction of the sympathetic nervous system or with other factors, to the development or maintenance of elevated blood pressure.

The Sympathetic Nervous System in Experimental Hypertension

Various models of experimental hypertension have been described but those, in most current use have been the model induced by excess of sodium with or without mineralocorticoids (Selye et al., 1943; Dahl et al., 1962), the one produced by renal artery stenosis (Goldblatt et al., 1934), or the one that issued from the development of two strains of spontaneously hypertensive rats: the Japanese strain (Okamoto, 1969) and the New Zealand strain (Phelan, 1968). Although none of these models can be matched exactly with human hypertension, the study of the mechanisms underlying the development of these various forms of hypertension may lead to the discovery of abnormalities which may be relevant to human diseases. Each experimental model probably corresponds to different facets of the multifactorial mechanism leading to human hypertension. Moreover, experimental hypertensive diseases share many characteristics with human hypertensive diseases, and a hyperfunction of the renal pressor system (Page, 1963), abnormalities in the sodium metabolism (Dahl, 1961; Knudsen and Dahl, 1966), and genetic factors (McKusick, 1960; Platt, 1963) have all been thought to play a role in the pathogenesis of both.

Desoxycorticosterone and Sodium Hypertension

Since 1965 our interest, in collaboration with Axelrod, Krakoff, and Mueller, has been mainly focused on the study of relationship between the sympathetic nervous system and the variation of blood pressure induced by various sodium intakes, ranging from sodium depletion to sodium loading and retention in the rat (de Champlain et al., 1966, 1967, 1968a, 1968b, 1969a, 1969b, 1970; Krakoff et al., 1967). These studies have permitted us to clearly establish that sodium metabolism directly or indirectly influences the activity of sympathetic fibers and the adrenal medulla, and that these functional changes may be responsible for the variations in blood pressure.

The selection of that model of study was mainly founded on the suggestion that the metabolism of sodium and other ions is abnormal in various forms of human and experimental hypertension (Raab, 1959; Tobian, 1960). The first indication that sodium was associated with elevated blood pressure came from the observation that a low sodium diet was efficient in lowering the blood pressure of hypertensive patients (Ambard and Beaujard, 1904; Allen and Sherrill, 1922). Other studies have shown that the plasma sodium (Halley et al., 1951; Albert et al., 1958) and total exchangeable sodium (Ross, 1956; Tomiga, 1961; Dahl et al., 1962; Hansen, 1968) are both significantly increased in patients with essential hypertension. An epidemiological study conducted among various populations has established a close correlation between the amount of sodium ingested in the diet and the incidence of hypertension in these populations (Knudsen and Dahl, 1966). Increase in sodium, potassium, and water content has also been a common finding in vascular tissues of animals made hypertensive by various experimental means (Table 8-2). Similarly, the sodium and water content of renal arteries of hypertensive patients was found increased (Tobian and Binion, 1952). More recent studies have shown that the calcium content in the ventricle (Tobian and Duke, 1969) and in the vessels (Hinde, 1966) of hypertensive rats is

Table 8-2   Ionic and water content of vessels of hypertensive rats

Authors	Tissue	Sodium	Potassium	Water
Desoxycorticosterone and Sodium				
Tobian and Binion (1954)	aorta	+	+	
Daniel and Dawkins (1957)	aorta	+	+	+
Gross and Schmidt (1958)	aorta	+	+	+
Fukuchi et al. (1964)	aorta	+	+	
Cier and Froment (1965)	aorta	+		
Demura et al. (1965)	aorta	+	+	
Hinke (1966)	caudal artery	+	+	
Renal hypertension				
Daniel and Dawkins (1957)	aorta	+	+	+
Tobian and Redleaf (1958)	aorta	+	+	
Freed (1961)	aorta	N	+	
Koletsky et al. (1959)	mesent. art.	+	+	
Heading and Randel (1964)	aorta	+	+	
Fukuchi et al. (1964)	aorta	+	+	
Demura et al. (1965)	aorta	+	+	
Cier et Froment (1965)	aorta	+		
Hagemeijer et al. (1966)	aorta	+	+	
Phelan and Wong (1968)	aorta	+	+	+
Van Cauwenberge and Rorive (1969)	aorta	+	+	+
Genetic hypertension				
Phelan and Wong (1968)	aorta	+	N	N
Nagaoka et al. (1969)	aorta	+	+	+

+ : Increased above normal levels
N : Normal levels

also increased. Therefore, ionic disturbances in vascular tissues involving sodium, potassium, and probably calcium appear to be an almost constant phenomenon associated with the rise in blood pressure. Whether these changes play a determinant role in the initiation of hypertension or are secondary to elevated blood pressure is still unsettled (Hollander et al., 1968). Nevertheless these changes could play a significant role in the chronic stage of hypertension since they are likely to influence either the contraction of arteriolar smooth muscle (Friedman et al., 1963; Bohr, 1964), or else the vascular reactivity to pressor substances or to nerve stimulation (Raab, 1959). Moreover, since many of the metabolic events responsible for impulse conduction and synaptic transmission as well as for the uptake, storage, release, and action of amines are dependent on ionic shifts (Bogdanski and Brodie, 1966, 1969; Daniel et al., 1970; Gillis and Paton, 1967; Horst et al., 1968; Iversen and Kravitz, 1966; Keen and Bogdanski, 1970), it is probable that an ionic disturbance would alter the function of the sympathetic nervous system in hypertensive diseases.

Uninephrectomized male Sprague-Dawley rats were used for our studies. Animals were made hypertensive by a weekly subcutaneous injection of desoxycorticosterone (DOCA) pivalate (10 mg/week) and by being given a solution of sodium chloride 1 per cent to drink *ad libitum*. Animals so treated showed a significant increase in blood pressure during the second week of treatment and reached levels between 180 to 200 mm Hg after six weeks of treatment (de Champlain et al., 1967). Animals were studied at various times after starting the treatment, up to 10 weeks after the beginning. The systolic blood pressure records and the various methods used in these studies have been previously published in detail (de Champlain et al., 1967). A systematic study of various functions of the sympathetic nerve endings was undertaken, especially in regard to the uptake, storage, turnover, subcellular distribution, and metabolism of norepinephrine in various peripheral organs of these hypertensive rats.

Uptake and Storage of Norepinephrine. The neuronal uptake of tritiated norepinephrine is normal in various sympathetically innervated peripheral organs of DOCA-hypertensive animals *in vivo* and *in vitro* (de Champlain et al., 1967). The uptake into the storage vesicles is also unimpaired in hearts of hypertensive animals (Krakoff et al., 1967). These findings as well as the observation that the fractional blood flow to various

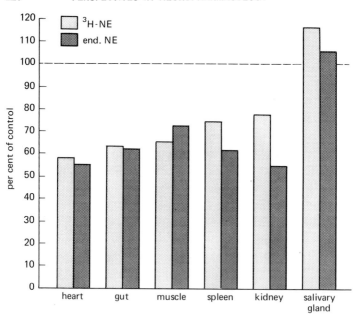

Figure 8-2   Retention of ³H-norepinephrine (³H-NE) one hour after intravenous injection of 25 μC of the tritiated amine and the endogenous norepinephrine levels (end. NE) in various tissues of DOCA-hypertensive rats. Each bar represents the mean of 10 to 16 values. The results are expressed as the percentage of the values found in normotensive control rats. With the exception of the heart and kidney in which the values were expressed per total organ, in all the other tissues the results were calculated per gram of wet tissue. (From de Champlain et al., 1967)

organs is normal in hypertensive animals gave assurance that exogenous-labelled norepinephrine could be used to study the functional dynamics of adrenergic nerves in this form of experimental disease (de Champlain et al., 1967).

One hour after injection, the amount of tritiated norepinephrine retained in the heart, intestine, skeletal muscle, spleen, and kidney is markedly reduced in hypertensive animals (Fig. 8-2). Endogenous norepinephrine levels are also significantly lower in the same tissues of hypertensive animals. In organs containing mainly a parenchymatous sympathetic innervation, such as the salivary gland and the vas deferens, the retention of norepinephrine as well as endogenous norepinephrine are normal. In other groups of normotensive animals receiving either DOCA or sodium alone these parameters do not differ from the control rats (de

Champlain et al., 1967). Although the heart and kidney of hypertensive animals show an hypertrophy of about 20 per cent, this cannot account for the reduction in the storage of norepinephrine since the amount of tritiated amine as well as the norepinephrine content are both reduced even when the values are expressed per total organ.

A highly significant inverse relationship can be observed between the systolic blood pressure and the capacity to retain tritiated norepinephrine in the heart (Fig. 8-3), spleen, and intestine. A similar inverse relationship was also made between the systolic blood pressure and the endogenous norepinephrine content of the heart of normotensive and hypertensive rats (de Champlain et al., 1967). Since these relationships are also significant in the heart of normotensive animals within the normal range of blood pressure, it appears that the greater decrease in norepinephrine retention or in endogenous norepinephrine levels observed in hypertension may be part of the same mechanism regulating the blood pressure in nor-

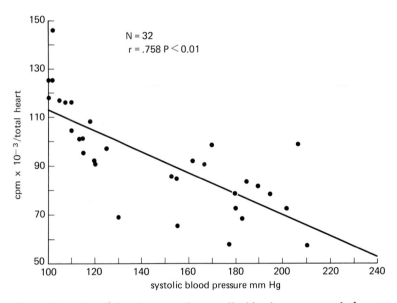

Figure 8-3 Correlation between the systolic blood pressure and the amount of tritiated norepinephrine retained in the hearts of normotensive and hypertensive rats one hour after the injection of 25 μC of ^{3}H-norepinephrine. The inverse relationship between the systolic blood pressure and the retention of ^{3}H-norepinephrine was not only significant for the normotensive and hypertensive animals combined but was also significant within each group of animals. (From de Champlain et al., 1967)

motensive animals. This defect in retention and storage of norepinephrine in DOCA- and sodium-hypertensive animals was confirmed recently
by others (Doyle, 1968; Kazda et al., 1969; Louis et al., 1970a) and in
one of these studies (Kazda et al., 1969) the inverse relationship between the capacity of the heart to retain tritiated norepinephrine and the
level of systolic blood pressure was also confirmed.

Turnover and Synthesis Rate of Norepinephrine. The study of the decay
of specific activity in the heart after injection of tracer doses of tritiated
norepinephrine was used to estimate the turnover and synthesis rate of

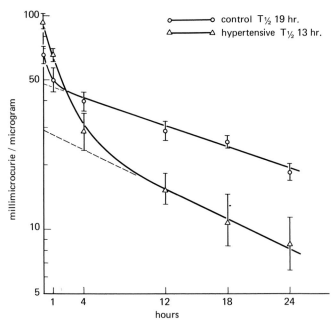

Figure 8-4   Decline in the specific activity of norepinephrine in the hearts of hypertensive and normotensive rats during the first 24 hours following the intravenous injection of 2 μC of tritiated norepinephrine. The specific activity is plotted semiloga-
rithmically against time, and the curves were derived from the weighted least squares
approximation of the logarithms of the data points. Five minutes after the injection
of tritiated norepinephrine, the accumulation was similar in the hearts of normotensive and hypertensive rats. However, because of lower endogenous norepinephrine
levels, the specific activity was significantly increased in the hearts of hypertensive
rats. The rapid initial fall in specific activity was significantly greater and more prolonged in the hearts of hypertensive animals. (From Krakoff et al., 1967)

norepinephrine (Costa et al., 1966). Compared with control animals, the specific activity of norepinephrine falls more rapidly in a distinct biphasic fashion in the hearts of hypertensive rats (Fig. 8-4). The half-life of norepinephrine calculated from the latter linear portion of the curve is shorter in the hearts of hypertensive rats (13 hours versus 19 hours for the controls). However, the calculated synthesis rate of norepinephrine is only slightly and not significantly increased: 32 ng/hr/heart for hypertensive rats and 29 ng/hr/heart for normotensive rats (Krakoff et al., 1967). An increase in the turnover rate was also found with other means of investigation. After inhibition of tyrosine hydroxylase by α-methyl tyrosine, the rate of decline of norepinephrine content is markedly accelerated in the heart, slightly accelerated in the spleen and intestine, and normal in salivary glands (de Champlain et al., 1969b). Moreover the tritiated norepinephrine formed from tritiated dopamine decreases significantly faster from the heart of hypertensive rats, thus indicating that the newly formed norepinephrine is utilized more rapidly in hypertensive rats (de Champlain, 1969b).

The increase in turnover rate could be secondary to the elevation of blood pressure or else it could contribute directly to the pathogenesis of hypertension. It appears from experiments made early in the course of treatment with DOCA and sodium that the increase in turnover rate precedes the development of hypertension. In animals treated for one week with DOCA and sodium, the capacity to retain norepinephrine is reduced by 26 per cent over a 24-hour period although the blood pressure is not significantly increased and endogenous norepinephrine levels are still normal in treated animals (Table 8-3). Using the same methodology Louis and his coworkers (1970a) found a slight but not significant reduction of about 20 per cent in the capacity of the heart to retain norepinephrine in similarly treated animals before the development of hypertension.

In view of these important changes in the turnover rate, the activity of tyrosine hydroxylase, which is the limiting step in the biosynthesis (Udenfriend, 1966), was indirectly estimated by measuring the capacity of the nerve fibers to convert ^{14}C-tyrosine into catecholamines. One hour after a single injection or at the end of a one-hour infusion of ^{14}C-tyrosine, the amount of ^{14}C catecholamines formed is slightly but not significantly increased in the hearts of hypertensive rats (Table 8-4). In the adrenal glands, however, the rate of conversion of tyrosine to catecholamines is

Table 8-3   Effect of one week treatment with DOCA and sodium on norepinephrine storage

	No	Syst. B.P. (mm Hg)	End. NE ng/heart	³H-norepinephrine mµc/heart
Control	10	112 ± 4.5	466 ± 12	38 ± 2.8
DOCA and sodium (one week)	10	120 ± 2.5	449 ± 29	28 ± 4.0*
Per cent change		+ 7.5	− 3.5	− 26

* $P < 0.05$

The treated group of rats was given one s-c injection 10 mg of a suspension of DOCA and a solution of NaCl 1 per cent to drink *ad libitum*. One week later, the animals were injected with 15 µC of ³H-norepinephrine i.v. and were killed 24 hours later. (Data taken from de Champlain et al. 1968a)

markedly increased in hypertensive animals. Since the endogenous norepinephrine and epinephrine levels are normal in the adrenal glands of hypertensive rats, an increase in the synthesis rate would necessarily be accompanied by an increased liberation of catecholamines into the circulation. Increased circulating levels of catecholamines could restore par-

Table 8-4   Catecholamine synthesis from ¹⁴C-tyrosine in heart and adrenal glands of hypertensive rats

	Endogenous NE µg/organ	¹⁴C-catecholamine (counts/min) after injection	after infusion
Heart			
Control	0.844 ± 0.050	110 ± 15	74 ± 12
Hypertensive	0.555 ± 0.035**	133 ± 12	88 ± 24
Per cent change	− 34	+ 20	+ 19
Adrenal glands			
Control	3.12 ± 0.34	517 ± 25	493 ± 64
Hypertensive	2.94 ± 0.63	1056 ± 200*	823 ± 136*
Per cent change	− 6	+ 105	+ 67

* $P < 0.05$
** $P < 0.01$

The heart and adrenal glands were examined for ¹⁴C-catecholamine either one hour after injection of 15 µC of ¹⁴C-tyrosine or after one-hour infusion of 20 µC of ¹⁴C-tyrosine. Groups of 6 or 7 animals were used with either technique. The specific activity of tyrosine was similar in normotensive and hypertensive rats. The systolic blood pressure of hypertensive animals was 215 ± 7.5 mm Hg compared with 118 ± 1.5 mm Hg in normotensive rats. The epinephrine content per pair of adrenal glands was 20.3 ± 1.9 µg for the hypertensive animals and 15.9 ± 0.8 µg for the normotensive rats. (Data taken from de Champlain et al., 1969b)

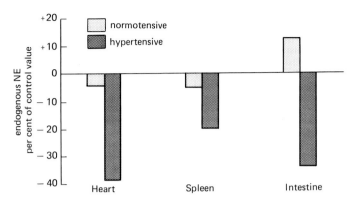

Figure 8-5   Effect of bilateral adrenalectomy on the endogenous norepinephrine levels of heart, spleen, and intestine of hypertensive and normotensive rats. The endogenous norepinephrine levels were measured one week after adrenalectomy and were expressed as the percentage change from control values in normotensive and hypertensive animals. Six to ten rats were used for each group of animals. In normotensive animals the effect of adrenalectomy was insignificant whereas this procedure resulted in marked reduction of the endogenous norepinephrine levels in the organs of hypertensive animals. (From J. de Champlain, and M. R. Corbeil, unpublished data)

tially the endogenous stores in adrenergic fibers in various organs of hypertensive rats and thus explain an increased turnover rate in these fibers without much change in their synthesis rate. One week after bilateral adrenalectomy, the endogenous norepinephrine levels in the heart, spleen, and intestine of normotensive rats are not different from the levels found before adrenalectomy (Fig. 8-5). In contrast, the already lower endogenous norepinephrine levels in the same organs of hypertensive rats are more considerably reduced one week after bilateral adrenalectomy, thus indicating that the endogenous norepinephrine stored in the adrenergic nerve fibers of hypertensive animals is in great part derived from circulating catecholamines coming from the adrenal medulla. This constitutes a unique condition, in which the neurotransmitter used in the nerve endings would originate in large part in an extraneuronal source. This mechanism also explains the increased turnover rate in the sympathetic nerve fibers of hypertensive rats without a significant increase in the synthesis rate.

Subcellular Distribution of Norepinephrine. When subcellular fractionation studies were made, it was found that the capacity of the storage vesicles of the heart of hypertensive rats to retain norepinephrine is profoundly impaired (Fig. 8-6). Although the initial uptake capacity of these vesicles is normal, the vesicles of hypertensive animals lose 45 per cent of their initial norepinephrine content within the following 4 hours whereas the storage vesicles of normotensive animals lose merely 8 per cent of their content during the same period. It appears therefore that there is a defect in the binding mechanism of norepinephrine within the storage vesicles in hypertensive rats. Such abnormality would allow more norepinephrine to leak out of its storage site and probably would increase the amount of physiologically active norepinephrine in the vicinity of receptors (Krakoff et al., 1967).

Studies on the intraneural distribution of norepinephrine confirmed that the proportion of soluble or free norepinephrine is proportionally

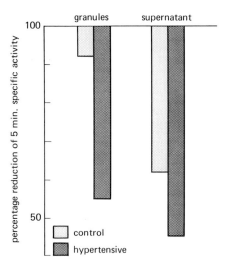

Figure 8-6   Decline in the specific activity of norepinephrine at the subcellular level in hearts of hypertensive and normotensive rats in the first 4 hours following the intravenous injection of 5 μC of tritiated norepinephrine. The hearts homogenized in isotonic sucrose were first centrifuged at 12,000 g for 10 minutes to remove the unbroken cells and mitochondria. The granular and supernatant fractions were obtained by further centrifugation at 105,000 g for one hour. Groups of rats were killed five minutes and four hours after the injection. At five minutes, the accumulation of tritiated norepinephrine in the granular fraction was similar in both groups of animals (39,000 counts/min/heart in normotensive and 40,600 counts/min/heart in hypertensive rats). The figure represents the changes in the specific activity from 5 minutes to 4 hours after the injections, expressed as the percentage change from the 5-minute value. (From Krakoff et al., 1967)

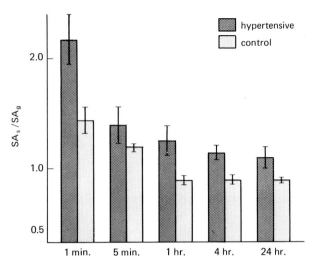

Figure 8-7 Subcellular distribution of norepinephrine in the hearts of hypertensive and normotensive rats at various intervals after the injection of 25 μC of the tritiated amine. Groups of 7 to 10 animals were used each time. This figure illustrates the intraneural distribution of norepinephrine expressed as the ratio of the specific activity of the supernatant fraction over the specific activity of the granular fraction (SA_s/SA_g). From one hour until 24 hours after the injection, this ratio remained constant in the hearts of control animals. In the hearts of the hypertensive rats, this ratio was always higher than that of the control animals and continued to decrease progressively during the first 24 hours after the injection. (From Krakoff et al., 1967)

greater in the hearts of hypertensive animals (Fig. 8-7). At various times after the injection of tritiated norepinephrine the ratio of soluble norepinephrine over the granule-bound norepinephrine in the heart is always greater in hypertensive rats than in normotensive rats. In the normotensive animals this ratio reaches equilibrium one hour after injection, whereas in the hypertensive rats the ratio continually decreases, thus indicating that the amount of norepinephrine coming out of the storage granules exceeds the elimination rate from the cytoplasm and from the extracellular space.

Metabolism of Norepinephrine. The increased norepinephrine turnover and the larger proportion of soluble norepinephrine in hypertensive rats were expected to yield a different pattern of metabolites due to a greater exposure of norepinephrine to the action of intraneuronal monoamine oxidase (MAO) and to the action of extraneuronal catechol-O-methyl

transferase (COMT). After injection of tritiated norepinephrine, norepinephrine is utilized and excreted more rapidly in the hypertensive animals
(Fig. 8-8). In the urinary collections made 4 to 24 hours after injection,
at a time when the tritiated compounds are derived exclusively from the
tritiated norepinephrine initially taken up and stored in the sympathetic
nerve fibers, the amount of tritiated amines and metabolites excreted in
the urine of hypertensive rats is approximately twice that excreted in the

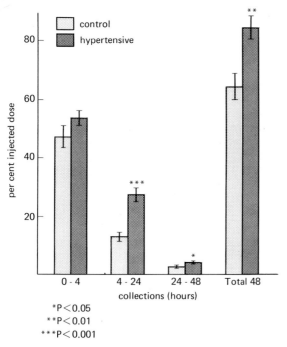

Figure 8-8   Urinary excretion of tritiated norepinephrine and metabolites following
an intravenous injection of 50 μC of d-1 tritiated norepinephrine to normotensive and
DOCA-hypertensive rats. Seven animals were used for each group of rats and the
results are expressed as percentages of the injected $\pm$ S.E.M. In the first 4 hours,
during which the major portion of the tritium excreted is derived from tritiated norepinephrine which was not taken up by nerve endings, no significant difference was
found between the amount excreted in normotensive and hypertensive rats. In the
following hours, however, when the excreted tritium compounds originated exclusively from the norepinephrine stored in the nerve endings mainly related to the
cardiovascular system, the amount of norepinephrine and metabolites excreted was
considerably greater in urine of DOCA-hypertensive rats. (Figure made from data
obtained by de Champlain et al., 1969a)

Table 8-5   Excretion of tritiated norepinephrine and metabolites in the kidney and urine of DOCA hypertensive rats

	Kidney 30 min after inject. (per cent)	Urine 4 to 24 hours after inject. (per cent)
Norepinephrine	+ 35	+ 100*
Deaminated catechols	+ 137**	+ 35*
Normetanephrine	+ 193**	+ 126**
Vanillylmandelic-acid	+ 119**	+ 75**
3-methoxy-4-hydroxyphenylglycol	+ 124**	+ 59**

* P < 0.05
** P < 0.01

The results are expressed as the percentage of change from control values in normotensive rats. In the study on the kidney, the animals were injected with 25 μC of tritiated norepinephrine and were killed 30 minutes later. For the urinary studies, rats were injected with 50 μC of tritiated norepinephrine and the urinary collection was made 4 to 24 hours after the injection. (Data taken from de Champlain et al., 1969a)

urine of normotensive rats. The pattern of metabolites in the kidney and urine of hypertensive rats indicates that norepinephrine, normetanephrine, deaminated catechols, vanillylmandelic-acid (VMA), and 3-methoxy-4-hydroxy-phenylglycol excretion are all markedly and significantly increased (Table 8-5). The increment in the excretion of free norepinephrine and O-methylated metabolites is highly suggestive that a larger amount of physiologically active norepinephrine available to react with the receptors is coming out of the adrenergic nerve fibers of hypertensive rats. These findings obtained after injection of tritiated amine are especially revealing since the use of such an approach permits a more accurate estimation of the metabolism of adrenergic fibers more specifically related to the cardiovascular system. These fibers are almost exclusively labelled by intravenous injection of tritiated norepinephrine whereas other important catecholamine-producing areas such as the brain, the vas deferens, and the adrenal medulla are insignificantly labelled due either to the blood-brain barrier or to a relatively small fractional blood flow distributed to these organs. Therefore, the information which can be obtained from urinary studies after injection of tritiated norepinephrine differs in significance from that obtained by measuring endogenous norepinephrine and metabolites. The urinary endogenous norepinephrine metabolites are the summation of the metabolic events occurring in the adrenal medulla as well as in all adrenergic fibers related or not to the cardiovascular system. Moreover, a dysfunction in a discrete area of the sympathetic nervous system can be diluted and hidden by metabolites coming from other areas which are functioning normally or in the opposite direction. These important distinctions may account for the discrepancy between our findings and the normal levels of endogenous normetanephrine and 3-methoxy-4-hydroxyphenylglycol in the urine of DOCA-hypertensive rats reported by Louis and coworkers (1970a).

The activity of the catecholamine degradative enzymes MAO and COMT is normal in all tissues of hypertensive animals with the exception of the hypertrophied heart, in which MAO activity is greatly increased (de Champlain et al., 1968b). Such a localized change in MAO activity cannot account for all the dysfunctions of the sympathetic nervous system described in the heart, adrenal medulla, and other organs. The increase in the MAO activity seems to be related exclusively to increased cardiac mass and is apparently independent of the changes in the metabolism and storage of norepinephrine in cardiac adrenergic fibers (de Champlain et al., 1968b).

Effect of Ganglionic Blockade on Norepinephrine Storage and on Blood Pressure. To determine whether the abnormal norepinephrine metabolism in hypertensive animals is due to a local metabolic defect at the nerve ending or to increased central sympathetic activity, the effect of ganglionic blockade on the norepinephrine storage was studied in these animals. One day after treatment of the hypertensive animals with a potent ganglion blocker the blood pressure falls within the normal range, and simultaneously the capacity of the hearts to retain norepinephrine is restored to normal (Fig. 8-9). It is also of interest to note in this study that the turnover rate is restored to normal in the treated hypertensive rat heart without any change in the MAO activity, thus ruling out the MAO increase as the cause of increased norepinephrine turnover in the heart of hypertensive rats (de Champlain et al., 1968a). These results also indicate that the neurogenic tone is increased in these animals and that this abnormality may contribute to the pathogenesis or to the maintenance of hypertension. However, an additional local metabolic defect at the site of adrenergic nerve ending cannot be excluded with this type of experiment due to the lack of knowledge on the direct effects of ganglionic blocking agent at this level.

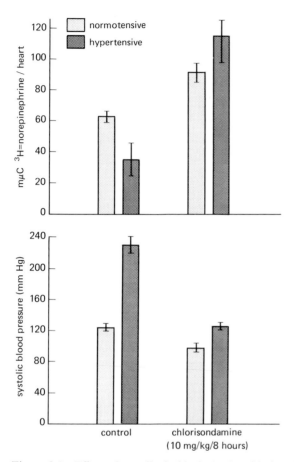

Figure 8-9   Effect of ganglionic blockade, by chlorisondamine, on norepinephrine storage and systolic blood pressure in normotensive and hypertensive rats. The animals were first injected with 25 μC of norepinephrine, and 15 minutes later the treatment with chlorisondamine (10 mg/kg every eight hours) was started. The rats were killed 24 hours after beginning of the treatment. Each group contained 7 to 8 rats, and the results are expressed as the mean $\pm$ S.E.M. This treatment lowered the blood pressure of the hypertensive animals to normotensive levels while it simultaneously restored the norepinephrine storage capacity of the heart to normal within 24 hours after the start of the treatment. (From de Champlain et al. 1968a)

Effect of Adrenalectomy and Sympathectomy on the Maintenance of Blood Pressure. Since the activity of the sympathetic system seems to be increased in hypertensive animals, it was of interest to determine the respective contributions of the adrenal medulla and the sympathetic fibers to the maintenance of hypertension. Chemical sympathectomy was produced in normotensive and hypertensive rats by intravenous injection of 6-hydroxydopamine (6-OH-DA). In studies with electron microscopy (Tranzer and Thoenen, 1967) and with fluorescent histochemistry (Malmfors and Sachs, 1968; de Champlain, 1971) this compound was found to destroy selectively the adrenergic terminal fibers. One week after either bilateral adrenalectomy or sympathectomy by one single injection of 6-OH-DA (100 mg/kg), the systolic blood pressure is reduced by 40 mm Hg in hypertensive rats with each procedure. In normotensive rats the blood pressure is decreased by about 30 mm Hg after sympathectomy but is decreased only slightly following adrenalectomy (Fig. 8-10). Although each procedure alone significantly reduces blood pressure in hypertensive rats, the levels of systolic blood pressure remain at hypertensive levels. Neither the sympathetic nerve fibers of the vascular system nor the

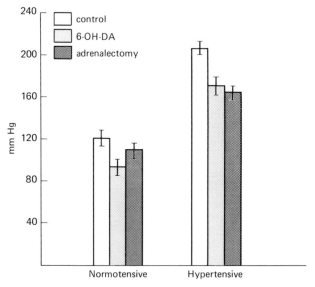

Figure 8-10   Effect of chemical sympathectomy and adrenalectomy on the systolic blood pressure of normotensive and hypertensive animals. One week after intravenous injection of 6-OH-DA (100 mg/kg) or one week after bilateral adrenalectomy, the blood pressure of the hypertensive rats was similarly reduced by about 40 mm Hg with either procedure. In normotensive animals, the hypotensive effect of the sympathectomy by 6-OH-DA was greater than the hypotensive effect of adrenalectomy alone. (From de Champlain, 1970)

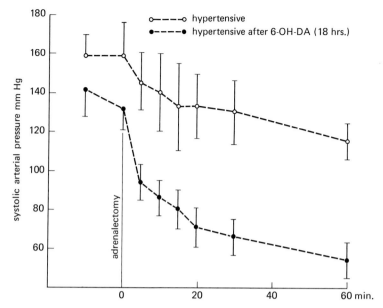

Figure 8-11 Effect of acute adrenalectomy in DOCA-hypertensive rats with and without pretreatment with 6-OH-DA. In untreated hypertensive rats (upper curve) acute adrenalectomy rapidly lowers blood pressure by about 40 mm Hg within 60 minutes. In hypertensive rats sympathectomized by treatment with 6-OH-DA (100 mg/kg, 18 hours previously) the systolic blood pressure was lower before adrenalectomy (lower curve). Acute adrenalectomy produced a rapid and severe hypotension in these animals by lowering the blood pressure more than 75 mm Hg within one hour. These acute experiments were carried on under pentobarbital anesthesia, and the blood pressure was recorded through canulation of the carotid artery. Each group contained 7 animals and each point is the mean ± S.E.M. (From J. de Champlain and M. R. Corbeil, unpublished data)

adrenal medulla alone could account entirely for the elevated blood pressure. However, it seems that both components of the sympathetic system have a synergetic influence on the maintenance of hypertension in these rats. In animals, previously sympathectomized, the removal of adrenal glands causes a rapid fall in blood pressure of greater magnitude than that occurring in untreated hypertensive animals after the same procedure (Fig. 8-11). The blood pressure of sympathectomized hypertensive animals falls to shock levels within minutes after bilateral adrenalectomy and none of the animals so treated has survived more than two hours after that procedure. The greater hypotensive effect of adrenalectomy in sympathectomized animals suggests that the fall in blood pressure after sympathectomy is probably minimized by a compensatory hyperfunction of the adrenal medulla. This is in agreement with the findings of Mueller et al. (1969), who reported a doubling of the synthesis rate of catecholamine in the adrenal medulla as early as 16 hours after sympathectomy by 6-OH-DA. A similar compensatory mechanism at the level of the sympathetic fibers was also reported following adrenalectomy (Westfall and Osada, 1969). Under normal conditions there seems to be a certain balance between the secretion of the adrenal medulla and the activity of the sympathetic nerve fibers, since the removal of either system immediately triggers a compensatory hyperactivity of the remaining system. In DOCA-hypertensive animals, this balance seems to be impaired since both components of the sympathetic system are simultaneously hyperactive. Their synergic effects might be responsible in great part for the maintenance of hypertension in these animals.

DOCA hypertension does not develop in rats treated from birth with weekly injections of 6-OH-DA (Table 8-6). Although the blood pressure was within normal range in sympathectomized rats given DOCA and sodium, their blood pressure was nevertheless significantly higher than that of control sympathectomized rats. This suggests that the sympathetic fibers may be essential for the development of hypertension, but the increase in blood pressure from hypotensive levels to normotensive levels

Table 8-6   Effect of sympathectomy on the development of DOCA hypertension

	Mean arterial pressure (mmHg)	Heart rate (beats/min)
Control	124 ± 5	403 ± 10
DOCA and sodium	154 ± 9*	358 ± 25
6-OH-DA	80 ± 7*	335 ± 18*
6-OH-DA + DOCA and sodium	115 ± 15	331 ± 25*

* $P < 0.05$

Animals treated with 6-OH-DA, received a weekly dose of 100 mg/kg subcutaneously from the day of birth for the following 13 weeks. When the animals weighed about 100 grams, they were uninephrectomized and two groups of them were given weekly subcutaneous injections of DOCA (10 mg/week) and saline 1 per cent to drink for 6 weeks. Because of the impossibility of measuring blood pressure by tail phlethysmography in the 6-OH-DA-treated rats, the mean blood pressure was measured by a cannula through the carotid artery in anesthetized animals. Groups of 8 animals were studied and the results are expressed as the mean ± S.E.M. (From J. de Champlain, M.-R. Corbeil, and A. Lacroix, unpublished data)

in sympathectomized animals indicates, however, that DOCA and sodium treatment can raise the blood pressure by means other than the sympathetic fibers, most probably through an increased liberation of catecholamines by the adrenal medulla. These findings are in agreement with those of Ayitey-Smith and Varma (1970), who have shown that DOCA and sodium hypertension could not be induced in totally immunosympathectomized rats. Animals only partially immunosympathectomized became hypertensive with the same treatment thus indicating the importance of a good evaluation of the degree of sympathectomy before reaching any conclusion on the role of the sympathetic nervous fibers (Ayitey-Smith and Varma, 1970; Varma, 1967). Willard and Fuller (1969) found that immunosympathectomy also prevented the development of hypertension produced by administration of triiodothyronine and sodium.

Recent studies have reached opposite conclusions on the role of the sympathetic fibers and adrenal medulla in the development and maintenance of DOCA and sodium hypertension in the rat. After treatment with 6-OH-DA, other investigators were unable to prevent the development of hypertension in DOCA- and sodium-treated rats (Finch and Leach, 1970a; Clarke et al., 1970). The efficiency of the sympathectomy was not evaluated in any of these studies and the negative findings may be the result of inadequate utilization of 6-OH-DA. In our studies, animals treated chronically were given weekly injections of 6-OH-DA (100 mg/kg) after finding that the regrowth of adrenergic fibers is rather rapid after their destruction by 6-OH-DA. Bundles of adrenergic fibers start to re-innervate the organs 5 to 7 days after treatment, and the innervation is almost normal within two months (de Champlain and Nadeau, 1971; de Champlain, 1971). With a schedule of weekly injections our animals were maintained at the highest degree of denervation possible, as indicated by endogenous norepinephrine levels less than 5 per cent of control values and by the absence of any detectable fluorescent adrenergic fibers in various organs. In the study of Finch and Leach (1970a) the animals were treated only once before starting the treatment with DOCA and sodium for 11 weeks. They found that the blood pressure started to rise with a slight initial delay in 6-OH-DA-treated rats but that the hypertensive levels reached after 11 weeks of treatment were identical to those of control hypertensive animals. The initial delay can be explained by the fact that their animals were probably initially denervated and that blood pressure rose to levels similar to those of control hypertensive rats when the sympathetic fibers had regrown. Moreover, their observation that the treatment of hypertensive rats with 6-OH-DA resulted in a rapid drop in blood pressure of about 50 mm Hg which lasted only two weeks is also of great interest since the re-innervation of organs is already advanced at this time and may be sufficient to re-establish the hypertension (de Champlain, 1971). Although these investigators concluded that the sympathetic nervous system was not necessary for the development of this type of hypertension, their studies nevertheless demonstrated remarkably well the importance of the sympathetic fibers in the evolution of DOCA and sodium hypertension. In addition, they also reported that the adrenal medulla was also unimportant in this form of hypertension since adrenal medullectomy, whether associated or not with 6-OH-DA treatment, did not interfere with the development of hypertension (Finch and Leach, 1970b). Adrenal medullectomy is known to produce, on its own, one type of experimental hypertension (Skelton and Brownie, 1967) and it is possible that in their experiment they were studying the development of adrenal regeneration hypertension rather than DOCA and sodium hypertension.

Relationship of Sodium Intake, Blood Pressure, and Catecholamine Metabolism. Among the various factors which may contribute to the dysfunction of sympathetic nervous system in DOCA-hypertensive rats, the sodium and/or related ions appear to be the most obvious choice. Since the sodium and related ions were found increased in vessels of DOCA-hypertensive rats (Table 8-2) and since the uptake, storage, and release of norepinephrine are ion-dependent (Potter and Axelrod, 1963; Stjarne and Von Euler, 1965; Bogdanski and Brodie, 1966, 1969; Daniel et al., 1970; Gillis and Paton, 1967; Horst et al., 1968; Iversen and Kravitz, 1966; Keen and Bogdanski, 1970), a closer look at the effect of sodium balance on catecholamine metabolism was justified.

During sodium depletion, a condition which is associated with a lowering of blood pressure, the retention of norepinephrine by the nerve endings is increased (Fig. 8-12). As for the hypertensive animals, the uptake of norepinephrine is normal in the hearts of sodium-depleted animals, but 24 hours later the norepinephrine remaining in the heart is significantly greater than in control rats, whereas it is reduced by about 50 per cent in hypertensive rats. The decrease in norepinephrine turnover during sodium depletion can also be correlated with the changes in blood

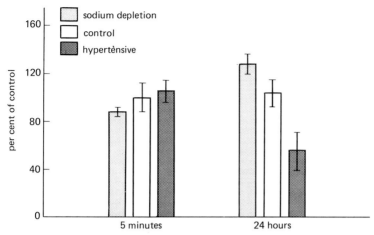

Figure 8-12   Uptake and retention of norepinephrine 5 minutes, and 24 hours, after the injection of 20 μC of tritiated norepinephrine in the hearts of control, sodium-depleted, and DOCA-hypertensive rats. The results are expressed as the percentage of the values observed in control animals. Each bar represents the mean of 6 to 10 animals. Although the initial uptake was normal in the hypertensive and sodium-depleted animals, the retention of norepinephrine (24 hours) was significantly increased during sodium depletion and markedly decreased in the hypertensive rats. (From de Champlain et al., 1969a)

pressure, thus suggesting that these changes and those observed in DOCA-hypertensive animals are probably part of the same mechanism which is influenced by the state of sodium balance. In various groups of rats receiving different sodium regimens the systolic blood pressure as well as the state of sodium balance could be inversely correlated with the capacity of the heart to retain tritiated norepinephrine (Fig. 8-13) or with the cardiac endogenous norepinephrine content (Fig. 8-14). The retention of tritiated norepinephrine and the endogenous norepinephrine content were highest during a state of negative sodium balance in sodium-depleted rats whereas they were lowest during a state of highly positive sodium balance in hypertensive rats.

The influence of sodium on the metabolism of norepinephrine and its importance in the pathogenesis of DOCA hypertension is strongly suggested by the observation that the withdrawal of sodium from the diet of hypertensive rats results in the lowering of blood pressure to within normotensive range while simultaneously restoring to normal the endogenous

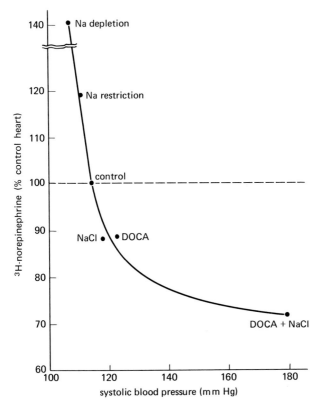

Figure 8-13   Relationship between systolic blood pressure and the capacity of the heart to retain tritiated norepinephrine in animals subjected to various sodium regimens for six weeks. NaCl refers to groups of rats given a solution of sodium chloride to drink. Sodium restriction was produced by giving the animals a sodium-free diet and distilled water. Sodium depletion was produced by giving a natriuretic (chlorothiazide) on the first day of the sodium free diet. The retention of norepinephrine was measured one hour after the intravenous injection of 25 μC of tritiated norepinephrine. Each point is the mean of 7 to 18 individual values expressed as the percentage of the value for normotensive control rats. (From de Champlain et al., 1968)

storage capacity and the turnover rate (Fig. 8-15). The effects of sodium balance could also be demonstrated at the site of the storage granules (Fig. 8-16). In the heart amine storage particles the capacity to retain tritiated norepinephrine and the endogenous norepinephrine content are slightly greater than control in sodium-depleted rats. The ratio of soluble

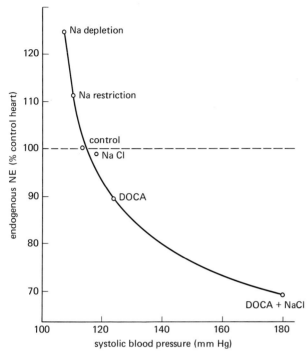

Figure 8-14   Relationship between systolic blood pressure and endogenous norepinephrine content of the hearts from the same groups of rats illustrated in Fig. 8-13. (From de Champlain et al., 1968a)

norepinephrine over granule-bound norepinephrine is significantly lower than normal in these animals, thus suggesting that a greater proportion of norepinephrine is bound and a smaller quantity of physiologically active norepinephrine is available to react with the receptors. In the hypertensive rats the withdrawal of sodium from the diet for two weeks lowers the blood pressure to normal and simultaneously restores the function of the storage vesicles. Moreover, the ratio of soluble norepinephrine to bound norepinephrine is also restored to normal, thus indicating that the correction of the sodium balance is accompanied by a normalization of the norepinephrine distribution in the subcellular compartments. The influence of sodium on norepinephrine metabolism is probably a determinant factor in the changes in storage and turnover of norepinephrine, which are closely associated with the development of hypertension or with the hypotensive effect of low sodium diet.

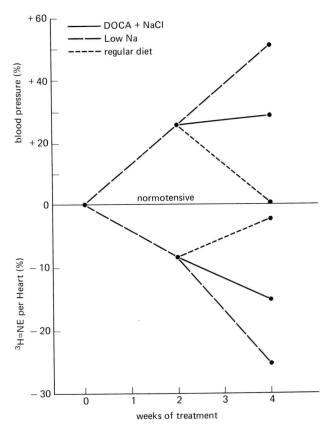

Figure 8-15 Comparative effects of sodium intake on blood pressure and on the capacity of the heart to retain norepinephrine. Each point is the mean of 6 to 8 values expressed as the percentage of increase or decrease compared with values in normotensive untreated animals. The upper part of the graph illustrates the changes in systolic blood pressure under treatment with various sodium regimens for 4 weeks. After 2 weeks of treatment with DOCA and saline (long dash lines), the blood pressure was significantly increased. At this point, the rats were divided in 3 groups, one group continued to receive DOCA and saline for the following 2 weeks and the blood pressure continued to rise progressively. In the other two groups, DOCA and saline treatment was stopped. One of these was shifted to a normal laboratory diet (full line) and in the following two weeks the blood pressure remained elevated at about the same level. Finally, the other group of hypertensive rats was given a sodium-free diet (short dash lines), and the blood pressure returned to normotensive levels within two weeks of the start of that diet. In the lower part of the graph is illustrated the retention of tritiated norepinephrine in the hearts of the same groups of animals 4 hours after intravenous injection of 25 μC of the tritiated amine. The changes in the capacity to retain norepinephrine vary in the opposite direction to the changes in blood pressure. The retention capacity is lowest when the blood pressure is highest, and this retention abnormality can be restored to normal simultaneously with the blood pressure in hypertensive rats treated with a sodium-deficient diet for 2 weeks. (From J. de Champlain, 1970)

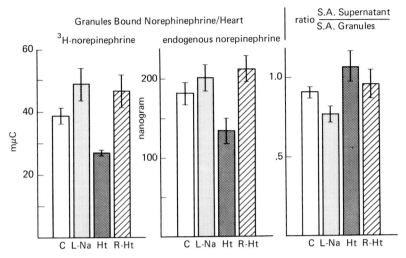

Figure 8-16   Subcellular distribution of exogenous and endogenous norepinephrine in the heart from groups of animals submitted to various sodium regimens. The letters under the bars identify the treatment: *C* stands for the control normotensive rats, *L-Na* stands for a group of normotensive rats submitted to a low sodium diet for 2 weeks, *Ht* stands for animals treated for 4 weeks with DOCA and saline, *R-Ht* stands for animals treated for the 2 weeks with DOCA and saline, then the treatment was stopped and the animals were put on a low sodium diet for 2 weeks. The mean systolic blood pressure was 118 mm Hg for the normotensive rat (C), 109 mm Hg for the sodium-restricted rats (L-Na), 183 mm Hg for the DOCA- and saline-treated rats (Ht), and 128 mm Hg for the hypertensive rats who were treated with a low sodium diet (R-Ht). As shown, the endogenous and tritiated norepinephrine content (24 hours after i.v. injection of 25 μC) of the heart granular fraction (105,000 g) were slightly higher in the sodium-restricted rats (L-Na) and markedly lower in DOCA-hypertensive rats (Ht). The endogenous and tritiated norepinephrine content of the granular fraction was restored to normal in the hypertensive animals treated with low sodium diet. The ratio of the specific activity of the supernatant over the specific activity of the granular fraction which was higher in hypertensive rats was lowered by treatment with low sodium diet. In the normotensive rats treated with a low sodium diet, this ratio was significantly lower, indicating a greater affinity of norepinephrine for the storage granules. (From studies by de Champlain et al., 1968a)

It is therefore possible that the changes in the ionic content of the nerve resulting from impaired sodium balance influence the storage and release of norepinephrine. Whether the ionic disturbance affects the binding or the transport of amine locally at the nerve ending, or whether it influences the sympathetic activity through a direct or reflex action on the central nervous system, is difficult to determine. The reversal of hypertension and the restoration of the norepinephrine storage capacity by an acute treatment with a ganglion blocker suggest that the central sympathetic activity is probably increased in hypertensive animals. However, ganglion blockers have also been found to be natriuretic (Gill et al., 1964), and it is possible that treatment with these drugs might affect the ionic content locally at the nerve ending. On the other hand, the sympathetic fibers are probably essential for the occurrence of a sodium accumulation in experimental hypertension. The severity of sodium retention, in man, after infusion of saline or administration of desoxycorticosterone is markedly reduced during treatment with ganglion blockers (Gill et al., 1964). Immunosympathectomy also prevents the increase in sodium concentration following a treatment with DOCA and sodium (Ayitey-Smith and Varma, 1970).

Although sodium has more often been the focus of recent studies of hypertension, it is possible that changes in other ions might have a more important influence than sodium on adrenergic mechanism. Recently, calcium content was found increased in the hearts of renal hypertensive rats (Tobian and Duke, 1969) and in the tail arteries of DOCA-hypertensive rats (Hinke, 1966). The changes in calcium might be influenced by the concentration of sodium through a sodium-calcium exchange pump (Baker et al., 1969). Since calcium is important for the uptake and binding of norepinephrine in nerve ending (Potter and Axelrod, 1963; Horst et al., 1968), for catecholamine liberation from the nerve endings and adrenal medulla (Rubin, 1969; Keen and Bogdanski, 1970), and for the effects of catecholamine on the effector cells (Daniel et al., 1970) it is possible that sodium might influence the catecholamine metabolism through changes in calcium concentration. However, further studies on calcium and other ions are needed for a better understanding of the links between catecholamines, ions, and hypertensive diseases.

Experimental Renal Hypertension

Ever since its description by Goldblatt and coworkers (1934), the pathogenesis of experimental renal hypertension, and later the pathogenesis of various forms of human hypertension, has been linked with an hyperactivity of the renin-angiotensin system (Page and McCubbin, 1968; Peart, 1965; Gross et al., 1965). However, direct measurement of renin, angiotensin, or aldosterone has failed to reveal any unequivocal increase in the levels of these substances in the plasma of most hypertensive patients (Genest et al., 1965; Boyd et al., 1969; Catt et al., 1969). Even in experimental hypertension increased levels of renin or angiotensin have not been found consistently during the initial phase of renal hypertension, and in the chronic phase of hypertension levels were found to be normal (Scornik and Paladini, 1959; Koletsky and Pritchard, 1963; Brown et al., 1966). Moreover, immunization of the animals against angiotensin before or after renal artery constriction did not modify the pattern of hypertension, although the immunization was sufficient to prevent the pressor response to angiotensin and renin (Hedwall, 1969; Heide and Aars, 1969; Johnson et al., 1970). Similarly, the injection of antibodies to renin did not lower acutely the blood pressure of renal hypertensive animals (Weiser et al., 1969; Hill et al., 1970). These studies strongly suggest that the renin-angiotensin system is not the sole factor implicated in the development or maintenance of renal hypertension.

In chronic renal hypertension, increased peripheral resistance and blood pressure are lowered by procedures or treatments interfering with the autonomic nervous system, thus suggesting that the chronic phase of renal hypertension probably depends on a sympathetic component (Gleen et al., 1938; Dock et al., 1942; Grollman et al., 1943; Ogden et al., 1946; Laverty and Smirk, 1961; Taquini, 1963). This hypothesis is also supported by the finding that although immunosympathectomy does not prevent the development of hypertension up to four weeks after renal artery stenosis, it does prevent the maintenance of hypertension in the following weeks (Dorr and Brody, 1964; Ayitey-Smith and Varma, 1970). The neurogenic component in chronic renal hypertension was suggested to be secondary—in major part—to a resetting of the baroreceptors in these animals (McCubbin and Page, 1963).

The turnover of norepinephrine appears to be increased in hearts of rats made hypertensive with renal artery stenosis, since the uptake of norepinephrine is normal but the retention is significantly reduced 24 hours after injection of tritiated norepinephrine (Table 8-7). An increased norepinephrine turnover rate was also observed in the heart of rats made hypertensive by renal encapsulation (Volicer et al., 1968) or by renal infarction (Henning, 1969). These changes in norepinephrine turnover are similar to those found in DOCA-hypertensive animals but, in contrast with this group, endogenous norepinephrine levels are normal in the heart, brain, skeletal muscle, spleen, intestine, and salivary glands of renal

Table 8-7   Changes in catecholamine turnover in experimental renovascular hypertension

	Blood pressure mm Hg	End. NE Heart (ng/heart)	Tritiated NE (mμC/Heart) 5 min	24 hours
Control	110 ± 2.5	1024 ± 25	787 ± 47	249 ± 30
Sham operated	109 ± 3.0	1140 ± 64	769 ± 131	227 ± 19
Hypertensive	185 ± 8.0**	1101 ± 37	784 ± 87	167 ± 12*

* $P < 0.05$
** $P < 0.01$

The rats were made hypertensive by application of a silver clip on the left renal artery. Sham operated animals had the same operation and their left renal pedicle was dissected. Eight weeks after this procedure, the animals were injected with 25 μC of ^{3}H-norepinephrine via the tail vein and were killed 5 minutes, and 24 hours, later. Each group of rats contained 8 to 10 animals and the results are expressed as the mean ± S.E.M. (From de Champlain, unpublished data)

hypertensive animals (de Champlain, unpublished data; Wegmann et al., 1962; Volicer et al., 1968; Robertson et al., 1968; Henning, 1969; Lefer and Ayers, 1969). Endogenous norepinephrine and epinephrine contents of the adrenal medulla are also normal in these animals (de Champlain, unpublished data; Wegmann et al., 1962). However, endogenous norepinephrine levels are decreased in the walls of various arteries and in the kidneys of hypertensive animals (Faradin et al., 1961; Wegmann et al., 1962; Lefer and Ayers, 1969). Although more studies on the metabolism of norepinephrine are required in the acute and chronic stage of this form of hypertension, it seems that the increase in turnover of norepinephrine may contribute to the maintenance of hypertension.

Recent studies have indicated that there may be a dysfunction in the liberation of norepinephrine upon nerve stimulation in this form of hypertension. In rats and dogs with renal hypertension stimulation of sympathetic fibers produces a greater vasoconstrictor response in various vascular territories (Aoki and Brodie, 1969; Moerman et al., 1969; Zimmerman et al., 1969; Brody et al., 1970). This enhanced response to nerve stimulation is not simply the consequence of supersensitivity of the adrenergic receptors but is also associated with the release of a larger quantity of norepinephrine at the nerve ending (Zimmerman et al., 1969). This phenomenon might be related to the increased number of small vesicles, which has been recently observed on electron microscopy, in the terminal adrenergic fibers of arteries of renal hypertensive animals (Burnstock et al., 1970; Graham et al., 1970).

The sodium and potassium content of aorta and other tissues is increased in renal hypertension (Table 8-2). These changes, however, are generally less marked than in DOCA-hypertensive animals. Although the ionic content may contribute to the increase in norepinephrine turnover and release in renal hypertension, other factors can also be implicated. The renin-angiotensin system has often been reported to be activated in the early phase of the renal hypertension, and in the light of recent findings on the effects of angiotensin on nerve transmission and on norepinephrine metabolism, it is likely that angiotensin could serve as a triggering mechanism for the hyperactivity of the sympathetic system (Lowe and Scroop, 1970). In presence of angiotensin, even at very low concentration, the response to sympathetic stimulation is potentiated in cutaneous and renal vascular beds (Zimmerman, 1967). Moreover, during angiotensin infusion, the sympathetic nerve releases a greater quantity of transmitter for a given number of nerve impulses (Zimmerman and Gisslen, 1968). Volicer and Visweswaram (1970) have also reported recently that infusion of nonpressor doses of angiotensin causes an increase in the norepinephrine turnover of the heart of the same magnitude of that than during renal hypertension. Finally, it was found that chronic treatment with angiotensin increases the number of small vesicles in the adrenergic nerve endings of the pineal gland (Panagiotis and Hungerford, 1966). The similarity between the changes in adrenergic function found in renal hypertensive animals and those found after angiotensin treatment is most striking and suggestive. Although angiotensin could contribute to the acute phase of renal hypertension, its role during the chronic stage is questionable. Whether angiotensin acts on adrenergic fibers directly or indirectly through the central nervous system or by contribution to the ionic disturbance (Villamil et al., 1970) remains to be demonstrated.

Genetic Spontaneous Hypertension

Recently two strains of spontaneously hypertensive rats have been developed by selective inbreeding: the New Zealand and the Japanese strains.

In the New Zealand strain the elevation of blood pressure does not seem to be due to a primary defect in kidney circulation or to the renin-angiotensin system (Phelan, 1968; Smirk and Phelan, 1965). Endogenous norepinephrine content is decreased in the heart, increased in brain and spleen, and is normal in skeletal muscle and adrenal gland (Robertson

et al., 1968). Phelan (1970) has recently reported that cardiac norepinephrine content is normal or increased in young hypertensive animals
and decreased in older hypertensive rats. Moreover, he also found that
the uptake and turnover of norepinephrine are normal in the hearts of
young hypertensive rats but that the turnover is decreased in older hypertensive rats, indicating that the sympathetic activity at least is variable
throughout the life span of these hypertensive rats. Sympathetic fibers
seem essential for the evolution of spontaneous hypertension, since immunosympathectomy prevents the development of hypertension in these
animals (Clark, 1969; Smirk, 1970). However, the adrenal gland is not
necessary for the development and maintenance of hypertension in this
strain of rat (Nolla-Panades and Smirk, 1964; Phelan, 1968). Although,
no evidence was found that sympathetic activity exceeds that of normotensive animals, the decrease in the turnover rate of norepinephrine from
young to old rats and the importance of an intact nervous system for the
development of hypertension leave open the possibility that the sympathetic nervous system may play a role in the pathogenesis of this form of
genetic hypertension.

The Japanese strain of spontaneous hypertensive rats differs from the
New Zealand in that it is a purer strain, the blood pressure levels are
higher, and hypertension is present in all the animals. Two series of studies have reached opposite conclusions on the role of the sympathetic
nervous system in these animals. In studies made by those who bred this
strain of animal, there are several indications of a dysfunction of the central vasomotor centers in spontaneously hypertensive rats. Under the
abnormal influence of the hypothalamus it was proposed that the pressor
centers of the medulla oblongata become hyperactive, thus increasing the
activity of the peripheral sympathetic fibers and adrenal medulla (Okamoto, 1969). Section of the neural connection between posterior hypothalamus and mesencephalon causes a greater fall in blood pressure in the
spontaneously hypertensive animals than in normotensive animals (Yamori and Okamoto, 1969). Transection experiments (*cerveau isolé* and
encéphale isolé) indicated that the ponto-bulbar portion of the brain stem
is responsible for the mechanism involved in the tonic maintenance of
high blood pressure in these animals (Okamoto et al., 1967). The hyperactivity of the motor centers seems to be a primary defect since the baroreceptors are functioning normally in these animals (Thant et al., 1969).
The observation that endogenous norepinephrine levels and the activity

of aromatic amino acid decarboxylase are both reduced in the brain stem and hypothalamus of hypertensive rats also gave support to the hypothesis of a dysfunction in the central vasomotor centers (Yamori et al., 1970).

Fluorescent histochemical observations on the superior cervical ganglia and on the adrenergic fibers related to the arteries have indicated that the ganglion cells and terminal fibers of the sympathetic system are hyperactive in the spontaneously hypertensive rats (Haebara et al., 1968; Matsumoto, 1969; Ichijima, 1969). Moreover, direct recording of the electrical activity of the left splanchinic sympathetic nerve of spontaneously hypertensive rats revealed that the peripheral sympathetic tone is markedly increased compared with control animals (Okamoto et al., 1967). Cardiac norepinephrine content is slightly elevated but the activity of monoamine oxidase and aromatic amino acid decarboxylase is normal in the heart. brain, and kidney (Ozaki, 1966). It is also interesting to note that hypertension starts to develop in these animals only after 5 weeks of age (Okamoto, 1969), at a time when the development of the sympathetic system is reaching maturity (Iversen et al., 1967; de Champlain et al., 1970; Sachs et al., 1970). Signs of hyperactivity could also be demonstrated in the adrenal medulla of these animals. The norepinephrine content of the adrenal medulla in the spontaneously hypertensive rats is about twice that of control rats (Ozaki et al., 1968), and the catecholamine synthesis and secretion rates are increased (Morisawa, 1968b). Moreover, under stress (Morisawa, 1968a) or after tyramine administration (quoted by Ozaki et al., 1968) noradenaline is secreted more readily from the adrenal medulla of spontaneously hypertensive animals. Electron microscopy and histochemical studies have also revealed that the number of norepinephrine storage granules is greater in the adrenal medullary cells (Maruyama, 1969) and that the area of the noradrenaline storing cell islets is about twice that of the control in the adrenal medulla of these hypertensive rats (Tabei, 1966). Finally, the adrenal gland seems to be necessary for the development and maintenance of hypertension in this strain of animals since adrenalectomy prevents the development of hypertension or decreases blood pressure within normotensive range in already hypertensive animals (Aoki, 1963; Ozaki, 1966).

In the same strain of hypertensive animals but using Wistar control rats of a different source, Louis and coworkers (1968, 1969a, 1969b, 1970a, 1970b) reported that norepinephrine turnover and synthesis rates are decreased in the hearts of spontaneously hypertensive rats. They concluded that these changes in norepinephrine metabolism are the result of a secondary compensatory mechanism rather than a primary factor in the development of this form of hypertension. This series of experiments raises the difficult problem of selecting the appropriate type of control animals to use in studies on highly inbred animals such as spontaneously hypertensive rats. Since the inheritance of spontaneous hypertension is incompatible with simple Mendelian inheritance and favors rather a polygenic mechanism (Louis et al., 1969c), the development of one genetic dominance such as an elevated blood pressure is likely to be associated with the development of other genetically linked behavioral characteristics. In two different strains of rats with opposite genetic susceptibility to experimental hypertension induced by salt, it was found that members of the sensitive strain were consistently less aggressive than those of the resistant strain (Ben-Ishay and Welner, 1969). Within the same colony it is difficult to attribute any biochemical changes to the primary characteristic of these animals without a careful evaluation of the influence of other genetically linked characteristics. In the studies of Louis and coworkers, the controls used were not from the original Wistar colony but were from the NIH colony. The interpretation of their results is even more difficult after the report by Neff and coworkers (1969) that there is as much as a twofold difference in the turnover of norepinephrine between various groups of rats, from the same strain, obtained from different sources. Recent studies on the vascular reactivity of the aorta of spontaneously hypertensive rats have also stressed the importance of choosing the right control rats for studies using these animals (Clineschmidt et al., 1970). Depending on the colony of Wistar rats used for controls (NIH or Carworth Farm), the aorta of spontaneously hypertensive rats had either a normal or decreased reactivity to norepinephrine. Therefore the evaluation of the sympathetic nerve functions in spontaneously hypertensive rats requires more studies with different types of control animals before a more definitive conclusion can be reached.

Other Forms of Experimental Hypertension

Norepinephrine turnover and synthesis rates are increased in the heart and adrenal medulla of rabbits made hypertensive by sino-aortic denervation (De Quattro et al., 1969). An increase in tyrosine hydroxylase activity was also observed in the heart and adrenal medulla of these animals. Since the endogenous norepinephrine content is normal in these organs, the increased synthesis rate indicates that larger amounts of norepinephrine are released from the adrenergic nerve endings and from the adrenal medulla in this form of hypertension.

Table 8-8   Endogenous norepinephrine levels and tritiated norepinephrine retention in cadmium hypertension (per cent)

	Endogenous NE	Retention of ^{3}H-NE—24 hours
Heart (total)	+ 18	− 50*
Spleen (per gram)	− 9	− 33*
Intestine (per gram)	− 26*	− 25*

* P < 0.02

Twelve hypertensive rats were compared with eight control animals. The cadmium hypertension was produced by giving the animals 50 to 200 parts per million of cadmium in drinking water for eight months. The systolic blood pressure of cadmium-treated rats varied between 160 to 200 mm Hg. Animals were injected with 25 μC of ^{3}H-norepinephrine i.v. and were killed 24 hours later. (From J. de Champlain and G. Denis, unpublished data)

In rats made hypertensive by cadmium administration (50 to 200 parts per million in drinking water for eight months) the endogenous norepinephrine content is normal in the heart and spleen but is decreased in the intestine (Table 8). The retention of tritiated norepinephrine was significantly reduced in these three organs 24 hours after injection of the tritiated amine, thus suggesting that the norepinephrine turnover rate is also increased in the sympathetic fibers of these hypertensive animals.

The Sympathetic Nervous System in Human Hypertension

For many years, the sympathetic nervous system has been suspected of playing a role in the pathogenesis of human hypertension, but until recently direct evidence supporting that hypothesis was lacking. Much direct and indirect evidence has been accumulating in favor of an increased sympathetic activity in hypertensive diseases of various etiologies. Hemodynamic studies have shown that the peripheral resistance is increased in all forms of human hypertension with the exception of labile hypertension (Frohlich et al., 1969), and that the cardiac output may be increased in the early phases of various forms of hypertension (Finkielman et al., 1965; Frolich et al., 1969). Increased activity in various autonomic functions, especially in regard to muscle tone activity and basal metabolism, was also observed in patients with essential hypertension (Von Eiff, 1970). The existence of an important neurogenic component in the maintenance of elevated blood pressure is also indicated by the observation that most hypotensive drugs interfere in some way with the function of the sympathetic system and that they produce greater falls in blood pressure in hypertensive than in normotensive patients (Doyle and Smirks, 1955; Green, 1962; Carlsson, 1966; Lucchesi and Whitsitt, 1969; Abrams, 1969).

Initial attempts to investigate more directly the sympathetic system by studying the urinary excretion of catecholamines and their metabolites in hypertensive patients failed to reveal any consistent indications of an hyperfunction of the sympathetic system in most cases of hypertension, with the exception of pheochromocytoma (Table 8-9). Until 1964, in most studies the excretion of norepinephrine, epinephrine, vanylmandelic-acid (VMA), and normetanephrine (NMN) was found normal or decreased. Nevertheless, in a few studies, a group of hypertensive patients (10 to 26 per cent) excreted quantities of norepinephrine or other cate-cholamines exceeding the upper range of control values (Table 8-9). The negative findings and discrepancies reported in these various studies may be explained by a variety of factors. In many of these studies, the determinations were made with bioassay techniques which lacked the sensitivity and specificity of more recent fluorometric methods. Many of these patients were receiving hypotensive medication or were submitted to low sodium diet at the time of the investigation. Moreover, the degree of arteriosclerosis and the impairment of renal functions was seldom evaluated in hypertensive patients, even though these factors could influence the pattern of urinary excretion since norepinephrine can be significantly reabsorbed by the renal tubule (Overy et al., 1967) and since norepinephrine excretion can be correlated with urinary flow or volume (de Schoepdryver and Leroy, 1961; Dawson and Bone, 1963; Hathaway et al., 1969). Ikoma (1965a) has shown the importance of evaluating renal function before interpreting urinary studies in hypertensive patients. He found that the excretion of catecholamines is significantly increased in essential hypertensive patients with normal renal function while it is decreased in those with impaired renal function. Since 1965, several other studies, carried out

Table 8-9   Urinary excretion of catecholamine and metabolites in hypertensive patients*

Authors	Number of Patients	Catechol- amine (NE and/ or E)	Per cent above Normal Range	VMA	NMN
Holtz et al. (1947)		increased			
Burn (1953)	8	normal			
Von Euler et al. (1954)	500	normal	16		
Goldenberg et al. (1954)	26	normal	22		
Hoobler et al. (1954)	14	normal			
Pekkarinen et al. (1955)	26	normal			
Griffiths and Collison (1957)	16	normal	20		
Birke et al. (1957)		decreased			
Moller et al. (1957)	100	decreased			
Yoshinaga et al. (1960)		decreased			
Von Studnitz (1960)	105			increased	
Gitlow et al. (1960)				normal	
Sunderman et al. (1960)	103	normal	16	normal	
Sjoerdsma (1961)				normal	normal
Crout et al. (1961)	118	normal		normal	normal
Goodall and Gogdonoff (1961)	500	normal	26		
Ritzel and Hunzinger (1963)	67	increased		normal	normal
Brunjes (1964)	73	decreased		decreased	decreased
Serrano et al. (1964)	99	normal	10		
Wolf et al. (1965)	53			slight incr.	slight incr.
Boak and Riek (1965)		increased			
Ikoma (1965a)	87	increased			
Stott and Robinson (1967)	20				increased
Nestel and Doyle (1968)	33	increased		increased	increased
De Quattro and Sjoerdsma (1968)	8	slight incr.	50	slight incr.	
Kuchel et al. (1970)	7	increased			

* These studies exclude patients with pheochromocytoma and were done mainly in patients with essential hypertension. The percentage above normal range refers to the percentage of hypertensive patients with excretion of catecholamine higher than the upper range of value for the control normotensive patients used in each study.

under more standardized conditions in unmedicated hypertensive patients with normal renal function, have consistently reported increased urinary levels of noradrenaline, VMA, or NMN in many patients with essential hypertension (Table 8-9). Moreover, a highly significant correlation was found between the systolic or diastolic blood pressure and the levels of norepinephrine in the urine of normotensive and hypertensive patients (Ikoma, 1965a; Nestel and Doyle, 1968). In contrast to the findings in

hypertension, the urinary catecholamines and the synthesis of norepinephrine are both decreased in cases of postural hypertension (Goodall,
1968; Hedeland et al., 1969). Moreover, the lowering of blood pressure
in hypertensive patients by treatment with hypotensive drugs or by low
sodium diet is also accompanied by a reduction of norepinephrine excretion. This striking correlation between blood pressure and urinary catecholamines in humans is in accordance with the inverse relationship found
between the turnover and storage of norepinephrine and the systolic blood
pressure in DOCA-hypertensive rats and in rats subjected to low sodium
diet.

Owing to very low circulating levels, studies on plasma catecholamines
have been less numerous in hypertensive patients. In studies using less
sensitive techniques, plasma catecholamine levels in hypertensive patients
were found either normal (Hoobler et al., 1954; Manger, 1962) or increased (Hirano et al., 1969). More recently, Engelman and coworkers
(1970), using a highly sensitive double isotope technique, reported that
circulating catecholamine levels in essential hypertension subjects were
about twice those of normotensive subjects.

The sympathetic response to tilting was originally found reduced in
hypertensive patients since the variations in urinary (Sundin, 1956) or
plasmatic (Hickler et al., 1959) catecholamines were considerably less
impressive in these patients than in normotensive subjects. In recent
studies made in young untreated hypertensive patients, however, mental
stress or tilting caused a greater increase in the excretion of norepinephrine in hypertensive patients than in normotensive subjects (Nestel,
1969; Nestel and Esler, 1970).

To evaluate more specifically the activity of the cardiovascular adrenergic fibers, the fate of tritiated norepinephrine was studied in hypertensive
patients. Gitlow and coworkers (1964) suggested that the storage and
binding of norepinephrine are reduced in the sympathetic fibers of patients with essential hypertension since tritiated norepinephrine declines
more rapidly in their plasma after intravenous infusion. After a single
intravenous injection of norepinephrine the amount of tritiated norepinephrine and metabolites excreted in the urine during the following 24 hours
is significantly greater in hypertensive patients, indicating again that the
turnover of noradrenaline is probably increased in the vascular sympathetic fibers (Gitlow et al., 1969). This abnormality in the pattern of
excretion of tritiated norepinephrine and metabolites in hypertensive

patients is strikingly similar to the pattern of urinary excretion in DOCA-hypertensive rats after an identical treatment (Fig. 8-8). De Quattro and Sjoerdsma (1968) failed, however, to detect any abnormality in the rate of disappearance of ^{3}H-norepinephrine from the plasma of hypertensive patients after administration of tritiated DOPA. However, with this technique, other organs in addition to those of the cardiovascular system are also labelled, thus complicating the interpretation of these studies.

In studies in which mean levels of catecholamine and metabolites were increased, still a population of hypertensive patients continued to have plasmatic or urinary levels within the normal range. It is unlikely that patients with essential hypertension constitute a homogeneous population of patients. A hypertensive patient is classified in the category of essential hypertension after all known causes of hypertension are excluded, and owing to the empiricism of this classification a variety of diseases of unknown etiology are most probably included in this group of patients. This may explain to a certain extent the wide range of variations of values obtained in this group. Concerning the role of the sympathetic system, it is also likely that the population of patients with essential hypertension is constituted by subgroups of diseases in which the sympathetic system may play a variable role in the pathogenesis and maintenance of hypertension. In one group of these patients, the hypertension may be associated with a hyperactivity of the sympathetic nervous system. In other patients with normal sympathetic activity and normal norepinephrine metabolism, the participation of the sympathetic activity to the hypertension cannot even be excluded because of the possibility of a hypersensitivity of the adrenergic receptors to normal amounts of the neurotransmitter in these patients. Changes in catecholamine metabolism may be a primary factor in some patients, while in others such changes may be secondary to hemodynamic disturbances or to circulating substances such as angiotensin. Moreover, the time of the study can be critical since the sympathetic nervous system may be responsible for only one stage of the disease. Arteriosclerosis and renal diseases, which often develop in the course of chronic hypertension, may modify considerably the parameter measured or else may also influence the activity of the sympathetic system so that the factors and mechanisms responsible for the maintenance of hypertension may change even during its evolution. Although there are numerous indications in favor of a role of the sympathetic nervous system in the pathogenesis and maintenance of human hypertension, a more careful and critical evaluation of the various factors and mechanisms is needed before reaching a final conclusion.

Conclusions

Evidence that the sympathetic nervous system may be implicated in various forms of experimental human hypertension has been reviewed and discussed. Although increased sympathetic activity was commonly detected by various means of study in different forms of experimental hypertension, the expression of this dysfunction varied from one type of hypertension to another. In DOCA-hypertensive animals, the increased norepinephrine turnover in the sympathetic fibers is associated with a decrease in the norepinephrine stores of various organs and with an hyperactivity of the adrenal medulla. In renal, neurogenic, and cadmium hypertension, the turnover rate of norepinephrine is increased but endogenous stores are normal. In spontaneously hypertensive rats, the turnover rate of norepinephrine is either normal or decreased, although definite signs of hyperactivity of the vasomotor centers and adrenal medulla have been observed. In most of these forms of hypertension, the absence of sympathetic fibers or adrenalectomy either prevented the development of hypertension or caused a marked reduction of the blood pressure, thus suggesting that the sympathetic nervous system (sympathetic fibers and adrenal medulla) may contribute, directly or indirectly, to the pathogenesis or maintenance of hypertension in these various experimental conditions.

Recent studies on human hypertension have also revealed signs of an increased sympathetic activity. Abnormalities found in the metabolism of norepinephrine in patients with essential hypertension are strikingly similar to those reported in certain forms of experimental hypertension. A highly significant inverse correlation between the turnover of norepinephrine and the level of blood pressure was observed in human as well as in experimental animals. In humans and in rats, elevated blood pressure is associated with an increased norepinephrine turnover rate and a decrease in storage, whereas low blood pressure is associated with a decreased turnover rate.

It is difficult at this point to determine whether the sympathetic nervous system plays a primary role in the pathogenesis of certain forms of hypertension or whether it contributes only to certain stages of the hypertensive disease. It is likely that both possibilities exist in human and experimental hypertension. In DOCA-hypertensive rats, it appears that the changes in norepinephrine turnover precede the rise in blood pressure, whereas in renal hypertension the sympathetic nervous system seems to be responsible for the maintenance of hypertension only in the chronic stage of the disease. The increase in the activity of the sympathetic nervous system in various forms of hypertension is not secondary to the rise in blood pressure since the usual baroreceptor response to elevation of blood pressure results rather in a decreased sympathetic activity. Even a normal sympathetic activity in hypertension constitutes an abnormality in this respect and indicates a resetting of the vasomotor reflexes. The increased norepinephrine turnover rate encountered in certain forms of hypertension does not necessarily indicate that the sympathetic dysfunction is localized exclusively in the efferent sympathetic fibers. The activity of these fibers may reflect a dysfunction occurring at any point on the vasomotor reflex arc.

There may be numerous triggering mechanisms leading to a dysfunction of the sympathetic system in the various forms of hypertension. In DOCA-hypertension it appears that sodium and/or other ions are probably the main factor influencing the metabolism of norepinephrine. In other forms of hypertension, ionic disturbances which are commonly found in vascular tissues in most hypertensive conditions could also be responsible for the change in sympathetic activity. Other factors such as angiotensin, mineralocorticoids, and other hormones could also contribute either directly or indirectly to a dysfunction of the sympathetic system. Although hypertension may be initiated by different etiological factors, it is possible that many of these factors increase the blood pressure indirectly by influencing the activity of the sympathetic system. The sympathetic nervous system would then serve as a common pathway for different etiological factors.

In various experimental and human hypertensive diseases, a greater amount of physiologically active norepinephrine seems to be present at the receptor site due to decreased storage or increased turnover at the nerve endings. However, more studies are needed before we understand the interrelationships of central and peripheral sympathetic system, ion metabolism, and receptor sensitivity in the mechanisms of hypertension.

References

Abrams, W. B. 1969. *Dis. Chest* 55:148.

Ahlquist, R. P. 1948. *Am. J. Physiol.* 153:586.

Albert, D. G., Morita, Y., and Iseri, L. T. 1958. *Circulation* 12:761.

Allen, F. M., and Sherill, J. W. 1922. *J. Metab. Research* 2:429.

Ambard, L., and Beaujard, E. 1904. *Arch. gén. Méd.* 1:520.

Aoki, K. 1963. *Jap. Heart J.* 4:443.

Aoki, V. S., and Brody, M. J. 1969. *Arch. Int. Pharmacodyn.* 177:423.

Axelrod, J. 1965. *Recent Prog. Hormone Res.* 21:597.

Axelrod, J. 1968. *Physiologist* 11:63.

Ayitey-Smith, E., and Varma, D. R. 1970. *Brit. J. Pharmac.* 40:175.

Baker, P. F., Blaustein, M. P., Hodgkin, A. L., and Steinhardt, R. A. 1969. *J. Physiol.* (Lond.) 200:431.

Bandick, N. R., and Sparks, H. V. 1970. *Am. J. Physiol.* 219:340.

Baum, T., and Shropshire, A. T. 1967. *Am. J. Physiol.* 212:1020.

Ben-Ishay, D., and Welner, A. 1969. *Proc. Soc. Exptl. Biol. Med.* 132:1170.

Bernard, C. 1851. *C.R. Soc. Biol.* 3:163.

Birke, G., Duner, H., von Euler, U. S., and Plantin, L. D. 1957. *Ztschr. Vitamin Hormon Ferment Forsch.* 9:41.

Boak, W. C., and Riek, L. I. 1965. *Clin. Res.* 13:202.

Bogdanski, D. F., and Brodie, B. B. 1966. *Life Sci.* 5:1563.

Bogdanski, D. F., and Brodie, B. B. 1969. *J. Pharmacol. Exptl. Ther.* 165:181.

Bohr, D. F. 1964. *Pharmacol. Rev.* 16:85.

Bohr, D. F., and Sitrin, M. 1970. *Circ. Research* suppl. II, 26-27:83.

Boyd, G. W., Landon, J., and Peart, W. S. 1969. *Proc. Roy. Soc. (Biol.)* 173:327.

Brody, M. J., Dorr, L. D., and Shaffer, R. A. 1970. *Am. J. Physiol.* 219:1746.

Brown, T. C., Davis, J. O., Olichney, M. J., and Johnston, C. I. 1966. *Circ. Research* 18:475.

Brown-Séquart, C. E. 1854. *C.R. Acad. Sci.* 38:72.

Brunjes, S. 1964. *New Eng. J. Med.* 271:120.

Burn, G. P. 1953. *Brit. Med. J.* 1:697.

Burnstock, G., Gannon, B., and Iwayama, T. 1970. *Circ. Research* suppl. II, 26-27:5.

Carlsson, A. 1966. In *Antihypertensive Therapy,* F. Gross (Ed.), Springer-Verlag, New York, p. 5.

Catt, K. J., Cain, M. D., Zimmet, P. Z., and Cran, E. 1969. *Brit. Med. J.* 1:819.

Cier, J. F., and Froment, A. 1965. *Pathol. Biol.* 13:1052.

Clark, D. W. J. 1969. *Proc. Univ. Otago Med. Sch.* 49:42.

Clarke, D. E., Smookler, H. H., and Barry, H., III. 1970. *Life Sci.* part I, 9:1097.

Clineschmidt, B. V., Geller, R. G., Govier, W. C., and Sjoerdsma, A. 1970. *Europ. J. Pharmacol.* 10:45.

Costa, E., Boullin, D. J., Hammer, W., Vogel, W., and Brodie, B. 1966. *Pharmacol. Rev.* 18:577.

Crout, J. R., Pisano, J. J., and Sjoerdsma, A. 1961. *Am. Heart J.* 61:375.

Dahl, L. K. 1961. *Am. J. Cardiol.* 8:571.

Dahl, L. K., Heine, M., and Tassinari, L. 1962a. *J. Exptl. Med.* 115:1173.

Dahl, L. K., Smilay, M. G., Silver, H., and Sparagen, S. 1962b. *Circ. Research* 10:313.

Daly, J. J., and Duff, R. S. 1960. *Clin. Sci.* 19:457.

Daniel, E. E., and Dawkins, O. 1957. *Am. J. Physiol.* 190:71.

Daniel, E. E., Paton, D. M., Taylor, G. S., and Hodgson, B. J. 1970. *Fed. Proc.* 29:1410.

Dawson, J., and Bone, A. 1963. *Brit. J. Psychiat.* 109:629.

de Champlain, J., Krakoff, L. R., and Axelrod, J. 1966. *Life Sci.* 5:2283.

de Champlain, J., Krakoff, L. R., and Axelrod, J. 1967. *Circ. Research* 20:136.

de Champlain, J., Krakoff, L. R., and Axelrod, J. 1968a. *Circ. Research* 23:479.

de Champlain, J., Krakoff, L. R., and Axelrod, J. 1968b. *Circ. Research* 23:361.

de Champlain, J., Krakoff, L. R., and Axelrod, J. 1969a. *Circ. Research* suppl. I, 24-25:75.

de Champlain, J., Mueller, R. A., and Axelrod, J. 1969b. *Circ. Research* 25:285.

de Champlain, J., Malmfors, T., Olson, L., and Sachs, C. 1970. *Acta Physiol. Scand.* 80:276.

de Champlain, J. 1970. In L-*DOPA and Parkinsonism,* A. Barbeau and F. H. McDowell (Eds.), F. A. Davis Co., Philadelphia, p. 269.

de Champlain, J. 1971. *Can. J. Physiol. Pharmacol.* 49:345.

de Champlain, J., and Nadeau, R. 1971. *Fed. Proc.* 30:877.

Demura, H., Fukuchi, S., Takahashi, H., and Goto, K. 1965. *Tohoku J. Exptl. Med.* 86:366.

De Quattro, V., and Sjoerdsma, A. 1968. *J. Clin. Invest.* 47:2359.

De Quattro, V., Nagatsu, T., Maronde, R., and Alexander, N. 1969. *Circ. Research* 24:545.

De Schaepdryver, A. F., and Leroy, J. G. 1961. *Acta Cardiol.* (Brus.) 16:631.

Dock, W., Shidler, F., and Moy, B. 1942. *Am. Heart J.* 23:513.

Dorr, L. B., and Brody, M. J. 1964. *Clin. Res.* 12:362.

Doyle, A. E., and Smirk, F. H. 1955. *Circulation* 12:543.

Doyle, A. E., Fraser, J. R. E., and Marshall, R. J. 1968. *Clin. Sci.* 18:441.

Doyle, A. E. 1968. *Lancet* 1:1399.

Edis, A. J., and Shepherd, J. T. 1970. *Arch. Intern. Med.* (Chicago) 125:716.

Eide, I., and Aars, H. 1969. *Nature* (Lond.) 222:571.

Engelman, K., Portnoy, B., and Sjoerdsma, A. 1970. *Circ. Research* suppl. I, 26-27:141.

Falck, B., Hillarp, N.-A., Thieme, G., and Torp, A. 1962. *J. Histochem. Cytochem.* 10:348.

Faradin, I., Benko, A., Winter, M., and Botos, A. 1961. *Experientia* 17:225.

Finch, L., and Leach, G. D. H. 1970a. *Brit. J. Pharmacol.* 39:317.

Finch, L., and Leach, G. D. H. 1970b. *Europ. J. Pharmacol.* 11:388.

Finkielman, S., Worcel, M., and Agrest, A. 1961. *Circulation* 31:356.

Freed, S. C. 1961. *Am. J. Cardiol.* 8:737.

Friedman, S. M., Nakashima, M., and Friedman, C. L. 1963. *Circ. Research* 13:223.

Frohlich, E. D., Tarazi, R. C., and Dustan, H. P. 1969. *Am. J. Med. Sci.* 257:9.

Fukuchi, S., Hanata, M., Takahashi, H., Demura, H., and Torikai, T. 1964. *Tohoku J. Exptl. Med.* 84:125.

Genest, J., de Champlain, J., Veyrat, R., Boucher, R., Tremblay, G. Y., Strong, C. G., Koiw, E., and Marc-Aurèle, J. 1965. *Circ. Research* suppl. II, 17:97.

Gill, J. R., Mason, D. T., and Bartter, F. C. 1964. *J. Clin. Invest.* 43:177.

Gillis, C. N., and Paton, D. M. 1967. *Brit. J. Pharmacol. Chemother.* 29:309.

Gitlow, S. E., Mendlowitz, M., Khassis, S., Cohen, G., and Sha, J. 1960. *J. Clin. Invest.* 39:221.

Gitlow, S. E., Mendlowitz, M., Wilk, E. K., Wilk, S., Wolf, R. L., and Naftchi, N. E. 1964. *J. Clin. Invest.* 43:2009.

Gitlow, S. E., Mendlowitz, M., Bertani, L. M., Wilk, E. K., and Glabman, S. 1969. *J. Lab. Clin. Med.* 73:129.

Glenn, F., Child, C. G., and Page, I. 1938. *Am. J. Physiol.* 122:506.

Goldblatt, H., Lynch, J., Hanzal, R. F., and Summerville, W. W. 1934. *J. Exptl. Med.* 59:347.

Goldenberg, M., Pines, K. L., Baldwin, E. F., Greene, D. G., and Roh, C. E. 1948. *Am. J. Med.* 5:792.

Goldenberg, M., Serlin, I., Edwards, I., and Rapport, M. M. 1954. *Am. J. Med.* 16:310.

Goodall, M., and Bogdonoff, M. 1961. *Am. Heart J.* 61:640.

Goodall, McC., Harlan, W. R., and Alton, H. 1968. *Circulation* 38:592.

Gordon, D. B., and Nogueira, A. 1962. *Circ. Research* 10:269.

Graham, J. D. P., Lever, J. D., and Spriggs, T. L. B. 1970. *Circ. Research* suppl. II, 26-27:25.

Green, A. F. 1962. *Advances Pharmacol.* 1:161.

Greisman, S. E. 1952. *J. Clin. Invest.* 31:782.

Griffiths, W. J., and Collison, S. 1957. *J. Clin. Path.* 10:120.

Grollman, A., Harrison, T. R., and Williams, J. R., Jr. 1943. *Am. J. Physiol.* 139:293.

Gross, F., and Schmidt, H. 1958. *Arch. Exptl. Path. Pharmak.* 233:311.

Gross, F., Brunner, H., and Ziegler, M. 1965. *Recent Prog. Hormone Res.* 21:119.

Guyton, A. C., Coleman, T. G., Fourcade, J. C., and Navar, L. G. 1969. *Bull. N.Y. Acad. Med.* 45:811.

Haebara, H., Ichijima, K., Tetsuzo, M., and Okamoto, K. 1968. *Jap. Circ. J.* 32:1391.

Hagemeijer, F., Rorive, G., and Schoffeniels, E. 1966. *Arch. Int. Physiol.* 74:807.

Halley, H. L., Elliott, H. C., Jr., and Holland, C. M., Jr. 1951. *Proc. Soc. Exptl. Biol. Med.* 77:561.

Hansen, J. 1968. *Acta Med. Scand.* 184:517.

Hathaway, P. W., Brehm, M. L., Clapp, J. R., and Bogdonoff, M. D. 1969. *Psychosom. Med.* 31:20.

Headings, V. E., and Rondell, P. 1964. *Univ. Michigan Med. Center J.* 30:167.

Hedeland, H., Dymling, J.-F., and Hokfelt, B. 1969. *Acta Endocr.* 62:399.

Hedwall, P. R. 1969. *Brit. J. Pharmacol.* 34:623.

Henning, M. 1969. *J. Pharm. Pharmacol.* 21:61.

Henningsen, B. 1969. *Z. Ges. Exp. Med.* 150:194.

Hickler, R. B., Hamlin, J. T., III, and Wells, R. E., Jr. 1959. *Circulation* 20:422.

Hill, R. W., Chester, J. E., and Wisenbaugh, P. E. 1970. *Lab. Invest.* 22:404.

Hinke, J. A. M. 1965. *Circ. Research* 17:359.

Hinke, J. A. M. 1966. *Circ. Research* suppl. I, 18-19:23.

Hirano, I. 1969. *Sapporo Med. J.* 36:159.

Hokfelt, B., Hedeland, H., and Dymling, J.-F. 1970. *Europ. J. Pharmacol.* 10:389.

Hollander, W., Kramsch, D. M., Farnelant, M., and Madoff, I. M. 1968. *J. Clin. Invest.* 47:1221.

Holz, P., Credner, K., and Kroneberg, G. 1947. *Arch. Exptl. Path. u. Pharmakol.* 204:228.

Hoobler, S. W., Agrest, A., and Warzynski, R. J. 1954. *J. Clin. Invest.* 33:943.

Horst, W. D., Kopin, I. J., and Ramey, E. R. 1968. *Am. J. Physiol.* 215:817.
Ichijima, K. 1969. *Jap. Circ. J.* 33:785.
Ikoma, T. 1965a. *Jap. Circ. J.* 29:1269.
Ikoma, T. 1965b. *Jap. Circ. J.* 29:1279.
Iversen, L. L., and Kravitz, E. A. 1966. *Mal. Pharmacol.* 2:360.
Iversen, L. L., de Champlain, J., Glowinski, J., and Axelrod, J. 1967. *J. Pharmacol. Exptl. Ther.* 157:509.
Jackson, W. B. 1958. *Am. Heart J.* 56:222.
Johnston, C. I., Hutchinson, J. S., and Mendelsohn, F. A. 1970. *Circ. Research* suppl. II, 26-27:215.
Kato, M., and Komata, K. 1969. *Tohoku J. Exp. Med.* 97:213.
Kazda, S., Pohlova, I., Bibr, B., and Kockova, J. 1969. *Am. J. Physiol.* 216:1472.
Keen, P. M., and Bogdanski, D. F. 1970. *Am. J. Physiol.* 219:677.
Knudsen, K. D., and Dahl, L. K. 1966. *Postgrad. Med. J.* 42:148.
Koletsky, S., Resnik, H., and Behrin, D. 1959. *Proc. Soc. Exptl. Biol. Med.* 102:12.
Koletsky, S., and Pritchard, W. H. 1963. *Circ. Research* 13:552.
Krakoff, L. R., de Champlain, J., and Axelrod, J. 1967. *Circ. Research* 21:583.
Kuchel, O., Cuche, J. L., Barbeau, A., Brecht, M., Boucher, R., and Genest, J. 1970. In l-*DOPA and Parkinsonism,* A. Barbeau and F. H. McDowell (Eds.), F. A. Davis Co., Philadelphia, p. 293.
Laverty, R. 1961. *Proc. Univ. Otago Med. Sch.* 39:23.
Laverty, R., and Smirk, F. H. 1961. *Circ. Research* 9:455.
Lee, R. E., and Holze, E. A. 1951. *J. Clin. Invest.* 30:539.
Lefer, L. G., and Ayers, C. R. 1969. *Proc. Soc. Exptl. Biol. Med.* 132:278
Linna, M. I., Aho, A., Pekkarinen, A., and Salmivalli, M. L. 1965. *Acta Pharmacol. et Toxicol.* 22:319.
Louis, W. J., Spector, S., Tabei, R., and Sjoerdsma, A. 1968. *Lancet* 1:1013.
Louis, W. J., Spector, S., Tabei, R., and Sjoerdsma, A. 1969a. *Circ. Research* 24:85.
Louis, W. J., Tabei, R., Spector, S., and Sjoerdsma, A. 1969b. *Circ. Research* suppl. I, 24-25:93.
Louis, W. J., Tabei, R., Sjoerdsma, A., and Spector, S. 1969c. *Lancet* 1:1035.
Louis, W. J. 1970. *Circ. Research* suppl. II, 26-27:49.
Louis, W. J., Krauss, K. R., Kopin, I. J., and Sjoerdsma, A. 1970. *Circ. Research* 27:589.
Lowe, R. D., and Scroop, G. C. 1970. *Am. Heart J.* 79:562.
Lucchesi, B. R., and Whitsitt, L. S.1969. *Prog. Cardiovasc. Dis.* 11:410.
Mallov, S. 1959. *Circ. Research* 7:196.
Malmejac, J. 1964. *Physiol. Rev.* 44:186.
Malmfors, T., and Sachs, C. 1968. *Europ. J. Pharmacol.* 3:89.
Manger, W. M. 1962. *Am. J. Cardiol.* 9:731.
Maruyama, T. 1969. *Jap. Circ. J.* 33:1271.
Matsumoto, M. 1969. *Jap. Circ. J.* 33:411.
McCubbin, J. W., and Page, I. H. 1963. *Circ. Research* 12:553.
McGregor, D. D., and Smirk, F. H. 1968. *Am. J. Physiol.* 214:1429.
McKusick, V. A. 1960. *Circulation* 22:857.
McQueen, E. G. 1956. *Clin. Sci.* 15:523.
Mellander, S., and Johansson, B. 1968. *Pharm. Rev.* 20:117.
Mendlowitz, M., and Naftchi, N. 1958. *J. Appl. Physiol.* 13:247.
Mendlowitz, M. 1967. *Am. Heart J.* 73:121.

Miller, N. E. 1969. *Science* 163:434.

Moerman, E. J., Herman, A. G., Bogaert, M. G., and de Schaepdryver, A. F. 1969. *Arch. Int. Pharmacodyn.* 178:492.

Moller, P., Buus, D., and Bierring, E. 1957. *Scand. J. Clin. Lab. Invest.* 9:331.

Morisawa, T. 1968a. *Jap. Circ. J.* 32:161.

Morisawa, T. 1968b. *Jap. Circ. J.* 32:177.

Moulton, R., Spencer, A. G., and Willoughby, D. A. 1958. *Brit. Heart J.* 20:224.

Mueller, R. A., Thoenen, H., and Axelrod, J. 1969. *Science* 163:468.

Nagaoka, A., Kikuchi, K., and Aramaki, Y. 1969. *Jap. J. Pharmacol.* 19:462.

Neff, N. H., Ngai, S. H., Wang, C. T., and Costa, E. 1969. *Mol. Pharmacol.* 5:90.

Nestel, P. J., and Doyle, A. E. 1968. *Austr. Ann. Med.* 17:295.

Nestel, P. J. 1969. *Lancet* 1:692.

Nestel, P. J., and Esler, M. D. 1970. *Circ. Research* suppl. II, 26-27:75.

Nolla-Panades, J. 1963. *Circ. Research* 12:3.

Nolla-Panades, J., and Smirk, F. H. 1964. *Austr. Ann. Med.* 13:320.

Norberg, K.-A. 1967. *Brain Research* 5:125.

Ogden, E., Collings, W. D., and Saperstein, L. A. 1946. *Exptl. Hypertension* 3:153.

Okamoto, K., Nosaka, S., Yamori, Y., and Matsumoto, M. 1967. *Jap. Heart J.* 8:168.

Okamoto, K. 1969. *Int. Rev. Exptl. Pathol.* 7:227.

Oono, Y. 1966. *Jap. Circ. J.* 30:267.

Overy, H. R., Pfister, R., and Chidsey, C. A. 1967. *J. Clin. Invest.* 46:482.

Ozaki, M. 1966. *Jap. J. Pharmacol.* 16:257.

Ozaki, M., Suzuki, Y., Yamori, Y., and Okamoto, K. 1968. *Jap. Circ. J.* 32:1367.

Page, I. H. 1963. *Arch. Int. Med.* 111:103.

Page, I. H., Kanebo, Y., and McCubbin, J. W. 1966. *Circ. Research* 18:379.

Page, I. H., and McCubbin, J. W. 1968. In *Renal Hypertension,* Chicago Year Book Medical Publishers Inc., Chicago.

Panagiotis, N. M., and Hungerford, G. F. 1966. *Nature* (Lond.) 211:374.

Peart, W. S. 1965. *Recent Prog. Hormone Research* 21:73.

Pekkarinen, A., and Pitkanen, M. E. 1955. *Scand. J. Lab. Clin. Invest.* 7:8.

Phelan, E. L. 1968. *New Zealand Med. J.* 67:334.

Phelan, E. L., and Wong, L. C. K. 1968. *Clin. Sci.* 35:487.

Phelan, E. L. 1970. *Circ. Research* suppl. II, 26-27:65.

Platt, R. 1963. *Lancet* I: 899.

Potter, L., and Axelrod, J. 1963. *J. Pharmacol. Exptl. Ther.* 142:299.

Raab, W. 1959. *Am. J. Cardiol.* 4:752.

Redleaf, P. D., and Tobian, L. 1958. *Circ. Research* 6:185.

Ritzel, G., and Hunzinger, N. A. 1963. *Klin. Wschr.* 14:419.

Robertson, A. A., Hodge, J. V., Laverty, R., and Smirk, F. H. 1968. *Austr. J. Exptl. Biol. Med. Sci.* 46:689.

Ross, E. J. 1956. *Clin. Sci.* 15:81.

Rubin, R. P. 1969. *J. Physiol.* 202:197.

Sachs, C., de Champlain, J., Malmfors, T., and Olson, L. 1970. *Europ. J. Pharm.* 9:67.

Scornik, O. A., and Paladini, A. C. 1959. *Am. J. Physiol.* 201:526.

Selye, H., Hall, C. E., and Rowley, E. M. 1943. *Can. Med. Ass. J.* 49:88.

Serrano, P. A., Figueroa, G., Tores, M. Z., and Raminez del Angel, A. 1964. *Am. J. Cardiol.* 13:484.

Sivertsson, R. 1970. *Acta Physiol. Scand.* suppl. 343:1.

Sjoerdsma, A. 1961. *Circ. Research* 9:734.
Skelton, F. R., and Brownie, A. C. 1967. *Meth. Achivm. Exp. Path.* 2:257.
Smirk, F. H., and Phelan, E. L. 1965. *J. Path. Bact.* 89:57.
Smirk, F. H. 1970. *Circ. Research* suppl. II, 26-27:55.
Spector, S., Fleisch, J. H., Maling, H. M., and Brodie, B. B. 1969. *Science* 166:1300.
Stjarne, L., and von Euler, U. S. 1965. *J. Pharmacol. Exptl. Ther.* 150:335.
Stott, A. W., and Robinson, R. 1967. *Clin. Chim. Acta* 16:249.
Sunderman, F. W., Jr., Cleveland, P. D., Law, N. C., and Sunderman, F. W. 1960. *Am. J. Clin. Path.* 34:293.
Sundin, T. 1956. *Acta Med. Scand.* suppl. 313, 154:48.
Tabei, R. 1966. *Jap. Circ. J.* 30:717.
Taquini, A. C. 1963. *Circ. Research* 12:562.
Thant, M., Yamori, Y., and Okamoto, K. 1969. *Jap. Circ. J.* 33:501.
Tobian, L., and Binion, J. T. 1952. *Circulation* 5:754.
Tobian, L., and Binion, J. T. 1954. *J. Clin. Invest.* 33:1407.
Tobian, L., and Redleaf, P. D. 1958. *Am. J. Physiol.* 192:325.
Tobian, L. 1960. *Physiol. Rev.* 40:280.
Tobian, L., and Duke, M. 1969. *Am. J. Physiol.* 217:522.
Tominaga, T. 1961. *J. Jap. Soc. Intern. Med.* 50:560.
Tranzer, J. P., and Thoenen, H. 1967. *Arch. Pharmacol. Exptl. Path.* 257:343.
Trendelenburg, U. 1965. *Pharmacol. Rev.* 15:225.
Udenfriend, S. 1966. *Pharmacol. Rev.* 18:43.
Van Cauwenberge, H., and Rorive, G. 1969. *Acquis. Med. Recent* p. 219.
Varma, D. R. 1967. *J. Pharm. Pharmacol.* 19:61.
Villamil, M. F., Nachev, P., and Kleeman, C. R. 1970. *Am. J. Physiol.* 218:1281.
Volicer, L., Scheer, R., Hilse, H., and Visweswaram, D. 1968. *Life Sci.* 7:525.
Volicer, L., and Visweswaram, D. 1970. *Life Sci.* 9:651.
Von Eiff, A. W. 1970. *Jap. Circ. J.* 34:147.
von Euler, U. S., Hellner, S., and Burkhold, A. 1954. *Scand. J. Clin. Lab. Invest.* 6:54.
von Euler, U. S. 1956. *Noradrenaline: Chemistry, Physiology and Pharmacology and Clinical Aspects,* Charles C Thomas, Springfield, Ill.
Von Studnitz, W. 1960. *J. Clin. Lab. Invest.* suppl. 48, 12:3.
Wegmann, A., Kako, K., and Bing. R. J. 1962. *Am. J. Physiol.* 203:607.
Weiser, R. A., Johnson, A. G., and Hoobler, S. W. 1969. *Lab. Invest.* 20:326.
Westfall, T. C., and Osada, H. 1969. *J. Pharm. Exptl. Ther.* 167:300.
Willard, P. W., and Fuller, R. W. 1969. *Nature* 223:417.
Wolf, R. L., Mendlowitz, M., Roboz, J., and Gitlow, S. E. 1965. *New Engl. J. Med.* 273:1459.
Yamori, Y., and Okamoto, K. 1969. *Jap. Circ. J.* 33:509.
Yamori, Y., Lovenberg, W., and Sjoerdsma, A. 1970. *Science* 170:544.
Yoshinaga, K., Sato, T., and Ishida, N. 1960. *Tohoku J. Exptl. Med.* 72:301.
Zimmerman, B. G. 1967. *J. Pharmacol. Exptl. Ther.* 158:1.
Zimmerman, B. G., and Gisslen, J. 1968. *J. Pharmacol. Exptl. Ther.* 163:320.
Zimmerman, B. G., Rolewicz, T. F., Dunham, E. W., and Gisslen, J. L. 1969. *Am. J. Physiol.* 217:798.
Zweifach, B. W., Rosenfeld, S., and Shorr, E. 1948. *Fed. Proc.* 7:139.

9

Influence of Neuronal and Extraneuronal Uptake on Disposition, Metabolism, and Potency of Catecholamines

GEORG HERTTING
JOSEF SUKO

During the last fifteen years, the availability of new biochemical and histochemical methods as well as electronmicroscopy has allowed a more thorough investigation of the function of the sympathetic nervous system. In addition, their combination with the methods of classical pharmacology led to a further elucidation of the various components influencing adrenergic mechanisms. The analysis of the modes of action of drugs upon sympathetic nervous function helped to reveal the possible sites of action of these drugs as well as the interaction of the various functional activities of sympathetic nerves. The use of isolated organs or subcellular structures eliminated the influence of many other interfering processes and permitted a more quantitative investigation of the single parameters of catecholamine synthesis, uptake, metabolism, release, and functional response. In addition drugs with a known mechanism of action could be used as tools to block some of these specific components and thus made possible the analysis of a previously masked mechanism. Quantitative differences between one or more of these parameters found in different tissues might reflect the adjustment of this regulatory system to the needs of the specific organ function. The knowledge of sympathetic mechanisms obtained in detail from *in vitro* experiments provides a basis for the understanding of the function of the sympathetic nervous system *in vivo*. It should be kept in mind that *in vivo* this system is under the additional control of centers, which integrate information of the functional status of the systems involved (for example, circulation, body temperature).

267

These control mechanisms maintain the organ function optimally adjusted to the momentaneous needs.

The present chapter will deal with the uptake processes of catecholamines associated with either adrenergic nerves or extraneuronal uptake sites in peripheral tissues. In addition, the main emphasis will lie on the interaction of uptake, binding, metabolism, and functional response to catecholamines. Since excellent comprehensive reviews have been published covering these subjects (Axelrod, 1963, 1965; Axelrod et al., 1969; Norberg et al., 1964; Stjärne, 1964; Kopin, 1964; Malmfors, 1965; Second Symposium on Catecholamines, 1966; Holtz et al., 1966; Iversen, 1967; Trendelenburg, 1963, 1969; Costa et al., 1970), this paper will discuss in greater detail some of the work done in our laboratory during the last years.

Historical Remarks

One of the first experiments, to our knowledge, that pointed to a neuronal uptake of catecholamines was performed as early as in 1932: Burn observed in the isolated, perfused hindleg of the dog a restoration of the vasoconstrictor effects after stimulation of the sympathetic chain following the infusion of epinephrine (E). It was of course impossible at that time to interpret this observation by replenishment of exhausted stores of a neurotransmitter.

After von Euler had established the role of norepinephrine (NE) as the transmitter of the sympathetic nervous system in mammals (von Euler, 1948; von Euler et al., 1956) the NE-depleting property of reserpine (Bertler et al., 1956) offered a promising tool for the study of the sympathetic nervous system. Thus, by using reserpine, Burn et al. (1958) showed that stimulation of sympathetic nerve fibers failed to cause vasoconstriction on the dog hindleg preparation. However, the response of the nerve stimulation was restored after perfusion of the hindleg with NE. The interpretation of this finding by the authors was that NE could accumulate in the drug-depleted postganglionic sympathetic fibers and so restore their function.

Axelrod and coworkers using tritium-labelled catecholamines demonstrated that injected NE as well as E was rapidly removed from the circulation and accumulated preferentially in organs as spleen, salivary glands, heart, and adrenals; a fraction of both catecholamines intravenously injected is almost instantly metabolized by catechol-O-methyl transferase (COMT) (Axelrod et al., 1959; Whitby et al., 1961). After being taken up the catecholamines were protected against metabolism and disappeared slowly from these organs.

The uptake of NE and E into tissues was markedly diminished by chronic postganglionic sympathetic denervation, suggesting the neuronal localization of the sites of uptake (Hertting et al., 1961a). It has been known for a long time that chronic, postganglionic sympathetic denervation leads to supersensitivity towards catecholamines (Cannon et al., 1949). Both observations were combined and it was concluded that uptake of circulating catecholamines is a very effective mechanism of inactivation, which limits the concentration of the free and active hormone at the receptor sites. Lack of uptake results in the persistence of higher catecholamine concentrations on the receptor sites, thus producing supersensitivity (Hertting et al., 1961a). Similarly cocaine, also known to produce supersensitivity towards catecholamines, was shown to inhibit uptake of NE into tissues with a high uptake capacity and consecutively to elevate NE blood levels (Whitby et al., 1960; Muscholl, 1960a, 1961).

It was shown that a number of drugs were capable of producing changes in NE tissue content and blood levels (Hertting et al., 1961b). When the drugs were given before the ^{3}H-NE was injected or after the amine had already been bound, it was possible to distinguish between "inhibition of uptake" and "release from binding sites" (Axelrod et al., 1962a). ^{3}H-NE, previously taken up, was released by sympathetic stimulation (Hertting et al., 1961c), suggesting that the uptake process was not merely a mechanism of inactivation but that it enabled the sympathetic neuron to reuse the transmitter in a very economic way. It was shown by Muscholl (1960b) and Dengler et al. (1961) that the incorporation of exogenous NE into tissues was due to a net uptake and not to an exchange with the endogenous transmitter.

Kinetic studies of the NE uptake process on tissue slices (Dengler et al., 1961) or the isolated perfused rat heart (Kopin et al., 1962a) demonstrated the presence of an active transport mechanism which accumulates the NE against a concentration gradient. The data from the experiments with the isolated perfused hearts suggested that the NE, after being taken up, is distributed into at least two different pools of different sizes and different turnover rates. In hearts pretreated with reserpine the NE, after being taken up, was deaminated before leaving the tissue.

This basic concept of the function of the postganglionic sympathetic nerves and the fate of their transmitter, based on these early findings, has since then been refined, completed, and extended by the work of numerous laboratories using different approaches to the problems. Many additional factors influencing the function of the sympathetic neuron as well as transmitter receptor interaction were established later, without substantially affecting this early concept.

Properties of the Sympathetic Neuron

Peripheral tissues contain all the enzymes necessary for the complete synthesis of the neurotransmitter NE (Chidsey et al., 1963a; Spector et al., 1963; Levitt et al., 1965; Roth et al., 1966a); the enzymes are located within the sympathetic neuron. Tyrosine hydroxylase has been suggested as the rate limiting step in NE synthesis (Levitt et al., 1965). Increase of noradrenaline utilization for a short time induced by a variety of pharmacological and other stimuli results in an immediate elevation of catecholamine synthesis due to an increased tyrosine hydroxylase activity (Roth et al., 1966a; Spector et al., 1967; Neff et al., 1966). This rapid adaption seems to be caused by a diminished end-product feedback inhibition and is not accompanied by an increase in the amount of enzyme *in vitro*. However, chronic sympatho-adrenal stimulation induced by such drugs as reserpine, 6-hydroxydopamine, or phenoxybenzamine resulted in an elevation of NE synthesis due to an increase in enzyme protein of tyrosine hydroxylase in adrenals and sympathetic ganglia (Mueller et al., 1969a; Mueller et al., 1969b). This enzyme induction is mediated trans-synaptically (Thoenen et al., 1969). The end-product of the synthesis, NE, is then stored in the granules or dense core vesicles of the sympathetic nerves (von Euler et al., 1965; Schümann, 1958; Potter et al., 1962a; Carlsson, 1965). These storage granules of sympathetic nerves are formed in the cell body and then transported down the axon to the terminals, where they are packed in the varicosities (Dahlström, 1966). There is an active transport of catecholamines into the granules, which is temperature-sensitive, stimulated by ATP and Mg^{++} ions and inhibited by reserpine (von Euler and Lishajko, 1963a; von Euler et al., 1963b; Stjärne, 1964). This intragranular NE is in balance with the extragranular but intraneuronal NE pool (Stjärne, 1964). Different compartments of the whole intraneuronal NE have been postulated according to different uptake rates (Iversen, 1963), different turnover rates (Axel-rod et al., 1961; Kopin et al., 1962a; Montanari et al., 1963; Brodie et al., 1966; Neff et al., 1969), different behavior towards releasing agents (Chidsey et al., 1963b; Crout, 1964; Potter et al., 1962b; Potter et al., 1963a; Stjärne, 1964), and different metabolic pathways of the NE re-leased (Kopin et al., 1962a; Kopin et al., 1962b; Kopin, 1964). Appar-ently the newly synthesized NE is associated with an available pool, since it is preferentially released by nerve stimulation (Kopin et al., 1968; Stjärne et al., 1970a). Monoamine oxidase (MAO), the enzyme respon-sible for deamination of NE, is mainly localized in mitochondria as shown for liver (Cotzias et al., 1951), adrenal gland (Blaschko et al., 1955), and brain (Bogdanski et al., 1957). On the other hand, in hearts, salivary glands (de Champlain et al., 1969), and splenic nerves (Roth et al., 1966b) MAO activity is also associated with microsomal fractions, indi-cating differences of the subcellular distribution of MAO in various tis-sues. In many tissues the MAO localized in sympathetic fibers represents only a minor portion of the total MAO activity. Under these circum-stances only small or negligible changes in total MAO activity can be detected after sympathetic denervation (Snyder et al., 1965; Potter et al., 1965), immunosympathectomy (Klingman, 1966), and 6-hydroxydopa-mine (Lowe et al., 1970). COMT, the enzyme mainly responsible for metabolic inactivation of circulating NE (Axelrod, 1959), is distributed in the cell sap of tissues and localized extraneuronally; however, an intra-neuronal localization has been postulated in brain (Alberici et al., 1965).

Neuronal uptake is referred to as transfer of NE across the neuronal membrane. This process seems to be mediated by an active transport mechanism as indicated by inhibition with metabolic inhibitors and tem-perature dependence (Kirpekar et al., 1968; Wakade et al., 1968).

Furthermore, the absolute requirement of sodium ions for the uptake process (Iversen et al., 1966; Bogdanski et al., 1966, 1969; Kirpekar et al., 1968; Horst et al., 1968), the inhibition by ouabain (Dengler et al., 1961), as well as high potassium (Bogdanski et al., 1969) concentration, suggests a possible link of the uptake system to the sodium pump of the axonal membrane (Bogdanski et al., 1969). The neuronal uptake process ("membrane pump") is kinetically characterized by a high affinity to NE but low capacity—"uptake I" (Iversen, 1963)—and becomes saturated at low amine concentrations.

This uptake mechanism operates most efficiently at the sympathetic nerve terminals, but is considerably less efficient on the axon membrane, where diffusion is of increasing importance (Stjärne et al., 1970b). A considerable amount of NE released by stimuli from the postganglionic sympathetic fiber is reaccumulated by the uptake process (Brown, 1965). In the nictitating membrane, blockade of neuronal uptake by cocaine potentiates the effect of NE released by nerve stimulation (Haefely et al., 1964). From the degree of potentiation these authors calculated that 95 per cent of released NE is inactivated by re-uptake. Re-uptake represents an economic way of maintaining the transmitter concentration within the intraneuronal pools. Endogenous NE does not seem to originate solely from the local synthesis within the sympathetic neuron. According to Kopin et al. (1963), 20 per cent of endogenous NE in the heart is derived by extraction from the plasma. Thus uptake and re-uptake of the transmitter are not only mechanisms of inactivation of liberated NE but in addition contribute to the maintenance of the intraneuronal stores.

The uptake process is markedly influenced by the perfusion rate of a tissue. The amount of injected NE taken up from the circulation is inversely related to the perfusion rate, as demonstrated on the isolated spleen (Hertting et al., 1963; Paton et al., 1965). The amount of NE leaving the spleen after electrical stimulation of the splenic nerves increases with the perfusion rate. When vasoconstriction is induced in an isolated spleen preparation shortly before nerve stimulation, practically no NE appears in the splenic outflow during and following stimulation. Therefore drugs which modify the perfusion rate of a tissue by changing blood pressure or peripheral vascular resistance will indirectly influence the rate of uptake or re-uptake of NE (Hertting, 1965). Neuronal uptake blockade accomplished by different means leads to an increase in sensitivity of these tissues towards NE and E. The coincidence of uptake blockade with supersensitivity has been shown for surgical denervation on the spleen (Hertting et al., 1967), the heart (Potter et al., 1965), and the nictitating membrane (Smith et al., 1966). Similar results were obtained after immunosympathectomy (Zaimis et al., 1965) or chemical sympathectomy with 6-hydroxydopamine (Haeusler et al., 1968, 1969). When the neuronal uptake mechanism is efficiently blocked by drugs such as cocaine (Whitby et al., 1960; Muscholl, 1960a), tissues similarly become supersensitive to catecholamines. In analogy to the events on the motor endplate, the terminology of "presynaptic" or "postsynaptic" type of supersensitivity was also used for the different types of supersensitivity

to catecholamines (Trendelenburg, 1966). Supersensitivity due to elimination of neuronal uptake was called "presynaptic," whereas a supersensitivity that was seemingly induced by changes in the responsiveness of
the effector cells was named "postsynaptic." The degree of potentiation
of the functional response to sympathomimetic amines by uptake blockade
in a certain tissue is determined by the affinity of the specific amine to the
uptake sites and its affinity and intrinsic activity to the receptor sites. In
tissues with a dense sympathetic innervation it is to be expected that uptake blockade will produce a more marked potentiation than in poorly
innervated tissues, where other mechanisms of inactivation are predominant.

Intricate experimental designs have been used to evaluate the relative
importance of the various mechanisms of inactivation of the transmitter
for the development of tissue supersensitivity. However, very often the
terms "uptake," "storage," and "metabolism" were used to explain supersensitivity towards NE induced by various means, while only the changes
in the tissue response were determined. Therefore we designed experimental conditions which allow comparison of the parameters of inactivation
(either by uptake or metabolism) as well as the effects produced by NE
infusions of short duration almost instantly as they occur in the organ.

Experiments with the Isolated Spleen
Effect of Chronic Postganglionic Sympathetic
Denervation, Reserpine, Cocaine, and Tyramine on Uptake,
Metabolism, and Action of Infused Norepinephrine

The following text and figures summarize the essence of our work and
data of more than eighty perfusion experiments (Hertting et al., 1966a,b;
Hertting et al., 1967; Suko et al., 1966).

Spleens of cats were isolated, placed in a plethysmograph, and perfused
with a constant flow rate (6.5 ml/min) with Krebs-Ringer solution containing ascorbic acid to prevent breakdown of the NE in the oxygenated
perfusion medium. Changes in the volume of the spleen and perfusion
pressure were recorded. Tritium-labelled dl-NE was infused within 2
minutes in amounts of either 54, 108, 216, or 432 nanograms into the
arterial cannula, and the perfusate was collected in fractions during and
after the NE infusion for 29 minutes. At the end of the experiment the
tissue was homogenized in perchlorate acid. Total radioactivity (TA),

³H-norepinephrine-noradrenaline (³H-NE) and its metabolites were measured in the tissue and the perfusate.

The following figures show schematically the fate of the infused ³H-NE in the various experiments. The total radioactivity (TA) is the sum of the radioactivity found in tissues and perfusates, and has been set at 100 per cent. The isolated ³H-NE and ³H-NE metabolites in the perfusate, collected over a period of 30 minutes, are expressed as percentages of TA.

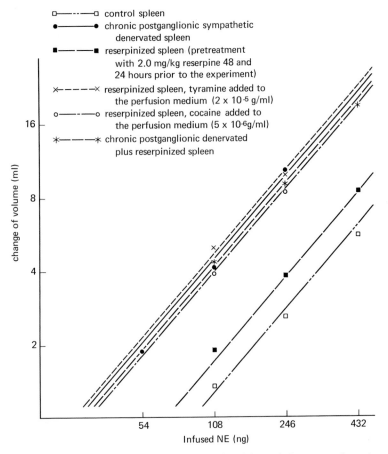

Figure 9-1   Spleens of cats were isolated, placed in a plethysmograph, and perfused at 37°C with Krebs-Ringer solution at a constant flow rate of 6.5 ml/min. dl-7-³H-norepinephrine (³H-NE) was infused into the arterial cannula within 2 minutes in amounts as indicated at the abscissa.

Although in some experiments there was a slight discrepancy between the sum of the identified compounds and the TA, the values listed in the figure have been corrected to add up to 100 per cent.

The parameter for the sensitivity of the preparations is the dose-response of the maximal changes in contraction volume (expressed in ml) to the different amounts of NE infused. The dose-response curve shows a linear regression in a double logarithmic system. The relative sensitivities were determined graphically (controls = 1.0), as seen at Fig. 9-1.

Maximal increase in sensitivity was seen after chronic postganglionic sympathetic denervation ("denervated spleen"). In these preparations the relative sensitivity was 3.0. The reserpinized spleen showed a small but significant increment in NE sensitivity to 1.3 only. Upon the addition of

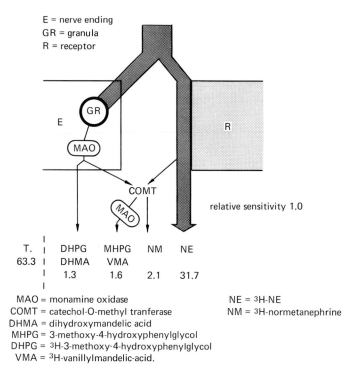

E = nerve ending
GR = granula
R = receptor

relative sensitivity 1.0

T.	DHPG	MHPG	NM	NE
63.3	DHMA	VMA		
	1.3	1.6	2.1	31.7

MAO = monamine oxidase   NE = 3H-NE
COMT = catechol-O-methyl tranferase   NM = 3H-normetanephrine
DHMA = dihydroxymandelic acid
MHPG = 3-methoxy-4-hydroxyphenylglycol
DHPG = 3H-3-methoxy-4-hydroxyphenylglycol
VMA = 3H-vanillylmandelic-acid.

Figure 9-2   Scheme of the fate of ^{3}H-NE infused into isolated perfused cat spleen (control). Values are expressed as per cent of radioactivity found in tissue (T) and perfusate. The perfusate was collected during and following ^{3}H-NE infusion for a period of 29 minutes. The relative sensitivity towards infused ^{3}H-NE of the control spleen was set arbitrarily at 1.0.

cocaine or tyramine to the perfusion medium of reserpinized spleens, the relative sensitivity of these organs was shifted to the maximum range as observed in denervated preparations. The relative sensitivity for reserpine-cocaine or reserpine-tyramine was 2.7 and 3.1, respectively. Cocaine did not further potentiate the response of the denervated spleens towards infused NE. The alteration in sensitivity observed either after denervation or after drugs was associated with a concomitant elevation of the concentration of NE in the corresponding perfusate sample.

Figure 9-2 shows the fate of ^{3}H-NE infused into the normal spleen. Of the ^{3}H-NE infused, 63.3 per cent of the radioactivity was found in the tissue at the end of the experiment, consisting exclusively of ^{3}H-NE; 31.7 per cent left the spleen unchanged; only small amounts of metabolites could be detected.

Figure 9-3 summarizes the results of spleens where the postganglionic sympathetic nerve fibers were cut 10 to 14 days prior to the experiment. The endogenous NE of these spleens decreased from 15.29 ± 1.32 μg/spleen to 0.22 ± 0.09 μg/spleen (1.44 %). Only 6.8 per cent of the infused activity was found in the perfused tissue, 84.9 per cent appeared unchanged in the perfusate.

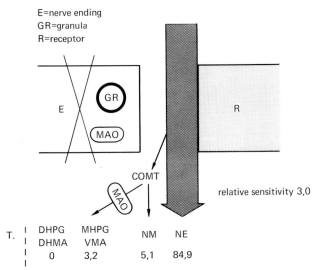

Figure 9-3   Scheme of the fate of ^{3}H-NE infused into chronic sympathetic denervated cat spleens. Experimental procedure and abbreviations as described in Figs. 9-1 and 9-2.

In innervated spleens of cats Gillespie et al. (1965) found 29 per cent of infused NE in the splenic outflow, in denervated organs over 80 per cent—values that are almost identical with ours.

There was a slight increase in the O-methylated metabolites, but neither dihydroxyphenylglycol nor dihydroxymandelic-acid was detectable. It can be deduced from the data of the denervated spleens that in this organ the sympathetic nerve terminals represent the mechanism responsible for the inactivation of physiological concentrations of NE. After their destruction greater concentrations of NE reach the receptor sites of the tissue and thus produce a greater action. The denervated spleens were 2.9 times as sensitive towards the infused NE as the normal tissue.

Spleens of the reserpine-treated animals (2.0 mg/kg 48 and 24 hours prior to the perfusion experiment; endogenous NE: 0.45 ± 0.05 μg/ spleen) retained 8.7 per cent of the infused activity only; 61.8 per cent of the ^{3}H-NE infused was found unchanged in the perfusate. But in contrast to the denervated or normal tissues, the NE also occurred in the fractions of the later sampling periods in considerable quantities; 21.4 per cent of the activity infused was identified as deaminated metabolites in the perfu-

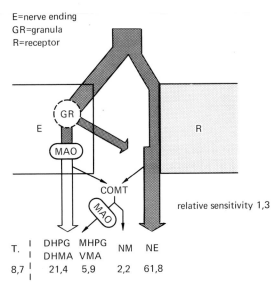

Figure 9-4   Scheme of the fate of ^{3}H-NE infused into isolated perfused spleens of reserpine-pretreated cats (2.0 mg/kg 48 and 24 hours prior to the experiment). Experimental procedure and abbreviations as in Figs. 9-1 and 9-2.

sate (Fig. 9-4). O-methylation, the sum of ³H-normetanephrine and the O-methylated-deaminated metabolites (³H-3-methoxy-4-hydroxyphenyl-glycol and ³H-vanillylmandelic-acid) had increased.

We interpret these findings as follows: The transport of NE across the neuronal membrane is either unimpaired or only slightly affected. Reserpine is known to interfere with the granular uptake and binding of NE (von Euler et al., 1963a; von Euler et al., 1963b; Stjärne, 1964). NE, which has been transported into the sympathetic nerve terminal, cannot be taken up into the granular stores and is therefore not protected against metabolic degradation by the intraneuronal MAO.

The intraneuronal MAO represents only a small fraction of the total MAO found in the tissue as shown by Klingman (1966) and Löwe et al. (1970). Because of the great efficiency of the neuronal uptake mechanism, which concentrates the substrate on the intraneuronally localized enzyme sites, this enzyme is almost exclusively responsible for the deamination of the transmitter, at least at physiological concentrations. A fraction of the NE, which has been taken up but not metabolized, leaks out from the nerves and appears in the later sampling portions. Because of lack of granular binding it seems possible that an intraneuronal gradi-

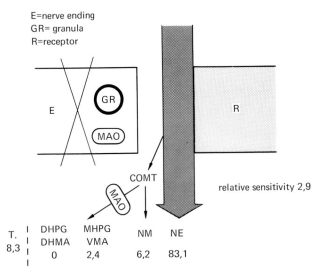

Figure 9-5 Scheme of the fate of ³H-NE infused into chronic sympathetic denervated cat spleens, pretreated with reserpine. Reserpine treatment as described in Fig. 9-4. Experimental procedure and abbreviations as in Figs. 9-1 and 9-2.

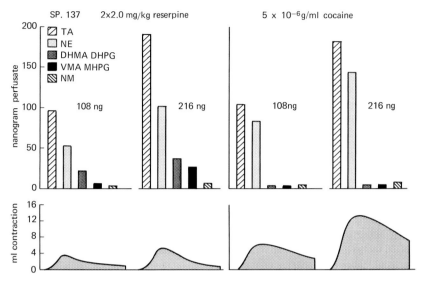

Figure 9-6   Total radioactivity (TA), ³H-NE, and ³H-NE metabolites in the per-fusate of an isolated perfused spleen of a reserpine-pretreated cat in the presence or absence of cocaine. Reserpine treatment as described in Fig. 9-4. Lower part: Contraction areas of the spleen recorded for 4 minutes. Upper part: 108 and 216 ng ³H-NE were infused within 2 minutes in the absence or presence of 5×10^{-6} g/ml cocaine in the perfusion medium. Bars represent the TA, ³H-NE, and ³H-NE metabolites of the perfusate collected for 29 min. following each infusion of ³H-NE.

ent of NE builds up, which in turn may decrease the transmembranal up-take (Trendelenburg et al., 1970). This mechanism could be responsible for the slight increase in sensitivity observed in our experiments in the reserpinized spleens.

When spleens are denervated prior to reserpine treatment, they cannot be differentiated with regard to sensitivity, pattern of metabolites, and distribution of activity in the corresponding perfusate samples from den-ervated, untreated tissues (Fig. 9-5). The denervated, reserpinized spleen shows the same degree of sensitivity towards NE, and the same pattern of metabolites, as the nonreserpinized denervated spleen. The effect of reserpine therefore, as demonstrated on NE metabolism, depends on the presence of the sympathetic neuron, provided that the neuronal NE uptake is unimpaired by other means. The figures of the following experiments should demonstrate these circumstances even more clearly.

Figure 9-6 shows a representative experiment of a series of reserpine-treated organs. Spleens received two consecutive infusions of 108 and 216 ng ^{3}H-NE, which were repeated in the presence of cocaine (5 $\times$ 10^{-6} g/ml) in the perfusion medium. The figure shows the contraction curves and the distribution of total radioactivity, ^{3}H-NE and its metabolites found in the perfusates, collected over the 29 minutes' sampling period. On the left side of the picture we find the typical characteristics of the reserpinized tissue already shown: the spleen cannot retain the infused ^{3}H-NE, most of the TA leaves the tissue to a large extent as deaminated metabolites. The blocking of the neuronal uptake by cocaine increases the tissue response and the amount of activity corresponding to the unchanged NE. Simultaneously, the deaminated metabolites decrease. However, the increase in the NE fraction produced by cocaine seems to be less pronounced than the increase in sensitivity.

The changes in TA and ^{3}H-NE uptake induced by cocaine in the re-

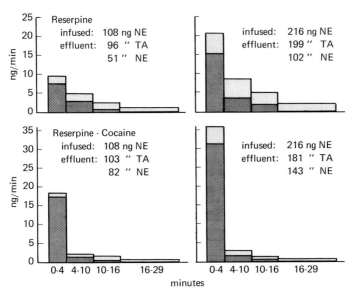

Figure 9-7 Total radioactivity and ^{3}H-NE in the various collection periods of the perfusate following ^{3}H-NE infusions into a reserpinized spleen in presence and absence of cocaine. The values are derived from the experiment given in Fig. 9-6. TA (black + white bars) and ^{3}H-NE (black bars) expressed as ng/NE-equivalents/min following the infusion of 108 and 216 ng ^{3}H-NE in the absence (upper part) and in the presence of 5 $\times$ 10^{-6} g/ml cocaine in the perfusion medium (lower part). The numbers represent the total amount of TA and ^{3}H-NE found in the perfusate, collected 29 minutes following each infusion of ^{3}H-NE.

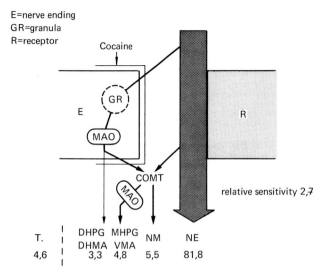

E=nerve ending
GR=granula
R=receptor

Figure 9-8   Scheme of the fate of ³H-NE infused into isolated perfused spleens of reserpine-pretreated cats in the presence of cocaine. Reserpine treatment as described in Fig. 9-4. Experimental procedure similar as described in Fig. 9-6. Abbreviations as described in Fig. 9-2.

serpinized spleen preparation become more related to the shift in NE sensitivity, when they are expressed as the rate of TA or NE leaving the spleen in the various subfractions. After infusion of ³H-NE for 2 minutes into a reserpinized spleen a considerable amount of TA and ³H-NE appears in the perfusate as late as 10 minutes (Fig. 9-7, upper part). The ³H-NE-metabolites (difference between TA and ³H-NE) represent a large part of activity in the effluent; their share increases in latter collection periods. In the presence of cocaine in the perfusion medium, ³H-NE leaves the spleen almost immediately during and shortly after the termination of the infusion. In addition the metabolites are markedly decreased (Fig. 9-7, lower part).

As compared with the corresponding fraction of the reserpinized tissue the ³H-NE practically doubles in the 4-minute fraction after the introduction of cocaine (32 ng versus 65 ng after the infusion of 108 ng; 66 ng versus 133 ng after the infusion of 216 ng). This is in accordance with the increase of the sensitivity of the spleen towards NE from 1.3 of the reserpinized preparation to 2.7 of the reserpinized-cocainized preparation. These events are picturized in the next figure (Fig. 9-8).

The neuronal uptake blocking property of cocaine is shared by a number of other compounds such as chlorpromazine, imipramine, desmethylimipramine, dibenzyline, bretylium, and guanethidine. Potentiation of the effects of administered NE or sympathetic stimulation can of course only be seen when uptake blocking drugs do not block simultaneously a specific type of adrenergic receptors (as dibenzyline) or interfere with the NE release of the transmitter from the sympathetic terminals (as bretylium or guanethidine). These "cocaine-like" neuronal-uptake blocking properties of drugs may considerably change the effect of NE released physiologically by blockade of the re-uptake of the transmitter.

It has been recognized for a long time that E was potentiated by cocaine (Froehlich et al., 1910); however, other compounds, which in their action differed only quantitatively from E, were abolished or diminished by cocaine pretreatment. This effect was first shown for tyramine by Tainter et al. (1926) and for tyramine and ephedrine by Burn et al. (1931), who called it the "cocaine paradox."

The group of compounds which were abolished by sympathetic denervation (Fleckenstein et al., 1953) or cocaine treatment (Fleckenstein et al., 1955) were named "neurosympathomimetics." It was postulated that these agents mimic the action of sympathetic stimulation or NE injection by releasing the transmitter from neuronal stores. This hypothesis was further supported by the fact that the action of tyramine and related drugs was abolished following reserpine treatment, which deprived the nerves of the neurotransmitter (Burn et al., 1958). Cocaine was shown to inhibit the sympathicomimetic effects by interfering with the tyramine-induced NE release (Lockett et al., 1960), presumably by preventing the tyramine from reaching the sites whence NE was liberated (Furchgott et al., 1963). The tachyphylaxis to tyramine was explained by the exhaustion of the NE stores available to tyramine release (Axelrod et al., 1962b).

The restoration of the tyramine-induced effects after reserpine pretreatment by infusion of NE was interpreted by Burn et al. (1958) as a refilling of the exhausted NE stores. But this explanation alone seemed insufficient in the face of careful comparisons between the amount of NE released and the sympathicomimetic effect produced by tyramine (Muscholl, 1960b; Crout et al., 1962).

Kuschinsky et al. (1960) found that the tyramine action on reserpinized rat atria was restored when NE was present in the incubation medium even in subthreshold concentrations. Lindmar et al. (1965) showed that tyramine produced a dose-dependent parallel shift of the NE dose-response curves on reserpinized rat atria. They concluded from their experiments that tyramine produces this increase in NE sensitivity by interference with the NE "removal." It had already been demonstrated that tyramine inhibits the accumulation of exogenous NE *in vivo* (Hertting et al., 1961b) and in the isolated perfused rat heart (Iversen, 1963). It can be understood that a drug with the combined properties of NE release and uptake blockade potentiates the effect of the released transmitter.

We investigated this "cocaine-like" action of tyramine on the isolated

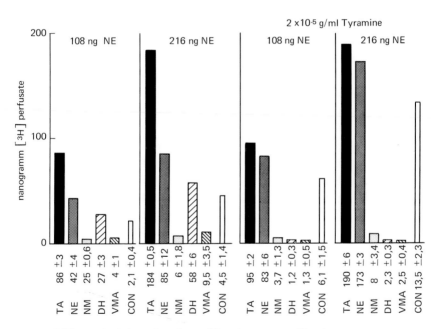

CON = maximal change in volume of the spleen, expressed in ml.
Abbreviations as described in Fig. 9-2.

Figure 9-9   The effect of tyramine on TA, ³H-NE, and ³H-NE metabolites in the perfusate following infusions of ³H-NE into spleens of reserpinized cats. Reserpine treatment as described in Fig. 9-4. 108 and 216 ng ³H-NE were infused within 2 minutes in the presence or absence of 2×10^{-5} g/ml tyramine in the perfusion medium. The values are means ± S.E.M. of TA, ³H-NE, and ³H-NE metabolites of the perfusates collected for 29 minutes following each individual infusion of ³H-NE.

perfused spleen. ^{3}H-NE was infused as described previously into reserpinized cat spleens in doses of 108 and 216 ng/2 min. TA, ^{3}H-metabolites as well as the splenic contraction were measured in the presence and absence of tyramine (2×10^{-5} g/ml) in the perfusion medium. Under this condition the effect of tyramine (Fig. 9-9) on infused ^{3}H-NE is indistinguishable from cocaine: both produce a maximal potentiation of splenic contraction, a marked increase of the concentration of ^{3}H-NE in the effluent as well as a considerable decrease of deaminated metabolites. Since tyramine is an excellent substrate of MAO the increase of ^{3}H-NE in the effluent could be due to a diminished deamination of NE by competition of tyramine and NE on the sites of the enzymes.

Therefore the action of tyramine was investigated on reserpinized spleens treated with the MAO inhibitor catron (10 mg/kg given 17 hours prior to the experiment). A representative experiment is given in Fig. 9-10. The lower part of the figure shows the TA, ^{3}H-NE and its ^{3}H-metabolites over the whole 29 minutes' collection period following each dose of 108 ng ^{3}H-NE infused within 2 minutes; the upper part compares the maximal splenic contraction with the ^{3}H-NE of the perfusate of the first 4 minutes' collection period. The blockade is not complete since deaminated metabolites can be demonstrated in the perfusate, although they are markedly diminished as compared with the spleen, which was reserpinized, but not treated with catron.

The total amount of ^{3}H-NE found in the 29 minutes' collection period is not very much changed by increasing concentrations of tyramine in the perfusion medium. A small rise of NE is observed, which corresponds to the decrease in the deaminated metabolites. There is, however, a definite increase in the effects produced by the ^{3}H-NE infused, which are accompanied by an increase of the ^{3}H-NE in the first 4 minutes' collection period. Basically we get the same picture as seen after cocaine in the reserpinized spleen preparation: the augmentation in tissue sensitivity is paralleled by an increase in the ^{3}H-NE concentration in the effluent of the first collection period. In the catron-treated reserpinized spleen much smaller concentrations of tyramine are necessary to induce these effects. Since tyramine in these experiments is not deaminated by the MAO, but the increase in the sensitivity of the tissue towards NE in the presence of tyramine is of the magnitude of the denervated or cocaine-treated tissue, this effect can be solely explained by a "cocaine-like" action of tyramine which inhibits the neuronal uptake of NE, as already proposed by Lind-

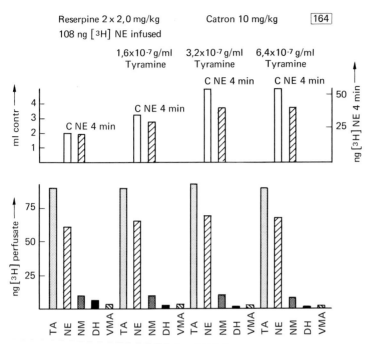

Figure 9-10   The effect of tyramine on splenic contraction, TA, ^{3}H-NE, and ^{3}H-NE metabolites in the perfusate following infusion of ^{3}H-NE into an isolated spleen of a cat pretreated with reserpine and catron. Reserpine treatment as described in Fig. 9-4. Catron (10 mg/kg) was given 17 hours prior to the experiment. 108 ng ^{3}H-NE was infused within 2 minutes in the absence or presence of increasing concentrations of tyramine in the perfusion medium. Lower part: Bars represent the TA, ^{3}H-NE, and ^{3}H-NE metabolites of the perfusate collected for 29 minutes following each individual infusion of ^{3}H-NE. Upper part: Maximal contraction of the spleen (expressed in ml) and ^{3}H-NE in the perfusate of the first 4-minute sampling period.

mar et al. (1965). Very similar interactions of tyramine, cocaine, and NE were observed on rat atria by Furchgott et al. (1963, 1968).

The essence of our results is given schematically in Fig. 9-11. Tyramine competes with the transport of NE into the nerve terminals, thus increasing the concentration on the receptor sites.

Our experiments with the isolated perfused spleen, in which the neuronal uptake and storage mechanisms for catecholamines were impaired either by denervation or drugs, demonstrate the essential role of the sympathetic nerve terminals for inactivation, metabolism, and tissue response of the neurotransmitter in this organ. This mechanism will be imperative

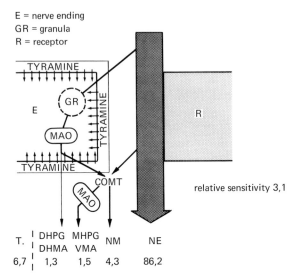

Figure 9-11   Scheme of the fate of ^{3}H-NE infused into isolated perfused spleens of reserpine-pretreated cats in the presence of tyramine. Reserpine treatment as described in Fig. 9-4. Experimental procedure similar as described in Fig. 9-9. Abbreviations as described in Fig. 9-2.

solely in structures where the sympathetic terminals are present in a favorable ratio and close proximity to the effector cells.

Experiments which excluded any possible influence on sympathetic nerve terminals on the catecholamine-tissue interaction, however, indicated that other mechanisms must exist that modify the fate of catecholamines.

The Extraneuronal Catecholamine Uptake

Reserpine-resistant accumulation of ^{3}H-NE was demonstrated in denervated tissues by Anden et al. (1963) and Fischer et al. (1965), suggesting an extraneuronal uptake.

Iversen (1965) described a second uptake process for catecholamines in the isolated rat heart (uptake II) which, in contrast to the intraneuronal uptake I, has a low affinity, but high capacity, for NE. Evidence for the extraneuronal localization of the uptake II has been presented by Ehinger et al. (1968), Farnebo et al. (1969), and Clarke et al. (1969). Avakian et al. (1968), Gillespie et al. (1970a), and Gillespie et al. (1970b) have shown that in the spleen and in isolated arteries of the rabbit ear, perfused with high concentrations of NE, this amine accumulated in the vascular smooth muscle.

Uptake I and uptake II differ in several aspects. Uptake I is stereo-chemically specific, preferring the l-isomer (Iversen, 1963; von Euler et al., 1965), whereas uptake II proved to have no stereochemical speci-ficity (Iversen, 1965). There are marked differences in affinities of vari-ous catecholamines to uptake I and uptake II and in the inhibition of both uptake processes by drugs or catecholamine metabolites.

Norepinephrine with a high affinity for uptake I is transported into the sympathetic fiber, isoprenaline, however, which has a very low affin-ity for uptake I is not taken up intraneuronally at all (Hertting, 1964). On the other hand isoprenaline is transported by the uptake II process (Callingham et al., 1966; Foster, 1969). Both mechanisms operate at the same time, and the uptake process which will become dominant depends on the affinity of the catecholamine to the two uptake processes as well as on the concentration used. It seems easily cognizable that in a specific tissue the relative importance of these two uptake mechanisms will depend on the ratio of the sympathetic nerve terminals—representing the uptake I —to the extraneuronal uptake II sites. Any changes of this ratio can be ex-pected to be reflected in changes of tissue sensitivity towards catechol-amines.

Bacq et al. (1961) observed that metanephrine potentiates the effects of NE as well as pre- or postganglionic stimulation on the nictitating mem-brane of the cat. Normetanephrine was less active. The sensitizing effect of the O-methylated catecholamine metabolites was demonstrable also after postganglionic sympathetic denervation. Langer et al. (1967), how-ever, characterize this effect of metanephrine on the nictitating membrane as an additive effect rather than a potentiation. Both metanephrine and normetanephrine are potent inhibitors of the uptake II process, as dem-onstrated by Iversen (1965) and Burgen et al. (1965).

Various steroid hormones were shown to increase the sensitivity of vascular smooth muscle to catecholamines (Zweifach et al., 1953; Le-comte et al., 1960; Kalsner, 1969a; Kalsner, 1969b). Iversen et al. (1970) demonstrated that these steroids are the most potent inhibitors of uptake II, with practically no influence on uptake I in the rat heart. The relative potency in inhibiting the uptake II agreed well with the rank order of the catecholamine potentiating effect. Drugs like cocaine, desimipramine, and phenoxybenzamine are very potent inhibitors of neuronal uptake. These drugs were even widely used to characterize the uptake I process. But they also have a definite inhibiting property on the uptake II mechanism, at least in the heart (Iversen, 1965). The evidence of the blockade of uptake II by drugs has also been demonstrated histochemically by Avakian et al. (1968), Clarke et al. (1969), and Gillespie et al. (1970a). In tissues in which uptake I predominates, the blockade of uptake II by the O-methylated metabolites, steroids, or drugs will be of minor importance. On the other hand, in tissues in which for anatomical reasons the sympathetic nerve terminals are dissociated from the receptor-bearing structures, as in the vascular bed, or in tissues in which uptake I was eliminated, uptake II will prevail and any interference with this mechanism now dominating will produce changes in tissue reactivity towards sympathomimetic amines. As already stated for uptake I, the inhibition of uptake II of a sympathomimetic amine by a drug will result in a potentiation of the sympathomimetic action only, when the drug used does not interfere with the receptor sites. Cocaine was shown to increase the maximum response of NE in a sympathetic nerve-free vascular muscle preparation, although this drug failed to produce a shift in the NE dose-response curve (Bevan et al., 1967). In doses much higher than required to block neuronal uptake, cocaine potentiated the effects of NE on nerve-free aortic strips (Kalsner et al., 1969). Similarly methoxamine, a drug which is not subject to intraneuronal uptake but with a higher affinity for uptake II (Burgen et al., 1965), was potentiated by cocaine (Kalsner et al., 1969). These data seem to indicate that in this preparation cocaine interferes with a second catecholamine inactivating mechanism, distinct from neuronal uptake. Although true kinetic data of this inactivation mechanism in the vascular smooth muscle are not available, its identity with uptake II can be assumed. To judge from the histochemical evidence, this uptake process of the vascular smooth muscle seems to be located within the smooth muscle cells, which contain the NE-degradating enzymes, the MAO, and the COMT. This concept may be identical with the model proposed by Levin and Furchgott (1970).

The alpha-mimetic response of splenic strips to isoprenaline, which as already mentioned is taken up solely by uptake II, was potentiated by high concentrations of cocaine (Davidson et al., 1970). These authors, however, found no change in the isoprenaline content between control and cocaine-treated strips. Since the isoprenaline determinations were made after an extensive washout, and since it is well known that the amines taken up by the uptake II mechanism are readily washed out, this lack of correlation between potentiation and uptake inhibition can easily be understood. On the tracheal chain Foster (1969) found a positive correlation between the potentiation of the isoprenaline effect and the inhibition of uptake due to cooling, or inhibitors of uptake II as metanephrine, phenoxybenzamine, and phentolamine. Cocaine, used in a concentration too low to interfere with uptake II, affected neither uptake nor tissue response.

It should be emphasized that since the distribution of uptake I and uptake II sites in diverse types of tissues varies, each tissue will have a very specific uptake pattern and therefore a very specific reaction to drugs interfering with these uptake processes. Any changes in the inactivation rate of the neurotransmitter are expected to influence the tissue response, blood flow, or the organ performance. Since the changes in the uptake pattern also influence the accessibility of the neurotransmitter to the enzymes localized in different tissue compartments, a reciprocal interaction of different proportions is to be expected between the uptake processes and metabolism.

Fate of ^{3}H-Dopamine Taken Up into the Rat Heart at Low or High Perfusion Concentrations

Kopin et al. (1962a) have shown that NE taken up into the rat heart at low perfusion concentrations was to a great extent protected against metabolic degradation; only a small fraction was metabolized, mainly by COMT. Lightman et al. (1969), using inhibitors of MAO and COMT, presented indirect evidence that NE taken up by uptake II is metabolized more rapidly.

According to the data by Iversen (1965) dopamine (DA) was expected to be taken up by both uptake I and uptake II mechanism. Since this amine is not only metabolized by MAO and COMT, but also transformed to NE by dopamine-β-hydroxylase, which is exclusively localized in the intraneuronal storage granules (Stjärne, 1966; Stjärne et al., 1967), the metabolic fate of DA taken up at various perfusion concentrations should give clues as to the distribution of this amine within the heart. Details of method and results are described in the paper of Hellmann et al. (1971a).

Hearts of rats were perfused at a constant flow rate of 8 to 10 ml with various concentrations of 7-^{3}H-DA at different time intervals. In the hearts—and in some experiments also in the perfusates—the following determinations were made: Total radioactivity (TA), activity of the alumina eluate (AL), which represents the sum of the amines and the deaminated catechols, as well as the ^{3}H-DA, ^{3}H-NE and their different metabolites. K_m and V_{max} values were determined graphically using the Lineweaver-Burk plot.

It was found that DA was accumulated by the isolated perfused rat heart by two distinct uptake mechanisms, characterized by different patterns and rates of metabolite production. A K_m of 0.68×10^{-6}M and a V_{max} of 1.45×10^{-9} mol/g/min were calculated for uptake I; for uptake II a K_m of 5.9×10^{-4}M and a V_{max} of 0.14×10^{-6} mol/g/min were found.

By using our kinetic data it can be calculated that at a perfusion concentration of 55×10^{-10} mol/ml the rates of uptake I and uptake II are about equal. The values obtained in the various experiments will always include different contributions by both uptake I and uptake II at each perfusion concentration used. Little mutual interference should be expected within the range of perfusion concentrations which typify the two uptake mechanisms because of the great difference in the kinetic data of the two uptake processes.

The Influence of Different Perfusion Concentrations on the Metabolism of ^{3}H-DA

As shown in Fig. 9-12, most of the DA taken up at this low DA perfusion concentration is stored unchanged. The concentration of the radioactive substances in the heart exceeds the perfusion concentration by a factor of 30. The total amount of products of metabolic degradation contributes only 2.6 per cent of the TA. NE is the main metabolite. The lack of O-methylation suggests that there is practically no extraneuronal uptake (Kopin et al., 1963). The low rate of deamination and the high rate of β-hydroxylation suggest that the DA, after being transported into the nerve terminals, is rapidly transferred into the dopamine-β-hydroxylase containing granules (Potter et al., 1963b). With increasing DA perfusion concentrations a progressively smaller percentage of the DA taken up by the heart is β-hydroxylated to NE (Fig. 9-13). O-methylation becomes

perfusion concentration 0047 x 10⁻¹⁰ mol/ml

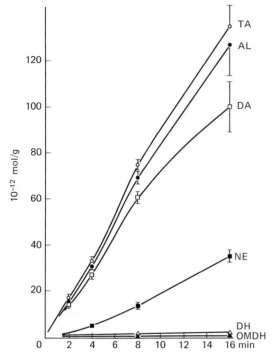

TA = total radioactivity
AL = radioactivity of the alumina eluate
        (sum of ³H-dopamine, ³H-epinephrine, and deaminated catechol metabolites

Figure 9-12   Metabolic fate of ³H-dopamine taken up at a perfusion concentration of 0.047×10^{-10} mol/ml into isolated pefused rat hearts. The values are expressed as 10^{-12} mol/g tissue. Each point represents a mean obtained from five hearts $\pm$ S.E.M. (From Hellmann et al., 1971a)

of considerable importance, as shown by the increase in the amount of O-methylated metabolites (sum of OM and OMDH). Deaminated products are the main metabolites. Since uptake I predominates at the perfusion concentration employed in this experiment, it can be concluded that this deamination occurs mainly intraneuronally. At the low perfusion concentrations DA, after being taken up into the sympathetic nerve, is rapidly transported into the storage granules, where it is protected from the intraneuronal MAO and serves as a substrate for the β-hydroxylating enzyme. With the increase of the DA concentration, but still within

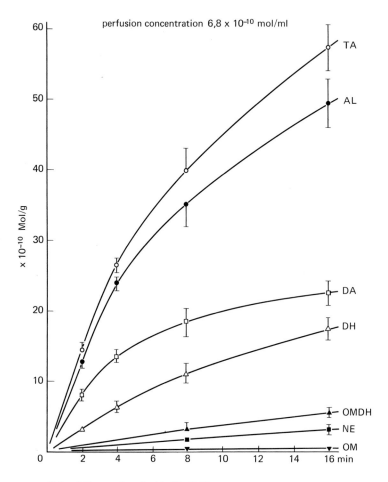

Abbreviations as described in Fig. 9-12.
O-methylated amine metabolites. (From Hellmann et al., 1971 a)

Figure 9-13   Metabolic fate of ³H-dopamine taken up at a perfusion concentration of 6.8 × 10⁻¹⁰ mol/ml into isolated perfused rat hearts. The values are expressed as 10⁻¹⁰ mol/g tissue. Each point represents a mean obtained from five hearts ± S.E.M.

the predominance of uptake I, transport across the neuronal membrane becomes faster than uptake into the granules, and an increasing pool of intraneuronal, but extragranular, DA builds up which is subject to deamination.

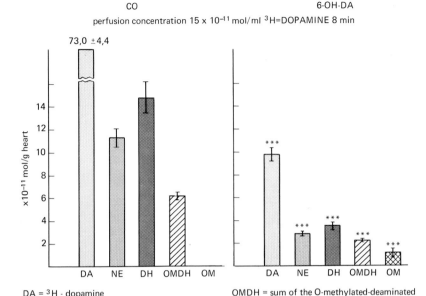

DA = ^{3}H - dopamine
NE = ^{3}H - norepinephrine
DH = sum of the deaminated catechol metabolites
*** P 0,001.

OMDH = sum of the O-methylated-deaminated
catechol metabolites.
OM = sum of the O-methylated amine metabolites

Figure 9-14   Rats were divided in control animals and those pretreated with 6-hydroxydopamine (6-OH-DA). The isolated hearts were perfused with 15×10^{-11} mol/ml ^{3}H-dopamine for 8 minutes. The values (means $\pm$ S.E.M.) are expressed as 10^{-11} mol/g heart.

This is confirmed by experiments, in which the sympathetic structures of the hearts were destroyed by treatment with 6-hydroxydopamine (6-OH-DA) (Hellmann et al., 1971b). In these experiments chemical sympathectomy was not complete, the endogenous NE of the hearts of the treated group was 18.4 per cent of the controls. It can be seen at Fig. 9-14 that in experiments with a low perfusion concentration the uptake of DA as well as β-hydroxylation is markedly diminished. Similarly, there is a considerable reduction in deaminated metabolites, indicating that at this perfusion concentration deamination has taken place intraneuronally. A similar reduction of catecholamine uptake and β-hydroxylation was observed after immunosympathectomy by Iversen et al. (1966); a reduction in tissue dopamine-β-hydroxylase after 6-OH-DA treatment was described by Molinoff et al. (1970). The residual endogenous NE as well as

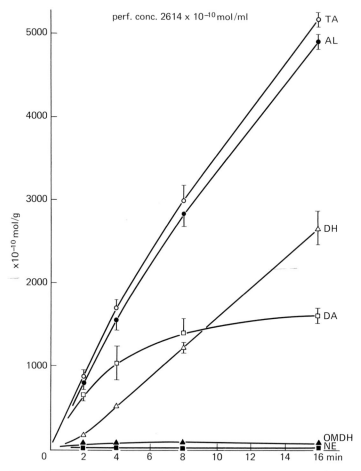

Figure 9-15   Metabolic fate of ³H-dopamine taken up at a perfusion concentration of 2.614 × 10⁻¹⁰ mol/ml into perfused rat hearts. The values are expressed as 10⁻¹⁰ mol/g tissue. Each point represents a mean obtained from five hearts ± S.E.M. Abbreviations as in Fig. 9-12. (From Hellmann et al., 1971a)

the remaining NE synthesis in the 6-OH-DA group indicate that some sympathetic nerves survived chemical sympathectomy.

In the experiments with a high perfusion concentration of DA the concentration of radioactive substances in the heart exceeds the DA perfusion concentration only by a factor of 2 (Fig. 9-15).

The fraction of DA converted to NE is negligible. The O-methylated metabolites represent only a small fraction of the TA present in the heart. Deamination is the dominant metabolic pathway. But in contrast to the experiments in the range of uptake I, in which the rate of deamination decreases with time, the rate of deamination tends to increase during the first minutes of perfusion with high DA concentration. This suggests that initially the more efficient uptake I decreases the concentration of DA on the uptake II sites. After uptake I has been saturated, uptake II takes over and deamination reaches its maximal rate.

In contrast to the experiments with a low perfusion concentration, chemical sympathectomy produced only slight changes in uptake and distribution of metabolites in experiments with a high perfusion concentration (Fig. 9-16). From the kinetic data given by Hellmann et al. (1971a) it can be calculated that at the perfusion concentration of 32.7×10^{-9} mol/ml DA the initial rate of uptake I would be about 20 per

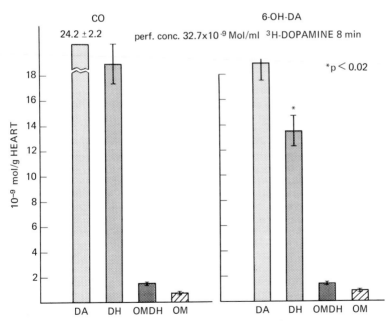

Figure 9-16   Rats were divided between control animals and those pretreated with 6-hydroxydopamine (6-OH-DA). The isolated hearts were perfused with 32.7×10^{-9} mol/ml ^{3}H-dopamine for 8 minutes. The values (means $\pm$ S.E.M.) are expressed as 10^{-9} mol/g heart. Abbreviations as in Fig. 9-14.

cent of the initial rate of uptake II. In the chemically sympathectomized group there is a small but insignificant decrease in DA. The TA and AL (not shown at Fig. 9-16) and the deaminated metabolites of this group, however, are significantly lowered in comparison with the untreated controls. The degree of diminution corresponds to the calculated fraction that can be attributed to uptake I, which has been eliminated in this group. The O-methylated metabolites remain unaffected by this treatment. The results from these experiments can be briefly summarized as follows:

DA is taken up by the rat heart by two different uptake mechanisms as defined by different kinetic constants and different patterns of metabolites.

At low perfusion concentrations DA is very efficiently concentrated by uptake I, the affinity of this uptake being about 870 times higher than for uptake II. At the lowest concentration employed, metabolism is negligible, a large fraction of the DA taken up is β-hydroxylated to NE. With an elevation of the DA perfusion concentration, but still within the range of uptake I, the rate of deamination increases. After partial chemical sympathectomy the uptake of DA, β-hydroxylation, and deamination of DA are markedly decreased, suggesting the neuronal localization of uptake I as well as of the site of deamination.

At high perfusion concentrations uptake I is saturated and uptake II becomes dominant, reaching a V_{max} about 100 times higher than uptake I. DA taken up by uptake II is deaminated very efficiently. DA uptake and deamination at uptake II concentrations are only slightly affected by chemical sympathectomy, suggesting the extraneuronal localization of this uptake process.

It can be concluded from our experiments, that deamination occurs intraneuronally as well as extraneuronally in both uptake I and uptake II experiments. Metabolism by COMT is not diminished by chemical sympathectomy, demonstrating the extraneuronal localization of this enzyme. Metabolism of catecholamines in the rat heart is therefore primarily determined by their distribution within the intra- and extraneuronal compartments and not only by their affinity to the enzymes. Their distribution on the other hand depends on the perfusion concentration used and on the relative affinity of the particular catecholamine to the uptake I and uptake II processes.

About the physiological significance of uptake II one can merely speculate. But it is quite conceivable that NE concentrations high enough to be subject to the uptake II process may occur in the synaptic gap during physiological NE release. In tissues with a scarce sympathetic innervation uptake II may be the dominant mechanism responsible for the inactivation of circulating catecholamines.

References

Alberici, M., De Lores Arnaiz, H. R., and De Robertis, E. 1965. *Life Sci.* 4:1951.

Anden, M. E., Carlsson, A., and Waldeck, B. 1963. *Life Sci.* 12:889.

Avakian, O. V., and Gillespie, J. S. 1968. *Brit. J. Pharmacol.* 32:168.

Axelrod, J., Weil-Malherbe, H., and Tomchick, R. 1959. *J. Pharmacol. Exp. Ther.* 127:251.

Axelrod, J. 1960. In *Ciba Foundation Symposium on Adrenergic Mechanism,* J. R. Vane, G. E. W. Wolstenhome, and M. O'Connor (Eds.), "The Fate of Adrenaline and Noreadrenaline," J. and A. Churchill, Ltd., London, p. 28.

Axelrod, J., Hertting, G., and Patrick, R. W. 1961. *J. Pharmacol. Exp. Ther.* 134:325.

Axelrod, J., Hertting, G., and Potter, L. T. 1962a. *Nature* 194:297.

Axelrod, J., Gordon, E. K., Hertting, G., Kopin, I. J., and Potter, L. T. 1962b. *Brit. J. Pharmacol.* 19:56.

Axelrod, J. 1963. In *The Clinical Chemistry of Monoamines,* H. Varley, and A. H. Gowenlock (Eds.), "The Formation, Metabolism, Uptake and Release of Noradrenaline and Adrenaline," Elsevier Publishing Company, Amsterdam, p. 5.

Axelrod, J. 1965. Academic Press Inc., New York, p. 597.

Axelrod, J., and Kopin, I. J. 1969. *Recent Prog. Brain Res.* 31:22.

Bacq, Z. M., and Renson, J. 1961. *Arch. Int. Pharmacol.* 130:385.

Bertler, A., Carlsson, A., and Rosengren, E. 1956. *Naturwissenschaften* 22:521.

Bevan, J. A., and Verity, K. A. 1967. *J. Pharmacol. Exp. Ther.* 157:117.

Blaschko, H., Hagen, P., and Welch, A. D. 1955. *J. Physiol.* 129:27.

Bogdanski, D. F., Weissbach, H., and Udenfriend, S. 1957. *J. Neurochem.* 1:272.

Bogdanski, D. F., and Brodie, B. B. 1966. *Life Sci.* 5:1563.

Bogdanski, D. F., and Brodie, B. B. 1969. *J. Pharmacol. Exp. Ther.* 165:181.

Brodie, B. B., Costa, E., Dlabac, A., Neff, N. H., and Smookler, H. H. 1966. *J. Pharmacol. Exp. Ther.* 154:493.

Brown, G. L. 1965. *Proc. R. Soc.* 162:1.

Burgen, A. S. V., and Iversen, L. L. 1965. *Brit. J. Pharmacol.* 25:34.

Burn, J. H., and Tainter, H. L. 1931. *J. Physiol.* 71:169.

Burn, J. H. 1932. *J. Physiol.* 75:144.

Burn, J. H., and Rand, M. J. 1958. *J. Physiol.* 144:314.

Callingham, B. A., and Burgen, A. S. V. 1966. *Mol. Pharmacol.* 2:37.

Cannon, W. B., and Rosenbluth, A. 1949. Macmillan & Co., New York.

Carlsson, A. 1965. *Handbuch der experimentellen Pharmakologie,* Springer Verlag, Berlin-Heidelberg-New York.

Champlain, de J., Müller, R. A., and Axelrod, J. 1969. *J. Pharmacol. Exp. Ther.* 166:339.

Chidsey, C. A., Kaiser, G. A., and Braunwald, E. 1963a. *Science* 139:828.

Chidsey, C. A., and Harrison, D. C. 1963b. *J. Pharmacol. Exp. Ther.* 140:217.

Clarke, D. E., Jones, C. J., and Linley, Z. A. 1969. *Brit. J. Pharmacol.* 37:1.

Costa, E., and Neff, N. H. 1970. *Handbook of Neurochemistry* 4:45.

Cotzias, G. C., and Dole, V. P. 1951. *Proc. Soc. Exp. Biol. Med.* 78:157.

Crout, J. R., Muskus, A. J., and Trendelenburg, U. 1962. *Brit J. Pharmacol.* 18:600.

Crout, J. R. 1964. *Arch. Exp. Path. Pharmak.* 248:85.

Dahlström, A. 1966. M.D. Thesis, Ivar Haeggström Tryckeri AB, Stockholm.

Davidson, W. J., and Ines, I. R. 1970. *Brit. J. Pharmacol.* 39:175.

Dengler, H. J., Spiegel, H. E., and Titus, E. O. 1961. *Science* 133:1072.

Dengler, H. J. 1965. In *Pharmacology of Cholinergic and Adrenergic Transmission. Effect of Drugs on Monoamine Uptake in Isolated Tissues,* Pergamon Press, London.

Ehinger, B., and Sporrong, B. 1968. *Experientia* 24:265.

Euler, U. S. von. 1948. *Acta Physiol. Scand.* 16:63.

Euler, U. S. von, and Hillarp, N. A. 1956. *Nature* 177:44.

Euler, U.S. von, and Lishajko, F. 1963a. *Acta Physiol. Scand.* 59:454.

Euler, U. S. von, Lishajko, F., and Stjärne, L. 1963b. *Acta Physiol. Scand.* 5:495.

Euler, U. S. von, and Lishajko, F. 1965. *Int. J. Neuropharmacol.* 4:273.

Faernebo, L. O., and Malmfors, T. 1969. *European J. Pharmacol.* 5:313.

Fischer, J. E., Kopin, I. J., and Axelrod, J. 1965. *J. Pharmacol. exp. Ther.* 147:181.

Fleckenstein, A., and Burn, J. H. 1953. *Brit. J. Pharmacol.* 8:69.

Fleckenstein, A., and Stöckle, D. 1955. *Arch. Exp. Path. Pharmak.* 224:401.

Foster, R. W. 1969. *Brit. J. Pharmacol.* 35:418.

Froehlich, A., and Loewi, O. 1910. *Arch. Exp. Path. Pharmak.* 62:159.

Furchgott, R. F., Kirpekar, S. M., Rieker, K., and Schwab, A. 1963. *J. Pharmacol. Exp. Ther.* 142:39.

Furchgott, R. F., and Sanchez-Garcia, P. 1968. *J. Pharmacol. Exp. Ther.* 163:98.

Gillespie, J. S., and Kirpekar, S. M. 1965. *J. Physiol.* 176:205.

Gillespie, J. S., and Muir, T. C. 1970a. *J. Physiol.* 206:591.

Gillespie, J. S., Hamilton, D. N. H., and Hosie, R. J. A. 1970b. *J. Physiol.* 206:563.

Haefely, W., Huerlimann, A., and Thoenen, H. 1964. *Brit. J. Pharmacol.* 22:5.

Haeusler, G., Thoenen, H., and Haefely, W. 1968. *Helv. Physiol.* 26:223.

Haeusler, G., Haefely, W., and Thoenen, H. 1969. *J. Pharmacol. Exp. Ther.* 170:50.

Hellmann, G., Hertting, G., and Peskar, B. 1971a. *Brit. J. Pharmacol.* 41:256.

Hellmann, G., Hertting, G., and Peskar, B. 1971b. *Brit. J. Pharmacol.* 41:270.

Hertting, G., and Schiefthaler, T. 1963. *Arch. exp. Path. Pharmakol.* 246:13.

Hertting, G., Axelrod, J., Kopin, I. J., and Whitby, L. G. 1961a. *Nature* 189:66.

Hertting, G., Axelrod, J., and Whitby, L. G. 1961b. *J. Pharmacol. Exp. Ther.* 134:146.

Hertting, G., and Axelrod, J. 1961c. *Nature* 192:172.

Hertting, G. 1964. *Biochem. Pharmacol.* 13:1119.

Hertting, G. 1965. *Pharmacology of Cholinergic and Adrenergic Transmission. Effect of Drugs and Sympathetic Denervation in NA Uptake and Binding in Animal Tissues,* Pergamon Press, London, p. 277.

Hertting, G., and Suko, J. 1966a. *Arch. Exp. Path. Pharmak.* 253:45.

Hertting, G., Suko, J., and Hellmann, G. 1966b. *Arch. Exp. Path. Pharmak.* 255:25.

Hertting, G., Suko, J., Widhalm, S., and Harbich, I. 1967. *Arch. Exp. Path. Pharmak.* 256.40.

Holtz, P., and Palm, D. 1966. In *Reviews of Physiology, Biochemistry and Experimental Pharmacology,* Springer Verlag, Berlin-Heidelberg.

Horst, W. D., Kopin, I. J., and Ramey, E. R. 1968. *Am. J. Physiol.* 215:817.

Iversen, L. L. 1963. *Brit. J. Pharmacol.* 21:523.

Iversen, L. L. 1965. *Brit. J. Pharmacol.* 25:18.

Iversen, L. L., and Kravitz, E. A. 1966a. *Mol. Pharmacol.* 2:360.

Iversen, L. L., Glowinski, J., and Axelrod, J. 1966b. *J. Pharmacol. Exp. Ther.* 151:273.

Iversen, L. L. 1967. In *The Uptake and Storage of Noradrenaline in Sympathetic Nerves,* Cambridge University Press, London and New York.

Iversen, L. L., and Salt, P. J. 1970. *Brit. J. Pharmacol.* 40:528.

Kalsner, S., and Nickerson, M. 1969. *Brit. J. Pharmacol.* 35:428.

Kalsner, S. 1969a. *Circul. Res.* 24:383.

Kalsner, S. 1969b. *Brit. J. Pharmacol.* 36:582.

Kirpekar, S. M., and Wakade, A. R. 1968. *J. Physiol.* 194:609.

Klingman, G., 1966. *Biochem. Pharmacol.* 15:1729.

Kopin, I. J., Hertting, G., and Gordon, E. K. 1962a. *J. Pharmacol. Exp. Ther.* 138:34.

Kopin, I. J., and Gordon, E. K. 1962b. *J. Pharmacol. Exp. Ther.* 138:351.

Kopin, I. J., and Gordon, E. K. 1963. *Nature* 199:1289.

Kopin, I. J. 1964. *Pharmacol. Rev.* 16:179.

Kopin, I. J., Breese, G. R., Krauss, K. R., and Weise, V. K. 1968. *J. Pharmacol. Exp. Ther.* 161:271.

Kuschinsky, G., Lindmar, R., Lüllmann, H., and Muscholl, E. 1960. *Arch. Exp. Path. Pharmak.* 240:242.

Langer, S. Z., Bogaert, M. G., and De Schaepdryver, A. F. 1967. *J. Pharmacol. Exp. Ther.* 167:517.

Lecomte, J., Dreese, A., and Cauwenberge, H. 1960. *Rev. Franc. Etudes Clin. et Biol.* 5:718.

Levin, J. A., and Furchgott, R. F. 1970. *J. Pharmacol. Exp. Ther.* 172:320.

Levitt, M., Spector, S., Sjoerdsma, A., and Udenfriend, S. J. 1965. *J. Pharmacol. Exp. Ther.* 148:1.

Lightman, S. L., and Iversen, L. L. 1969. *Brit. J. Pharmacol.* 37:638.

Lindmar, R., and Muscholl, E. 1965. *Arch. Exp. Path. Pharmak.* 252:122.

Lockett, M. F., and Eakins, K. E. 1960. *J. Pharm. Pharmacol.* 12:513.

Lowe, M. C., and Horita, A. 1970. *Nature* 228:175.

Malmfors, T. 1965. *Studies on Adrenergic Nerves,* Almquist & Wiksells, Stockholm-Uppsala.

Molinoff, P. B., Weinshilboum, R., and Axelrod, J. 1970. *Fed. Proc.* 29:278.

Montanari, R., Costa, E., Beaven, N. A., and Brodie, B. B. 1963. *Life Sci.* 4:232.

Mueller, R. A., Thoenen, H., and Axelrod, J. 1969a. *J. Pharmacol. Exp. Ther.* 169:74.

Mueller, R. A., Thoenen, H., and Axelrod, J. 1969b. *Science* 163:468.

Muscholl, E. 1960a. *Arch. Exp. Path. Pharmak.* 240:8.

Muscholl, E. 1960b. *Arch. Exp. Path. Pharmak.* 240:234.

Muscholl, E. 1961. *Brit. J. Pharmacol.* 16:352.

Neff, N. H., and Costa, E. 1966. *Fed. Proc.* 25:259.

Neff, N. H., Ngai, S. H., Wang, C. T., and Costa, E. 1969. *Mol. Pharmacol.* 5:90.
Norberg, K. A., and Hamberger, B. 1964. *Acta Physiol. Scand.* 63 suppl. 238.
Paton, D. H., and Gillis, C. N. 1965. *Nature* 208:391.
Potter, L. T., and Axelrod, J. 1962a. *Nature* 194:581.
Potter, L. T., Axelrod, J., and Kopin, I. J. 1962b. *Biochem. Pharmacol.* 11:254.
Potter, L. T., and Axelrod, J. 1963a. *J. Pharmacol. Exp. Ther.* 140:199.
Potter, L. T., and Axelrod, J. 1963b. *J. Pharmacol. Exp. Ther.* 142:299.
Potter, L. T., Cooper, T., Willman, V. L., and Wolfe, D. E. 1965. *Circul. Res.* 16:468.
Roth, R. H., Stjärne, L., and von Euler, U. S. 1966a. *Life Sci.* 5:1071.
Roth, R. H., and Stjärne, L. 1966b. *Acta Physiol. Scand.* 68:342.
Schümann, H. J. 1958. *Arch. Exp. Path. Pharmak.* 233:296.
Second Symposium on Catecholamines. 1966. G. H. Acheson (Ed.), *Pharmacological Reviews*, p. 18.
Smith, C. B., Trendelenburg, U., Langer, S. Z., and Tsai, T. H. 1966. *J. Pharmacol. Exp. Ther.* 151:87.
Snyder, S. H., Fischer, J., and Axelrod, J. 1965. *Biochem. Pharmacol.* 14:363.
Spector, S., Sjoerdsma, A., Zaltsman-Nirenberg, P., Levitt, K., and Udenfriend, S. 1963. *Science* 139:1299.
Spector, S., Gordon, R., Sjoerdsma, A., and Udenfriend, S. 1967. *Mol. Pharmacol.* 3:549.
Stjärne, L. 1964. *Acta Physiol. Scand.* 62 suppl. 228.
Stjärne, L. 1966. *Acta Physiol. Scand.* 67:441.
Stjärne, L., and Lishajko, F. 1967. *Biochem. Pharmacol.* 16:1719.
Stjärne, L., Roth, R. H., and Giarman, N. J. 1968. *Biochem. Pharmacol.* 17:2008.
Stjärne, L., and Wennmalm, A. 1970a. *Acta Physiol. Scand.* 80:428.
Stjärne, L., Roth, R. H., Bloom, F. E., and Giarman, N. J. 1970b. *J. Pharmacol. Exp. Ther.* 171:70.
Suko, J., and Hertting, G. 1966. *Arch. Exp. Path. Pharmak.* 253:87.
Tainter, M. L., and Chang, D. K. 1926. *J. Pharmacol. Exp. Ther.* 30:193.
Thoenen, H., Müller, R. A., and Axelrod, J. 1969. *J. Pharmacol. Exp. Ther.* 169:249.
Trendelenburg, U. 1963. *Pharmacol. Rev.* 15:225.
Trendelenburg, U. 1966. *Pharmacol. Rev.* 18:629.
Trendelenburg, U. 1969. *Recent Prog. in Brain Res.* 31:73.
Trendelenburg, U., and Draskoczy, P. R. 1970. *J. Pharmacol. Exp. Ther.* 175:521.
Wakade, A. R., and Furchgott, R. T. 1968. *J. Pharmacol. Exp. Ther.* 163:123.
Whitby, L. G., Hertting, G., and Axelrod, J. 1960. *Nature* 187:604.
Whitby, L. G., Axelrod, J., and Weil-Malherbe, H. 1961. *J. Pharmacol. Exp. Ther.* 132:193.
Zaimis, E., Berk, L., and Callingham, B. 1965. *Nature* 206:1221.
Zweifach, B. W., Shorr, E., and Black, M. M. 1953. *Ann. N.Y. Acad. Sci.* 56:626.

10

Chemical Sympathectomy: A New Tool in the Investigation of the Physiology and Pharmacology of Peripheral and Central Adrenergic Neurons

H. THOENEN

Destruction or functional elimination of an organ in order to characterize its physiological role is one of the oldest and most commonly used methods in biological research. This principle has been widely applied in the investigation of the physiology and pharmacology of the sympathetic nervous system. Beyond the elucidation of the general homeostatic function of the sympathetic nervous system, denervation experiments were of crucial importance in the localization of the sites of synthesis, storage, and enzymatic degradation of the physiological adrenergic transmitter. Moreover, denervation played a predominant role in the assessment of the importance of uptake into the adrenergic neuron as a mechanism of norepinephrine inactivation after exogenous application or endogenous liberation by nerve impulses (for references see Thoenen, 1971a; Trendelenburg, 1971).

Surgical denervation is still the method of choice for experiments designed to study the effect of deprivation from sympathetic innervation in single organs or groups of organs with a simple topographical sympathetic innervation such as the iris, salivary gland, and nictitating membrane, which are exclusively innervated from the superior cervical ganglion. However, for general sympathectomy or for denervation of organs with a more complex or less easily accessible innervation, the surgical procedure is too cumbrous, too time-consuming, and virtually impracticable in small animals. These limitations in the applicability of surgical denervation explain the great interest in methods which bring about a selective destruction of sympathetic nerves by other means (for references see Thoenen, 1971a).

In 1959, Senoh and co-workers (Senoh et al., 1959a,c; Senoh and Witkop, 1959b) reported that 6-hydroxydopamine might be formed from dopamine as an autoxidation product or metabolite. Neither the quantitative aspects, nor the sites of formation, nor possible physiological implications of this product of an aberrant metabolic pathway have been clarified so far. However, pharmacological studies with 6-hydroxydapomine have shown that this amine produces an extremely long-lasting depletion of norepinephrine from peripheral sympathetically innervated organs (Porter et al., 1963; Stone et al., 1963; Laverty et al., 1965). The mechanism of this long-lasting depletion was the subject of extensive speculation (Porter et al., 1963, 1965; Laverty et al., 1965) until electron microscopic studies revealed that 6-hydroxydopamine produces a destruction of adrenergic nerve terminals (Tranzer and Thoenen, 1967a, 1968).

Meanwhile, the morphological alterations have been studied in more detail, their biochemical counterparts investigated, and their main functional consequences characterized. It is the aim of this chapter to present the actual state of knowledge in this field, to delineate the new experimental possibilities provided by the particular action of this amine, and to discuss its possible mechanism of action at the molecular level.

Peripheral Sympathetic Nervous System

Morphology

The peculiar properties of 6-hydroxydopamine were detected in the course of studies designed to localize, at the ultramorphological level, phenylethylamines which act as false adrenergic transmitters (Tranzer and Thoenen, 1967a,b, 1968). The chemical isomer of 6-hydroxydopamine, 5-hydroxydopamine, is a potent depletor of norepinephrine and acts, together with its O-methylated and/or β-hydroxylated metabolites, as a false adrenergic transmitter (Thoenen et al., 1967). After administration of doses of 5-hydroxydopamine which reduce the norepinephrine content of peripheral sympathetically innervated organs of rat and cat to less than 10 per cent, all the vesicles of adrenergic nerve terminals are completely filled with a dense osmiophilic material, whereas the vesicles of cholinergic nerve endings remain empty (Fig. 10-1). The high selectivity of the accumulation of the osmiophilic material in the storage vesicles of adrenergic nerve terminals, together with the blockade of this accumulation by reserpine,

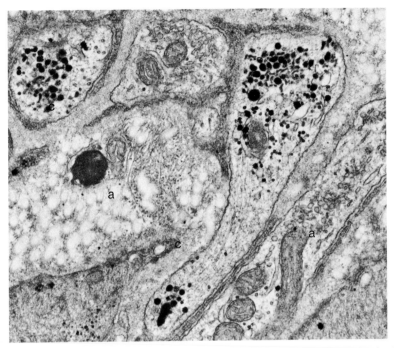

Figure 10-1   Ultramorphological localization of 5-hydroxydopamine in the iris of the cat. The animal was treated with 4 × 20 mg/kg of 5-hydroxydopamine (given within 48 hours; last dose 4 hours before killing of the animal). The norepinephrine content of the iris was reduced to less than 10 per cent of control values. a = adrenergic nerve terminals; c = cholinergic nerve terminals. (From Tranzer and Thoenen, 1967b)

provide strong evidence that the dense osmiophilic material represents the ultramorphological visualization of a false adrenergic transmitter (Tranzer and Thoenen, 1967b; Tranzer et al., 1969).

The ultramorphological changes produced by doses of 6-hydroxydopamine which reduce the norepinephrine content of sympathetically innervated organs to a similar extent as does 5-hydroxydopamine are completely different; a selective destruction of adrenergic nerve terminals occurs (Tranzer and Thoenen, 1967a, 1968).

In cats, 30 minutes after administration of large doses of 6-hydroxydopamine, the typical degenerative changes are not yet apparent, but 6-hydroxydopamine can be visualized in the storage vesicles of the adrenergic nerve terminals (Tranzer and Richards, 1971). This is possible since 6-hydroxydopamine can be located by a single fixation with OsO₄, whereas the physiological transmitter norepinephrine is only very poorly preserved by this procedure. In this way 6-hydroxydopamine just accumulated can be distinguished from the residual amounts of the physiological transmitter still present at the time of the experiment. After the injection of low doses of 6-hydroxydopamine there seems to be a preferential accumulation in the large ($\sim$1000 Å) vesicles, at least in the domestic fowl (Bennett et al., 1970; Cobb and Bennett, 1971).

By one hour after intravenous administration of large doses of 6-hydroxydopamine in cats, very distinct, fine structural alterations become apparent. Some cytoplasmic areas of the adrenergic nerve terminals appear very light, whilst others become dense. The vesicles contain less osmiophilic material than after 30 minutes, and generally the cellular structures are more or less ill-defined (Tranzer and Richards, 1971). These alterations progress gradually and, after 2 to 3 days, both in cat and rat (Tranzer and Thoenen, 1967a, 1968; Thoenen and Tranzer, 1968), most of the adrenergic nerve terminals appear as dark amorphous masses or are in the process of lysis (Fig. 10-2). They can only be recognized as residues of adrenergic nerve terminals by their topographical localization between smooth muscle cells or surrounding Schwann cells. In many instances the Schwann cells seem to engulf the degenerating nerve terminals, and the plasma membranes of the two cells are hardly discernible (Tranzer et al., 1969). These ultramorphological changes resemble very closely those encountered after surgical denervation (Van Orden et al., 1967).

The ultramorphological changes are strictly confined to the adrenergic nerve terminals. The surrounding Schwann cells, smooth muscle cells, and particularly the cholinergic nerve endings do not exhibit any ultramorphological alterations (Tranzer and Thoenen, 1967a, 1968; Tranzer et al., 1969). The contrast between adrenergic and cholinergic nerve endings is most impressively demonstrated in organs such as iris and vas deferens, where the two kinds of autonomous nerves are located in close proximity, sometimes enclosed by the same Schwann cell (Fig. 10-2). After 5 to 10 days, the degenerated adrenergic nerve terminals finally disappear, whereas the cholinergic nerves appear perfectly normal throughout this period of observation. The completeness of destruction and the time course of regeneration vary from organ to organ and from species to species (Thoenen and Tranzer, 1968; Malmfors, 1971; Thoe-

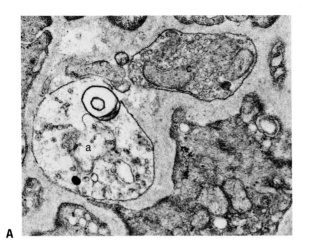

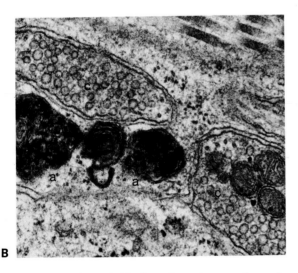

Figure 10-2 Effect of 6-hydroxydopamine on adrenergic nerve endings in the cat iris (A) and the rat heart (B). Twenty-four to 48 hours after administration of the last dose of 6-hydroxydopamine (4 × 20 mg/kg given intraperitoneally within 48 hours in cats, 2 × 50 mg/kg given intravenously within 24 hours in rats), the adrenergic (a) nerve endings are at various stages of degeneration. Cholinergic (c) nerve terminals do not show any signs of morphological alterations. From Thoenen and Tranzer, 1968; Tranzer and Thoenen, 1968)

nen, 1971a). In the nictitating membrane of the cat, for instance, the normal morphological pattern, together with a normal level of norepinephrine, is reached again after 12 to 14 weeks (Tranzer and Thoenen, 1968; Häusler et al., 1969; Tranzer et al., 1969).

In the sympathetic ganglia of adult cats and rats, the cell bodies corresponding to the destroyed nerve terminals show neither light microscopic nor electron microscopic alterations (Tranzer and Thoenen, 1968; Tranzer et al., 1969; Tranzer and Richards, 1971). Moreover, in the superior cervical and mesenteric ganglia of the cat, neither close arterial nor intraganglionic injections of high doses of 6-hydroxydopamine were able to produce morphological alterations (Tranzer and Richards, 1971). The ultramorphological findings that only nerve terminals are destroyed in adult animals are in agreement with fluorescence microscopic observations in rats and mice, which demonstrated that treatment with 6-hydroxydopamine produces a preferential disappearance of the terminal network in the iris, whereas the fluorescence in the more proximal parts of the axon persists or even increases (Malmfors and Sachs, 1968). This increase in fluorescence could be taken to indicate that the storage vesicles produced in the intact cell body are transported down the axon and pile up in the "amputation stump" as observed after crushing or ligating adrenergic nerves (Kapeller and Mayor, 1967, 1969; Geffen and Ostberg, 1969).

In contrast to adult animals, the treatment of newborn mice and rats with 6-hydroxydopamine results in severe damage of the cell bodies of adrenergic neurons in peripheral sympathetic ganglia, as recently reported by Angeletti and Levi-Montalcini (1970). Daily injections of 50 mg/kg of 6-hydroxydopamine for 10 days after birth have produced a virtually complete destruction of the neuronal cell bodies in all sympathetic ganglia studied so far. The sequence, ultrastructural localization, and time course of the degenerative events occurring after administration of 6-hydroxydopamine are entirely different from those produced by the nerve growth factor antiserum. After treatment of newborn animals with nerve growth factor antiserum, the early lesions detectable at the ultramorphological level are mainly located in the nuclear and nucleolar compartment, whereas those occurring after 6-hydroxydopamine are primarily located in the cytoplasm. Lacunar spaces are scattered throughout the cytoplasm, the shape of the mitochondria is altered, and cell membranes have partially disappeared (Angeletti and Levi-Montalcini, 1970). In 2-week-old chicks, the morphological alterations produced by 6-hydroxydopamine seem to be classifiable between those occurring in adult and newborn mammals. The main lesions are located in the terminal parts of the neurons, and only minor but clearly discernible changes such as necrosis and lysis of single mitochondria are present in the perikaryon (Cobb and Bennett, 1971).

According to Angeletti and Levi-Montalcini (1970), who have studied very intensely the biological effects of the nerve growth factor and its antiserum (Levi-Montalcini and Angeletti, 1966, 1968), the destruction of neuronal cells in sympathetic ganglia accomplished by repeated administration of 6-hydroxydopamine to newborn animals is more complete than that achieved by nerve growth factor antiserum.

The differences between the effect of 6-hydroxydopamine in newborn and adult animals provide the unique possibility of using the amine as a tool for "irreversible chemical sympathectomy" if administered to newborn, and "reversible chemical sympathectomy" if administered to adult animals (Thoenen, 1971b).

Biochemical Effects of 6-Hydroxydopamine on Peripheral Adrenergic Neurons

The prominent finding of the initial pharmacological studies with 6-hydroxydopamine was the efficient and very long-lasting depletion of norepinephrine from peripheral sympathetically innervated organs of various species (Porter et al., 1963; Stone et al., 1963; Laverty et al., 1965). Originally it was proposed that 6-hydroxydopamine might damage the amine storage sites in the adrenergic nerve terminals (Porter et al., 1963; Laverty et al., 1965) or act as a false adrenergic transmitter (Porter et al., 1965) with an extremely long biological half-life resulting from a high affinity to the storage sites.

After electron microscopic studies had provided a satisfactory explanation for the peculiar long-lasting norepinephrine depletion, the question arose as to whether the reduction of the norepinephrine content represents a reliable measure for the extent of the destruction of adrenergic nerve terminals and for the time course of their regeneration. The relevance of this assumption is supported by the recent finding that—at least in the rat heart—there is a good correlation between the 6-hydroxydopamine-induced reduction of the norepinephrine content and the activity of tyrosine hydroxylase (Thoenen, 1971b), an enzyme which is selectively located within adrenergic neurons (Sedvall and Kopin, 1967; Mueller et al., 1969a). Both 24 hours and one week after administration of a single dose (1 millimole/kg) of 6-hydroxydopamine, the percentage reduction in nor-

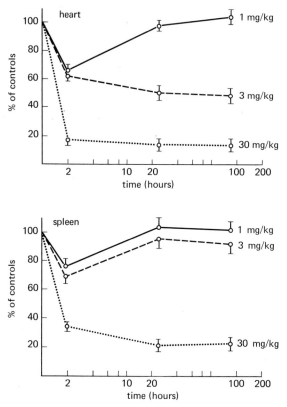

Figure 10-3 The effect of single doses of 6-hydroxydopamine on the norepinephrine content of the rat heart and spleen. Six-hydroxydopamine was injected intravenously in 0.001 N HCl. The norepinephrine content is expressed in per cent of controls injected with 0.001 N HCl only. (From Thoenen and Tranzer, 1968)

epinephrine content and tyrosine hydroxylase activity were very similar (Thoenen, 1971b), as was the rate of recovery observed over several weeks after repeated administration of 6-hydroxydopamine (Mueller and Thoenen, unpublished results).

That the uptake of 6-hydroxydopamine into the adrenergic nerve terminals is a prerequisite for its destructive effect can be deduced from the fact that desmethylimipramine and related compounds, which interfere with the transport of norepinephrine and other phenylethylamines through the neuronal membrane of adrenergic neurons (Hertting et al., 1961; Axelrod et al., 1962; Iversen, 1965), prevent the norepinephrine depletion by 6-hydroxydopamine (Stone et al., 1964) and abolish the corresponding fluorescence microscopic changes (Malmfors and Sachs, 1968). Moreover, a critical dose of 6-hydroxydopamine seems to be necessary to produce the characteristic long-lasting norepinephrine depletion and hence destruction of adrenergic nerve terminals. This can be deduced from the time course of norepinephrine depletion after administration of single doses of 6-hydroxydopamine (Fig. 10-3). In the rat heart, 1 mg/ kg of 6-hydroxydopamine produced only a transient reduction of the norepinephrine content, and control levels were reached again after 24 hours. However, 3 mg/kg produced a depletion which showed no tendency to recover for up to one week. In the spleen, the long-lasting depletion occurred only after administration of 30 mg/kg, demonstrating that the dose of 6-hydroxydopamine critical for this effect varies considerably from organ to organ. These organ differences depend most probably on the varying blood supply, both with respect to the organ mass and, above all, the density of the adrenergic innervation. The denser the innervation, the smaller is the share of the amine delivered by the bloodstream to a single nerve ending.

The assumption that the destruction of adrenergic nerve terminals depends on a critical dose of 6-hydroxydopamine has been confirmed in a series of morphological studies (Cobb and Bennett, 1971; Malmfors, 1971) and is further supported by biochemical experiments performed with tritiated 6-hydroxydopamine (Thoenen and Tranzer, 1968). Thirty minutes after administration of 1, 3, and 30 mg/kg of ^{3}H-6-hydroxydopamine the quantity of ^{3}H-amines (6-hydroxydopamine and possible metabolites) retained by the rat heart and spleen correspond to the doses injected. However, after 2 hours and, even more strikingly, after 24 hours the quantity of ^{3}H-amines retained was inversely related to the dose initially administered (Fig. 10-4). These results suggest that 6-hydroxydopamine, given in low doses, is taken up and stored in adrenergic nerve terminals without producing detectable damage to structural elements. The norepinephrine content recovers rapidly, no changes in tyrosine hydroxylase activity are detectable (Thoenen et al., 1970), and the 6-hydroxydopamine accumulated can be liberated as a false adrenergic transmitter, as shown in the isolated perfused spleen of the cat (Thoenen and Tranzer, 1968). Higher doses of 6-hydroxydopamine, however, result in damage to structural elements, and as soon as a critical stage of damage is reached complete degeneration of the nerve terminals occurs.

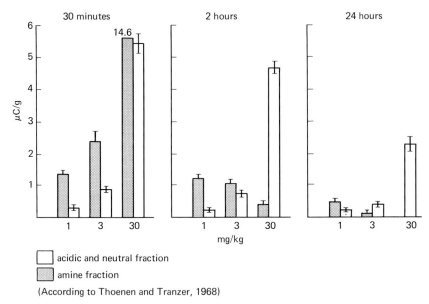

acidic and neutral fraction
amine fraction

(According to Thoenen and Tranzer, 1968)

Figure 10-4   Uptake and retention of ^{3}H-6-hydroxydopamine in the rat heart. The animals were injected intravenously with 1, 3, or 30 mg/kg of ^{3}H-6-hydroxydopamine. They were killed 30 minutes, 2 hours, or 24 hours later. The radioactivity present in the supernatant of hearts homogenized in 0.4 N perchloric acid was separated into acidic and basic (amine) fractions on Dowex 50 WX4 columns.

Consequently, the same happens to the storage sites which are also no longer available for the accumulation of 6-hydroxydopamine. This explains the paradoxical retention of ^{3}H-amines after administration of ^{3}H-6-hydroxydopamine, that is, large amounts of retained ^{3}H-amines after low doses of ^{3}H-6-hydroxydopamine and small amounts after high doses.

As was to be expected from experiments after surgical denervation and immunosympathectomy (for references see Thoenen, 1971a), the uptake and retention of intravenously injected ^{3}H-norepinephrine in sympathetically innervated organs was greatly reduced after repeated administration of 6-hydroxydopamine. However, the reduction of ^{3}H-norepinephrine was somewhat less than that of endogenous norepinephrine (Thoenen and Tranzer, 1968). This is in accordance with observations of Hertting and Schiefthaler (1964) in the heart of cats after surgical denervation. These findings might be explained either by a relatively higher contribution of extraneuronal uptake of ^{3}H-norepinephrine after destruction of the main part of adrenergic neurons or by an increased uptake by the residual intact nerve terminals. The latter possibility seems to be very plausible since the number of nerve endings available for the removal of circulating norepinephrine is reduced and therefore the surviving nerve terminals are exposed for a longer time to higher concentrations of ^{3}H-norepinephrine. In addition to the reduced uptake and retention of intravenously injected ^{3}H-norepinephrine there was also a relative increase of the O-methylated and/or deaminated metabolites of ^{3}H-norepinephrine (Thoenen and Tranzer, 1968). Jonsson and Sachs (1970) made very similar observations *in vitro* when tissues of animals treated with 6-hydroxydopamine were incubated with ^{3}H-norepinephrine.

In recent experiments, Hertting and Peskar (1971) studied the effect of chemical sympathectomy on the uptake and retention of ^{3}H-norepinephrine and ^{3}H-dopamine in the isolated perfused heart of the rat. They found that uptake I was greatly reduced for both amines whereas uptake II was unchanged. These findings further support the concept that uptake I depends on intact adrenergic nerves whereas uptake II involves extraneuronal sites (for references see Lightman and Iversen, 1969). Furthermore, they found that not only uptake I of dopamine was greatly reduced but also the transformation of dopamine into norepinephrine. This is in agreement with the recent observation of Molinoff et al. (1970) that 6-hydroxydopamine results not only in a reduction of the *in vitro* tyrosine hydroxylase activity in the rat heart but also in a reduction of dopamine-β-hydroxylase activity.

After administration of high doses of 6-hydroxydopamine, which lead to an extensive destruction of peripheral adrenergic nerve terminals in adult rats and cats, neither light nor electron microscopic alterations could be detected in the corresponding cell bodies (Tranzer and Thoenen, 1968; Tranzer and Richards, 1971). However, recent biochemical investigations have brought forth evidence that, in spite of the absence of morphological alterations, 6-hydroxydopamine is, also in adult animals, not devoid of any damaging effect on the cell bodies of adrenergic neurons. In previous studies it has been shown that 6-hydroxydopamine produces an induction of tyrosine hydroxylase in the rat adrenal medulla (which is not destroyed by 6-hydroxydopamine), resulting from a reflex increase in the activity of the splanchnic nerves supplying the adrenals (Mueller et al., 1969a; Thoenen et al., 1969a). A series of different drugs, which interfere by other mechanisms with the postganglionic adrenergic transmission, share this property with 6-hydroxydopamine (Thoenen et al., 1969a). However, in contrast to the latter, they induce tyrosine hydroxylase not only in the adrenal medulla but also in sympathetic ganglia. This dissociation between neurally mediated enzyme induction in adrenal medulla and sympathetic ganglia could be interpreted as damage to the ganglionic cell bodies caused by 6-hydroxydopamine, although of minor degree when compared with that of the nerve terminals. This assumption is supported by the observation that treatment with high doses of 6-hydroxydopamine not only failed to produce the expected transsynaptic induction of tyrosine hydroxylase in sympathetic ganglia of the rat, but also prevented the induction of this enzyme—at least transiently—by subsequent exposure to cold or administration of reserpine (Thoenen, 1971b), both of which cause an efficient trans-synaptic induction of tyrosine hydroxylase (Mueller et al., 1969b; Thoenen, 1970) and dopamine-β-hydroxylase (Molinoff et al., 1970; Thoenen et al., in preparation) in the superior cervical and stellate ganglia of the rat. It cannot yet be decided whether this transient block of enzyme induction is due to a direct effect of 6-hydroxydopamine on the cell body or to a transient functional impairment resulting from the destruction of the corresponding adrenergic nerve terminals.

In accordance with the morphological findings of Angeletti and Levi-Montalcini (1970) in newborn mice and rats, recent biochemical studies have shown that, in adult rats treated from birth for 2 weeks with 6-hydroxydopamine (150 mg/kg/day subcutaneously), not only the size of the superior cervical and stellate ganglia was markedly reduced, but also the activity of tyrosine hydroxylase, an enzyme which is selectively located in adrenergic neurons (Sedvall and Kopin, 1967; Mueller et al., 1969a). Both the total activity of the enzyme (expressed in terms of DOPA formed/pair ganglia/hour) and the "specific activity" (expressed in terms of DOPA formed/mg protein/hour) were markedly reduced (Fig. 10-5). The total enzyme activity is a measure for the number of surviving adrenergic neurons and the "specific activity" for the changes in the ratio between neuronal and non-neuronal cells. Similar results were obtained for dopamine-β-hydroxylase (Thoenen and Kettler, unpublished observations).

At present, the reason for the differing effect of 6-hydroxydopamine on the ganglionic cell bodies of newborn and adult animals can as yet only be a matter for speculation. Among other possibilities, differences in the

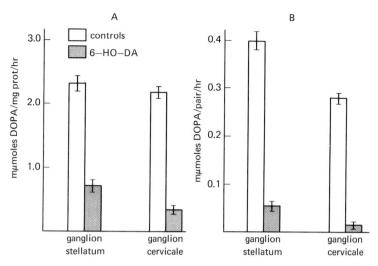

Figure 10-5   Tyrosine hydroxylase activity in stellate and superior cervical ganglia of adult rats treated as babies with 6-hydroxydopamine. The animals were injected subcutaneously for 14 days with 150 mg/kg of 6-hydroxydopamine starting on the day of their delivery. Tyrosine hydroxylase was assayed according to Mueller et al. (1969b). In Fig. 10-5A, the enzyme activity is expressed in terms of mμmoles DOPA formed/hour/mg protein (specific activity), in Fig. 10-5B, in terms of mμmoles DOPA formed/hour/pair of ganglia (total activity)

blood supply to the ganglia or differences in the efficiency of 6-hydroxy-dopamine transport into the adrenergic cell bodies have to be considered. The fact that in adult cats neither close arterial infusion nor even intra-ganglionic injection of 6-hydroxydopamine produce morphological changes (Tranzer and Richards, 1971) favors the latter possibility.

Functional Consequences of Acute and Chronic
Administration of 6-Hydroxydopamine

Morphological and biochemical studies have shown that small doses of 6-hydroxydopamine produce only a short-lasting depletion of norepineph-rine from peripheral sympathetically innervated organs, without causing any detectable damage to structural elements of adrenergic neurons. Under these experimental conditions the functional alterations are also only short-lived. The injection of 6-hydroxydopamine is followed by a short sympathomimetic response resulting from the displacement of norepinephrine. Six-hydroxydopamine is accumulated in the storage vesicles of the adrenergic nerve terminals (Bennett et al., 1970; Tranzer and Richards, 1971) and can be liberated as a false adrenergic transmitter (Thoenen and Tranzer, 1968).

In contrast, the administration of large doses of 6-hydroxydopamine is followed by a very long-lasting sympathomimetic effect which is accompanied by a gradual deterioration of adrenergic nerve function, particularly that of the neuronal membrane. In the perfused cat heart, isolated 30 minutes after intravenous injection of 40 mg/kg 6-hydroxydopamine, the heart rate was increased to about 200/min, as compared with an average of 110/min in controls (Häusler, 1971). This increased frequency persisted even *in vitro* for at least 2 hours and it could be brought to normal by administration of propranolol. It could also be prevented by pretreatment with reserpine 16 hours prior to the injection of 6-hydroxydopamine. The increased heart rate was accompanied by a very marked elevation of the norepinephrine concentration in the perfusion fluid. This prolonged spontaneous norepinephrine output, which could hardly be further increased by sympathetic nerve stimulation, is calcium-dependent (Häusler, 1971). This calcium dependence excludes a tyramine-like, indirect sympathomimetic effect, which does not require calcium, at least not for the liberation of norepinephrine from adrenergic nerve terminals (Lindmar et al., 1967; Thoenen et al., 1969b). Moreover, the calcium dependence also does not support the idea of a mere norepinephrine leakage from the damaged adrenergic nerve terminals. The most plausible explanation for the prolonged 6-hydroxydopamine-induced release of norepinephrine seems to be that of an increased calcium permeability of the neuronal membrane of the adrenergic nerve terminals. The conditions would therefore resemble those produced normally by electrical nerve stimulation, administration of acetylcholine or KCl (Häusler et al., 1968). This assumption is further supported by the fact that there is an increase in spontaneous junction potentials in the smooth muscle of the vas deferens after administration of 6-hydroxydopamine (Furness et al., 1970), which represents the electrophysiological manifestations of an increased quantal release of norepinephrine from adrenergic nerve terminals.

The fact that the liberation of norepinephrine into the perfusion fluid of the isolated cat heart by electrical stimulation of postganglionic sympathetic nerves was greatly reduced 30 and completely abolished 60 minutes after administration of 6-hydroxydopamine, and also that the asynchronous retrograde firing after injection of acetylcholine or KCl into the per-fusion cannula was markedly reduced, could be taken to indicate that all the observed phenomena (increased quantal release of norepinephrine, reduced responsiveness to sympathetic nerve stimulation, abolition of ret-rograde firing after injection of acetylcholine or KCl) are due to a depo-larization of the neuronal membrane of the adrenergic nerve terminals. However, depolarization of adrenergic nerve terminals results in abolition of their neuronal amine uptake, and (Hamberger and Malmfors, 1967), at least in the cat nictitating membrane, the norepinephrine transport seems to be completely intact up to 3 hours after administration of 6-hydroxydopamine. A distinct impairment of this membrane function, characteristic of the adrenergic nerve terminal, was observed much later, 14 hours after administration of 6-hydroxydopamine, when the isolated nictitating membrane was no longer contracted (Häusler, 1971). At that time the preparation showed a supersensitivity to norepinephrine which was as high as that of controls in the presence of optimal concentrations of cocaine. It can be concluded that there is a dissociation between the appearance of the impairment of the different membranal functions of the adrenergic nerves. An increased calcium permeability seems to be the first detectable alteration, and this is followed by the failure to generate and/or conduct nerve impulses. The amine-transport through the neu-ronal membrane seems to be a rather resistant function, still entirely in-tact 3 hours after administration of high doses of 6-hydroxydopamine (Häusler, 1971).

The prolonged sympathomimetic effect of high doses of 6-hydroxy-dopamine is also very impressively demonstrated by the time course of the contraction of the nictitating membrane of conscious cats (Trende-lenburg and Wagner, 1971): A maximal contraction occurs immediately after the injection of the amine and about 11 hours are required until half relaxation is reached again. Supersensitivity to norepinephrine de-velops during the falling phase of the contraction, and this process re-sembles the events observed after surgical denervation where prejunc-tional supersensitivity to norepinephrine develops parallel to the decrease of the denervation contraction (Langer, 1966; Smith et al., 1966; Langer et al., 1967).

Repeated administration of high doses of 6-hydroxydopamine leads to an extensive destruction of peripheral adrenergic nerve terminals in vari-ous species. However, there are considerable differences from one organ

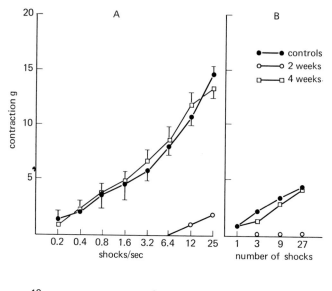

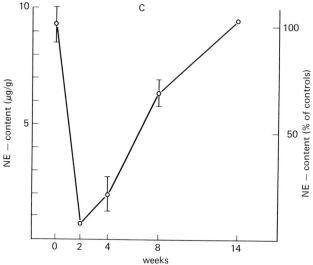

A = frequency response curve
B = stimulus number response curve
    (stimuli applied at a frequency of 1.6/sec)
C = time course of norepinephrine content.
    (The times indicated refer to the last dose of 6-hydroxydopamine.)

Figure 10-6 Contractile response of the isolated nictitating membrane to sympathetic nerve stimulation in comparison with its norepinephrine content at various times after treatment with 6-hydroxydopamine (2 × 20 mg/kg, injected intravenously within 24 hours, one week later 2 × 50 mg/kg). (According to Häusler et al., 1969)

to the other in the extent of this destruction and, accordingly, also in the functional impairment (for references see Thoenen, 1971a). After chemical sympathectomy of adult cats (intravenous administration of 2×20 mg/kg of 6-hydroxydopamine within 24 hours, followed by 2×50 mg/kg one week later; animals used one week after the last dose) the response of both the isolated perfused heart and the isolated nictitating membrane to sympathetic nerve stimulation was greatly reduced (Häusler et al., 1969). Similarly, in chemically sympathectomized rats the blood pressure response to tyramine and to electrical stimulation of the peripheral sympathetic nervous system, using the method of Gillespie and Muir (1967), was markedly reduced (Finch and Leach, 1970). While there is a good correlation between the number of reappearing nerve terminals estimated from electron microscopic pictures and the recovery of the norepinephrine content of the corresponding organs (Tranzer and Thoenen, 1968; Thoenen, 1971a), a complete recovery of the response to sympathetic nerve stimulation is reached when the regeneration of nerve terminals is far from complete (Häusler et al., 1969) (Fig. 10-6). This "premature" recovery of function is most probably of complex origin. It cannot yet be decided whether the newly regenerated terminals are able to release a higher quantity of norepinephrine per arriving nerve impulse. However, as long as the regeneration of the nerve terminals is not complete, there is a supersensitivity to norepinephrine (Häusler et al., 1969), resulting most probably from a decreased uptake of norepinephrine into the nerve terminals (Trendelenburg, 1971), and in some organs there is an additional nonspecific supersensitivity of the effector cells (for references see Thoenen, 1971a).

In general, the damaging effect of 6-hydroxydopamine is strictly confined to the adrenergic neurons. However, after intravenous injection of rats with extremely high doses of 6-hydroxydopamine (200 mg/kg), there occurred transient damage to the α-adrenergic receptors of the mesenteric artery (Häusler, 1971). Thirty minutes to 20 hours after injection of 6-hydroxydopamine the dose-response curve of norepinephrine in the isolated perfused mesenteric artery was shifted to the right and the maximum was greatly depressed (Häusler, 1971). However, there was a partial recovery after 2 days and a full recovery after 5 days. That the depression of the dose-response curve for norepinephrine results from a noncompetitive blockade of α-receptors and not from a nonspecific action of 6-hydroxydopamine on vascular smooth muscle can be deduced from the fact that neither the vasoconstrictor effect of KCl nor that of Ca^{++} in depolarized preparations was reduced after administration of 6-hydroxydopamine (Häusler, 1971). Furthermore, when phentolamine, a rapidly reversible α-adrenergic blocking agent, was given 30 minutes prior to the injection of 6-hydroxydopamine, there was an almost complete protection from damage by 6-hydroxydopamine of the α-adrenergic receptors of the vascular smooth muscle.

Central Nervous System

Morphology

As a result of its poor penetration through the blood-brain barrier 6-hydroxydopamine has no significant effect on brain monoamines after systemic administration (Porter et al., 1963; Laverty et al., 1965). However, intracerebral or intraventricular injection of 6-hydroxydopamine elicits characteristic long-lasting biochemical and morphological alterations (Ungerstedt, 1968; Bloom et al., 1969; Burkard et al., 1969; Uretsky and Iversen, 1969, 1970). The details of the fluorescence and electron microscopic changes have been reviewed very recently (Bloom, 1971; Richards, 1971; Ungerstedt, 1971) and therefore the main emphasis will be put on the differences between peripheral and central nervous system.

Neither ultramorphological nor permanent biochemical defects have been observed in peripheral sympathetic ganglia after systemic administration of 6-hydroxydopamine to adult animals. This lack of an effect on the cell bodies of adrenergic neurons seems to be the basis for the complete or almost complete regeneration of destroyed adrenergic nerve terminals, although the time course of their regeneration varies very considerably from organ to organ and species to species (Thoenen, 1971a). In the central nervous system—at least in the rat—there is neither morphological (Bloom, 1971; Ungerstedt, 1971) nor biochemical (Uretsky and Iversen, 1970; Iversen and Uretsky, 1971) evidence for regeneration of destroyed nerve terminals, even in studies extended over more than two years (Ungerstedt, 1971). The failure of the central adrenergic neurons to regenerate their destroyed nerve endings may—at least partially —be due to direct damage to the corresponding cell bodies. In areas of the lateral brain stem, known to contain numerous noradrenergic cell bodies

(Dahlström and Fuxe, 1964), the intracisternal administration of 6-hydroxydopamine leads to an accumulation of autofluorescent, orange-yellow material in the perikaryon of many neurons (Bloom, 1971). The electron microscopic counterparts of these fluorescence microscopic findings are highly dystrophic areas, characterized by extremely electron-dense cytoplasm, partially destroyed mitochondria and remnants of endoplasmic reticulum. These structures are frequently contacted by synaptic terminals which appear quite normal (Bloom, 1971). It is worthy of note that the dystrophic perikaryal structures remain unchanged for months, whereas the degenerated nerve terminals, such as those in the periphery, are removed within a few days by ingestion into surrounding glia or other phagocytotic cells (Bloom, 1971). However, the damage to neuronal cell bodies cannot fully account for their failure to regenerate the destroyed nerve terminals, since completely intact (morphologically speaking, at least) neuronal cells also lack the ability to regenerate their destroyed nerve endings in the central nervous system (Bloom, 1971; Ungerstedt, 1971).

There is a further marked difference between the effect of 6-hydroxydopamine in the periphery and the central nervous system: in the periphery there is a good correlation between the ultramorphological and biochemical alterations, whereas, in the brain, distinct dissociations have been reported to occur under specific experimental conditions. Bartholini et al. (1970, 1971) reported that a single dose of 200 μg of intraventricularly injected 6-hydroxydopamine elicits a permanent reduction of the norepinephrine content and tyrosine hydroxylase activity in various areas of the brain without detectable ultramorphological changes. These findings are in accordance with previous observations of Bloom et al. (1969) that, within a certain dose range, 6-hydroxydopamine produces a long-lasting depletion of dopamine from the nucleus caudatus without any electron microscopic alterations. All these experimental data show that, in the central nervous system, permanent damage to structural elements may occur without detectable ultramorphological alterations. In the context of this dissociation between ultramorphological and biochemical findings in the brain, it must be borne in mind that the detection of ultramorphological changes in the brain is much more difficult than in the periphery: minor changes can easily go unnoticed and can be compromised by borderline adequacy of perfusion fixation (Bloom, 1971). Even in brain regions with the highest density of adrenergic neurons, their nerve terminals represent at most 3 per cent of the total number (Richards, 1971). Furthermore, nerve terminals with a more or less normal appearance have been shown to be engulfed by surrounding glia cells, which is indirect evidence for major damage to these nerve endings, in spite of a normal morphology (Bloom, 1971).

It is not surprising that a continuous spectrum of damage is encountered, i.e. functional impairment only, biochemically detectable alterations of structural elements and morphological changes. However, it is an extraordinary finding that structural elements of nerve cells such as tyrosine hydroxylase, and DOPA-decarboxylase are *permanently* reduced without any morphological manifestation. It seems that, in the central nervous system, the replacement of damaged elements is very limited, since there is neither any regeneration of destroyed nerve terminals, nor any removal and replacement of single damaged cell constituents in otherwise still functioning neurons, as demonstrated by the persistence of morphological damage to single elements in the cell body (Bloom, 1971) and the persistent reduction of enzymes in neurons without detectable morphological alterations (Bartholini et al., 1971). These findings could be of considerable importance with respect to the permanent changes of structural elements which are involved in the regulation and determination of interneuronal pathways (Glassman and Wilson, 1970).

Biochemical Effects of 6-Hydroxydopamine in the Central Nervous System

Like the systemic administration in the periphery, the effect of intraventricular or intracisternal injection of 6-hydroxydopamine seems to be confined virtually selectively to noradrenergic or dopaminergic neurons. Doses of 6-hydroxydopamine which produce an efficient and long-lasting depletion of norepinephrine and dopamine have no significant effect on the content of 5-hydroxytryptamine and γ-aminobutyric acid of the rat brain (Burkard et al., 1969; Uretsky and Iversen, 1969, 1970). There are also considerable differences in the degree of catecholamine depletion between different brain regions (Bloom et al., 1969; Uretsky and Iversen, 1970; Bartholini et al., 1971). After administration of two doses of 250 μg of 6-hydroxydopamine the region most severely depleted was the cerebral cortex, in which the norepinephrine content was reduced to 3 per cent of that of controls. The region least affected was the medulla-pons area in which the norepinephrine content was reduced to 35 per cent only (Iversen and Uretsky, 1971). The total amount of norepinephrine in the medulla-pons region normally accounts for only 15 per cent of that found in the whole brain, but after administration of 6-hydroxydopamine almost 50 per cent of the residual norepinephrine is localized in this region. The regional differences in the efficiency of norepinephrine depletion by 6-hydroxydopamine may partially result from differences in the concentrations of 6-hydroxydopamine to which the single neurons are exposed, depending on their localization with respect to the site of drug injection. However, this cannot fully explain the poor effect on the medulla-pons region, since there is a much more efficient norepinephrine depletion in the spinal cord (Iversen and Uretsky, 1971), which is even more remote from the site of injection. It is possible that the relative resistance of the medulla-pons region results from differences in the ratio between nerve terminals and cell bodies. This region is particularly rich in adrenergic cell bodies (Dahlström and Fuxe, 1964), and it seems that not only in the periphery but also in the central nervous system there is preferential damage to nerve terminals (Bloom, 1971; Ungerstedt, 1971). It has not yet been established whether these differences in susceptibility result mainly from a more efficient amine transport in the nerve terminals or whether differences in the volume/surface ratio are also of importance.

There are not only considerable differences in the extent of catecholamine depletion between different brain regions, but also between the extent of norepinephrine and dopamine depletion. After repeated intraventricular administration of large doses of 6-hydroxydopamine, the norepinephrine content of the whole rat brain was reduced to 10 per cent, whereas that of dopamine was diminished to 25 per cent only (Iversen and Uretsky, 1971). These differences in the ability of 6-hydroxydopamine to deplete the two catecholamines can be used for a more or less selective depletion of norepinephrine. After administration of three doses of 25 μg of 6-hydroxydopamine, the norepinephrine content of the rat brain was reduced to 25 per cent, whereas the dopamine content was only diminished to 90 per cent (Iversen and Uretsky, 1971). On the other hand, the particularly effective protection of noradrenergic neurons from the effect of 6-hydroxydopamine by protriptyline (Stone et al., 1964) can be used for a relatively selective destruction of dopaminergic neurons. In rats pretreated with 15 mg/kg of protriptyline two hours prior to the intraventricular injection of 100 μg of 6-hydroxydopamine it was possible to achieve a substantial depletion of dopamine (reduced to 50 per cent of controls) without any significant change in norepinephrine content (Evetts and Iversen, 1970).

As in the periphery, there is generally also a good correlation between the permanent reduction of the catecholamine content and the reduction of tyrosine hydroxylase (Uretsky and Iversen, 1970; Bartholini et al., 1971; Iversen and Uretsky, 1971), which is a characteristic marker enzyme for neurons which synthesize and store catecholamines. DOPA-decarboxylase or, more correctly, "aromatic amino acid decarboxylase," is also diminished after administration of 6-hydroxydopamine, although to a lesser degree than tyrosine hydroxylase (Uretsky and Iversen, 1970). This is consistent with other observations which indicate that only part of DOPA-decarboxylase is located in catecholamine neurons, and that this enzyme is also associated with serotonin neurons and endothelial cells of cerebral blood vessels (Iversen and Uretsky, 1971).

The fact that both catechol-O-methyltransferase and monoamine oxidase activity in the rat hypothalamus and striatum is not diminished after intraventricular administration of 6-hydroxydopamine suggests that the greater part of these enzymes is not associated with catecholamine neurons (Uretsky and Iversen, 1970).

Both in the periphery and the central nervous system there is, in general, a close parallelism between the permanent reduction of the norepinephrine content, the reduction of tyrosine hydroxylase, and the diminution of ^{3}H-norepinephrine uptake (Thoenen and Tranzer, 1968; Uretsky and Iversen, 1970; Iversen and Uretsky, 1971; Jonsson, 1971; Thoenen, 1971). All these parameters represent quantitative biochemical counterparts to the damage to structural elements in catecholamine neurons. However, in contrast to the periphery, in the central nervous system there seems to exist the possibility that, under particular experimental conditions, permanent damage to structural elements occurs without detectable ultramorphological changes (Bartholini et al., 1970, 1971).

Functional Consequences of Intraventricular Administration of 6-Hydroxydopamine

In the investigation of the peripheral sympathetic nervous system, the lesioning of a given group of neurons to study the consequences of their elimination and, thus, delineation of their physiological function, has found wide application (for references see Thoenen, 1971a). In the central nervous system the application of this principle is greatly limited by the topographical complexity of the neuronal systems. Therefore, the possibility of achieving a selective destruction of a single population of neurons is of even greater interest in the brain than in the periphery. This is particularly the case with dopaminergic and noradrenergic neurons, which are suspected to play an important role in a great variety of regulatory functions.

The results achieved so far with 6-hydroxydopamine have not completely fulfilled the initial optimistic expectations. Although 6-hydroxydopamine is able to eliminate the noradrenergic and dopaminergic nerve terminals in large areas of the brain, this elimination is not complete and the main part of cell bodies and nonterminal axons survive (Bloom, 1971; Richards, 1971; Ungerstedt, 1971). In view of the extraordinary capacity of the brain to compensate for the loss of destroyed components, the surviving elements may provide a baseline function of the central noradrenergic and dopaminergic neurons. The incompleteness of destruction and the redundancy of neuronal circuits which may compensate for the lost original pathways have to be borne in mind if one wishes to interpret the functional consequences of intraventricular injection of 6-hydroxydopamine. The situation becomes even more complex when one considers the possibility that 6-hydroxydopamine may also involve receptor sites. Recent experiments have provided evidence for this by demonstrating that intraventricularly injected 6-hydroxydopamine impairs for several days the otherwise easily reproducible hypothermic effect of intraventricularly injected norepinephrine (Nakamura and Thoenen, in preparation).

During the first hours after intraventricular injection of 6-hydroxydopamine the behavior of rats resembles that after administration of reserpine, i.e. they have a hunched back, and raised fur, and show a decreased motor activity. The initially reduced water and food intake returns to normal after three to four days (Evetts et al., 1970). One week to ten days after administration of 6-hydroxydopamine a depression of motor and exploratory behavior can be consistently observed only after two doses of 250 μg 6-hydroxydopamine, whereas a single dose has no significant effect (Burkard et al., 1969; Evetts et al., 1970). One of the most prominent changes in behavior is the increased irritability of rats on being handled. This effect is already evident after a single dose of 250 μg of 6-hydroxydopamine, but becomes more pronounced after one to two further doses (Evetts et al., 1970). The longest period of increased irritability observed so far was more than a month (Nakamura, personal communication).

The stimulation of motor activity by (+)-amphetamine is not significantly changed by prior administration of 2×250 μg 6-hydroxydopamine, which reduces the total catecholamine content of the brain to 20 to 25 per cent (Evetts et al., 1970). These results, together with others, suggest that there is no simple relationship between the level of cerebral catecholamines and the magnitude of the response to (+)-amphetamine (Evetts et al., 1970), although there is good evidence that catecholamines play an important role in the stimulation of motor activity by (+)-amphetamine (Smith, 1963; Stein, 1964; Weissman et al., 1966). The influence of intraventricular treatment of rats with 6-hydroxydopamine on the subsequent administration of neuroleptic and antidepressive drugs is rather complex and the interpretation ambiguous. For details on this subject the reader is referred to the study of Jalfre and Haefely (1971).

It can be concluded that the intraventricular administration of 6-hydroxydopamine has revealed many interesting morphological and biochemical aspects of central catecholamine neurons. However, the use of this method has serious limitations for the elucidation of the role played by the systems of noradrenergic and dopaminergic neurons in the normal functions of the brain and for the action of neuropsychotropic drugs. The local, intracerebral injection of 6-hydroxydopamine for elimination of well-defined systems of dopaminergic and noradrenergic neurons seems to be more promising (Ungerstedt, 1968; 1971), since it avoids some of the pitfalls inherent in the more general but incomplete effect of intraventricular administration. However, also for the local, intracerebral administration of 6-hydroxydopamine it remains to be established whether the effect is strictly confined to dopaminergic and noradrenergic neurons and to what extent receptive structures of catecholamines are also involved. As already stated above, there is strong evidence that norepinephrine receptors involved in temperature regulation are temporarily damaged, and the accumulation of spontaneously fluorescent material in Purkinje cells after accidental local injection of 6-hydroxydopamine into the cerebellum (Bloom, 1971) seems to indicate that also noncatecholamine neurons may also be damaged by 6-hydroxydopamine if sufficiently high local concentrations are reached.

Attempts To Achieve Destruction of Central Adrenergic Neurons by Systemic Administration of 6-Hydroxydopa

After the discovery that 6-hydroxydopamine produces a selective destruction of adrenergic nerve terminals in the periphery, the next logical step was to study the effect of 6-hydroxy-DOPA, which could be expected to cross the blood-brain barrier by means of transport mechanisms for L-amino acids, to be decarboxylated in the brain, and thus to destroy central adrenergic neurons. The results obtained so far with 6-hydroxy-DOPA are very disappointing (Ong et al., 1969; Berkowitz et al., 1970; Corrodi et al., 1971), since the amino acid is considerably more toxic than the corresponding amine (Thoenen, unpublished results), and the nor-epinephrine depletion achieved in the brain is much less efficient than that obtained by intraventricular injection of 6-hydroxydopamine, even when sublethal doses of 6-hydroxy-DOPA are used (Table 10-1). Furthermore, the lack of a decrease in tyrosine hydroxylase activity (one week after the last dose of 6-hydroxy-DOPA there is even a slight increase) suggests that the relatively small reduction of the norepinephrine content does not result from a destruction of adrenergic neurons. This poor effect of 6-hydroxy-DOPA could also not be improved by concomitant administration of inhibitors of DOPA-decarboxylase (Corrodi et al., 1971;

Table 10-1 Effect of 6-hydroxy-DOPA on norepinephrine content and tyrosine hydroxylase activity of the rat brain

Brain region	Norepinephrine content in per cent of controls		Tyrosine hydroxylase in per cent of controls	
	24 hours	1 week	24 hours	1 week
Medulla oblongata	38 ± 1.0***	65 ± 3***	96 ± 6	114 ± 2**
Hypothalamus	54 ± 2.7***	79 ± 4**	92 ± 9	110 ± 8
Residual parts of the brain	24 ± 2***	43 ± 2***	88 ± 8	115 ± 4*

The animals were pretreated with 2×0.5 millimoles of 6-hydroxy-DOPA, injected intravenously within 24 hours. The rats were killed 24 hours or one week after the last dose. Twenty to 30 per cent of the animals died within a week after administration of the last dose.

   * P <0.05
  ** P <0.01
 *** P <0.001

Thoenen, unpublished results) which mainly act in the periphery and which, if given together with L-DOPA, lead to a much greater increase in the brain catecholamines than L-DOPA alone (Bartholini and Pletscher, 1967; Lotti and Porter, 1970).

The high toxicity of 6-hydroxy-DOPA—the animals do not die immediately after administration of the drug but general condition deteriorates progressively in the following days—most probably results from the fact that 6-hydroxy-DOPA is as easily oxidized as 6-hydroxydopamine and that the damage caused by the very reactive oxidation products is not mainly confined to the adrenergic nerve terminals, as is the case with 6-hydroxydopamine, since the amino acid is not selectively accumulated there. The rapid oxidation of 6-hydroxy-DOPA could also explain the failure of the combination of 6-hydroxy-DOPA with a peripheral inhibitor of DOPA-decarboxylase (Corrodi et al., 1971), since 6-hydroxy-DOPA is most probably more rapidly oxidized than decarboxylated. Therefore, peripheral inhibition of DOPA-decarboxylase does not lead to higher concentrations of 6-hydroxydopamine after decarboxylation.

Various derivatives of 6-hydroxy-DOPA and 6-hydroxydopamine have been synthesized with the aim of achieving a better destruction of central adrenergic neurons than with 6-hydroxy-DOPA after systemic administration. However, of all derivatives tested so far none has been as efficient as intraventricularly injected 6-hydroxydopamine (Langemann and Thoenen, unpublished results).

Reversible and Irreversible Chemical Sympathectomy: Comparison with Surgical and Immunological Methods

The differences between the effect of 6-hydroxydopamine in adult and newborn animals provide the unique possibility of achieving either an "irreversible chemical sympathectomy" by treatment of newborn animals or a "reversible chemical sympathectomy" by treatment of adult animals.

Both for reversible and irreversible peripheral chemical sympathectomy, the repeated administration of 6-hydroxydopamine proved to be superior to a single, even very high dose of 6-hydroxydopamine (Thoenen, 1970, 1971). This is in agreement with the observations made in the central nervous system (Uretsky and Iversen, 1969, 1970). In adult animals the differences in the efficiency of reversible denervation most probably result from differences in blood supply to the single organs, both with respect to their mass and particularly with respect to their norepinephrine content, which reflects the density of their innervation (Thoenen and Tranzer, 1968). The denser the innervation, the smaller is the share of 6-hydroxydopamine delivered by a given blood volume to a single nerve ending. In this context, the poor effect of 6-hydroxydopamine on the adrenergic nerves in the mesenteric vessels of the rat is remarkable (Häusler et al., 1971) and most probably results from the particular localization of adrenergic nerves in the blood vessels, especially the arteries (Lever and Esterhuizen, 1961; Fuxe and Sedvall, 1965). They are mainly found in the adventitio-medial junction. In the rat, the blood supply to the adventitia by vasa vasorum is negligible (Wolinsky and Glagov, 1967), and therefore 6-hydroxydopamine has to reach the nerve terminals in the adventitia by diffusion from the vascular lumen through intima and media which may represent considerable diffusion barriers.

Table 10-2 shows that marked differences in the degree of norepinephrine depletion are not only present in animals treated as adults with

Table 10-2   Changes in norepinephrine content after repeated administration of 6-hydroxydopamine to adult and newborn rats

Organ	Norepinephrine content in per cent of controls			
	2×50 mg/kg[a] 2×100 mg/kg (adults)	4×100 mg/kg[b] (adults)	10×100 mg/kg[c] (newborn)	14×150 mg/kg[d] (newborn)
Heart	7.6 ± 0.8	6.2 ± 1.0	1.9 ± 0.7	<1.0
Spleen	5.1 ± 0.9	3.7 ± 0.7	<1.0	<1.0
Salivary gland	—	8.0 ± 0.8	<1.0	<1.0
Mesenterium	—	31.8 ± 4.4	—	24 ± 6.0
Vas deferens	18.8 ± 1.8	10.5 ± 1.3	73.0 ± 9.0	32 ± 3.0
Adrenals	95.7 ± 6.9	94.0 ± 2.4	105.0 ± 2.8	130 ± 19

The treatment of groups a and b was begun when the animals weighed 100 to 110 g. Group a was injected intravenously with 2×50 mg/kg of 6-hydroxydopamine within 24 hours. One week later, 2×100 mg/kg were administered. Group b was injected four times with 100 mg/kg 6-hydroxydopamine at one-week intervals. Group c was treated intraperitoneally for ten days from birth with 100 mg/kg 6-hydroxydopamine given daily. Group d was treated subcutaneously for fourteen days from birth with 150 mg/kg 6-hydroxydopamine given daily. The animals of groups a and b were killed one week after the last dose of 6-hydroxydopamine, and those of groups c and d as soon as they had reached a weight of 120 to 140 g. The values given represent the mean $\pm$ S.E. of 6 to 7 experiments. The values given for the adrenals refer to the sum of norepinephrine plus epinephrine.

6-hydroxydopamine (reversible sympathectomy), but also in those treated as newborn rats. In both cases the catecholamine content of the adrenals is not significantly changed and the tissues least affected are the vas deferens and the mesentery. With the information available so far it cannot be decided for certain whether the long-lasting norepinephrine depletion in adult rats treated as babies with 6-hydroxydopamine is a measure for the permanent destruction of the whole adrenergic neuron, or whether it results from a "mixed effect," i.e. destruction of cell bodies including nerve terminals and nerve terminals only. This "mixed effect" could be suspected from the fact that the reduction of tyrosine hydroxylase (which is a biochemical measure for the extent of the destruction of adrenergic neurons)—both in the superior cervical and stellate ganglion (Fig. 10-5) —is smaller than the reduction of the norepinephrine content in the salivary gland and heart (Table 10-2), organs which are innervated from these two ganglia. It could therefore well be that the possible regeneration of nerve endings was not yet complete when the animals had reached a weight of 120 to 140 g. Experiments are in progress which will establish whether a further recovery of the norepinephrine content occurs in these organs as the animals increase in age.

It is worthy of note that the adrenal medulla and the adrenergic nerves supplying the vas deferens are both more or less resistant to 6-hydroxydopamine (Table 10-2) and immunosympathectomy (Levi-Montalcini and Angeletti 1966). The hypothesis might therefore be drawn up that there is a common reason for the resistance in baby rats of these specific neurons to 6-hydroxydopamine and nerve growth antiserum. As regards the nerve growth antiserum, it has been shown that the ganglia are highly susceptible to it for only a relatively short period during their development (Levi-Montalcini and Angeletti, 1966). Since the effect of 6-hydroxydopamine seems to depend mainly on the transport of 6-hydroxydopamine through the neuronal membrane, it remains to be established whether there is a parallel development (and disappearance) of the transport mechanism for phenethylamines in ganglionic cell bodies and susceptibility to nerve growth antiserum. This would explain the generally similar susceptibility of sympathetic ganglia of newborn animals to nerve growth antiserum and 6-hydroxydopamine.

Surgical denervation is still the method of choice for studying the effect of deprivation from sympathetic innervation in single organs, possibly in comparison with intact contralateral innervation. In spite of a very marked, long-lasting depletion of norepinephrine from iris and nictitating membrane of the cat by repeated administration of 6-hydroxydopamine, the completeness of surgical denervation is not achieved by this procedure (Thoenen and Tranzer, 1968; Häusler et al., 1969). However, for denervation of organs such as the heart with a more complex and less easily accessible adrenergic innervation, chemical or immunological sympathectomy are preferable above all for experiments which require a large number of small animals (for references see Thoenen, 1971a). In spite of an extensive destruction of adrenergic nerves, neither the immunological nor the chemical procedure achieves a complete general sympathectomy, and therefore the applicability of both methods has its limitations. Angeletti and Levi-Montalcini (1970), who have extensive experience using both methods, reported that the destruction of adrenergic cell bodies by repeated administration of 6-hydroxydopamine is more complete than that produced by nerve growth antiserum. It is not yet established whether permanent chemical sympathectomy is, in any case, superior to immunosympathectomy. However, it is a unique property of 6-hydroxydopamine that it can be used for reversible and irreversible sympathectomy in the periphery, and also that an extensive destruction of central noradrenergic and dopaminergic neurons can be achieved by intraventricular or intracerebral administration.

Compensatory Mechanisms

The destruction of adrenergic nerves leads to an increased response of the denervated organ to exogenously administered norepinephrine. This so-called denervation supersensitivity is composed of two qualitatively and quantitatively different components. One of them resembles remarkably the supersensitivity occurring after administration of cocaine. This cocaine-like component develops very rapidly and is the consequence of the abolition of what is generally the most important mechanism of inactivation of endogenously liberated and exogenously administered norepinephrine, i.e. uptake into the adrenergic nerve terminals. The second component develops slowly over several weeks. It is nonspecific and does not develop in every sympathectomized organ. There is strong evidence that this second component results from alterations in the cells of the effector organ. The time course of the development of these two components of denervation supersensitivity, their relative importance in various organs and species, and their mechanism of action have been reviewed recently (Thoenen, 1971a; Trendelenburg, 1971) and shall not be presented in detail here.

From a teleological point of view, the supersensitivity to the physiological transmitter norepinephrine can be considered as a compensatory mechanism, which helps to maintain the homeostasis of autonomic functions after destruction of greater parts of the sympathetic nervous system by surgical, immunological, or chemical procedures. Although the denervated organs no longer receive the nerve impulses which normally control their activity, they may still take part in some general reaction of the organism due to their increased response to the circulating transmitter substances.

Both chemical (permanent and reversible) and immunological sympathectomy leave the adrenal medulla unaffected (Levi-Montalcini and Angeletti, 1966; Thoenen and Tranzer, 1968; Angeletti and Levi-Montalcini, 1970; Thoenen, 1971b). It seems that the adrenals take over—at least partially—the function of the extensively destroyed sympathetic nervous system by an augmented delivery of catecholamines to the circulation, promoted by an increased reflex activity of the splanchnic nerves supplying the adrenal medulla. Under these experimental conditions, the turnover of catecholamines and their rate of synthesis from tyrosine are increased. The increased rate of synthesis is accompanied by a trans-synaptic induction of tyrosine hydroxylase, the rate-limiting enzyme in the synthesis of norepinephrine and epinephrine (for references see Mueller et al., 1969a; Thoenen et al., 1969a; Mueller, 1971). Furthermore, an increase in the *in vitro* activity of dopamine-β-hydroxylase has been observed after administration of 6-hydroxydopamine (Molinoff et al., 1970), whereas the *in vitro* activity of DOPA-decarboxylase, an enzyme which is not selectively located in adrenergic neurons or chromaffin cells, is not augmented (Thoenen et al., in preparation).

Mechanism of Action

The results presented so far show that the uptake of a critical amount of 6-hydroxydopamine into the adrenergic nerves is a prerequisite for the destructive action of this amine (Tranzer and Thoenen, 1968; Malmfors, 1971; Thoenen, 1971b). The fact that 6-hydroxydopamine, when given to adult animals, destroys the nerve terminals only, whereas, in newborn animals primarily the cell bodies are involved, most probably results from a shift in the transport-efficiency for phenylethylamines from the cell body to the periphery in the course of the development from birth to adult life.

Whereas the accumulation of 6-hydroxydopamine by the neuronal membrane pump seems to be an indispensable prerequisite for chemical sympathectomy (Stone et al., 1964; Malmfors and Sachs, 1968; Evetts and Iversen, 1970), the uptake into the storage vesicles does not seem to be necessary, since administration of reserpine prior to the injection of 6-hydroxydopamine neither prevented the characteristic ultramorphological changes (Bennett et al., 1970; Tranzer and Richards, 1971) nor the reduction of tyrosine hydroxylase in the rat heart (Thoenen et al., 1970).

These experimental data allow an assessment of the importance of the accumulation and subcellular distribution of 6-hydroxydopamine in adrenergic neurons for its specific effect, but they do not yield any information on the mechanism of action at the molecular level.

In previous preliminary experiments it has been shown that, after administration of ^{3}H-6-hydroxydopamine, a considerable part of the radioactivity present in sympathetically innervated tissues is not extractable by repeated homogenization in $HClO_4$ (Thoenen and Tranzer, 1968). In view of the extreme ease with which 6-hydroxydopamine is oxidized, we have put forward the working hypothesis that oxidation products of 6-hydroxydopamine undergo covalent binding with nucleophilic groups of biological macromolecules (Fig. 10-7). Since 6-hydroxydopamine is accumulated in adrenergic neurons, the highest density of covalent bindings, and therefore the highest degree of denaturation and impairment of function of macromolecules, occurs there. Degeneration becomes manifest as soon as a critical degree of damage is reached.

In more recent experiments it has been shown that destruction of adrenergic nerve terminals prior to administration of ^{3}H-6-hydroxydopamine results not only in a very marked reduction of the total amount of radioactivity retained by the denervated organs but also in a proportional reduction of the nonextractable radioactivity, demonstrating that the main part of radioactivity bound under normal conditions is located in adrenergic nerve terminals (Saner and Thoenen, 1971a). In spectroscopic studies

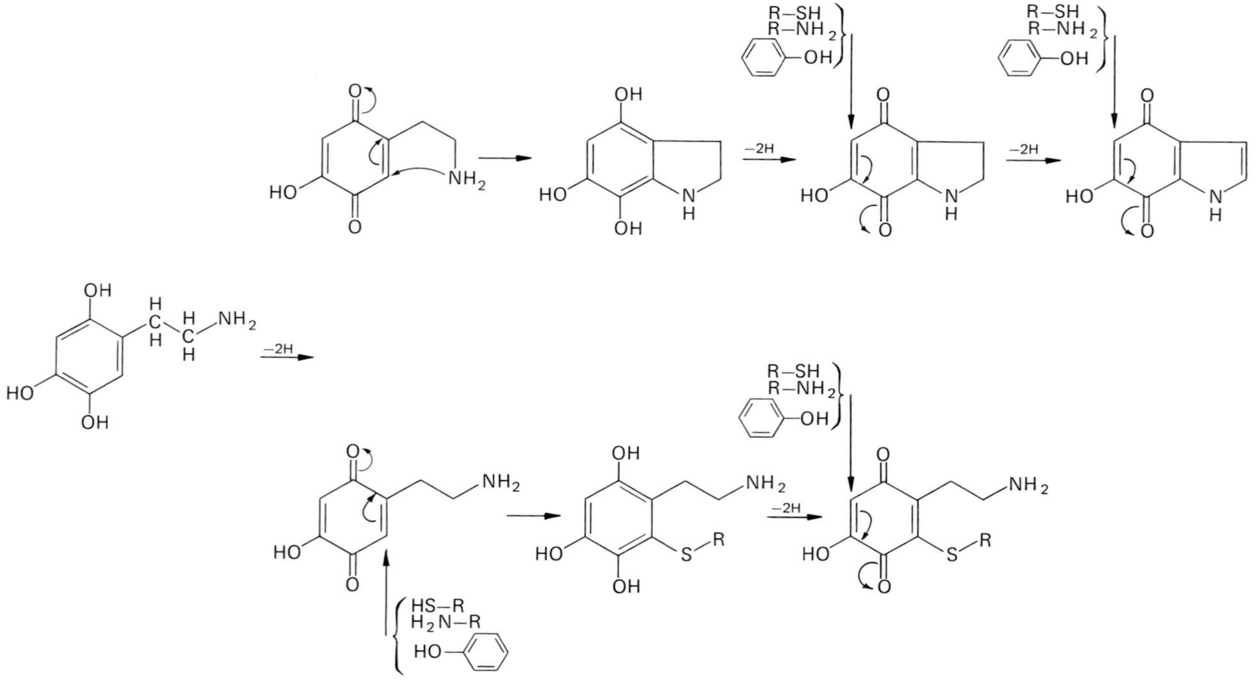

Figure 10-7 Hypothetical mechanism of action of 6-hydroxydopamine. Six-hydroxydopamine is oxidized to its p-quinone derivative which can undergo further transformation to indoline and indole derivatives. Both the original p-quinone and the indoline-indole derivatives can form covalent bindings with nucleophilic groups of biological macromolecules.

in vitro it has been shown that the oxidation products postulated in our working hypothesis are formed *in vitro* and that their formation is pH-dependent, i.e. oxidation is favored at neutral and alkaline pH levels (Saner and Thoenen, 1971b).

The involvement of nucleophilic groups of macromolecules in the covalent binding of ^{3}H-6-hydroxydopamine was studied *in vitro* using bovine albumin as a macromolecular model. Like the formation of oxidation products the covalent binding of ^{3}H-6-hydroxydopamine to bovine albumin was pH-dependent. The covalent binding of radioactivity was saturable. At a 0.5 mM concentration of bovine albumin, saturation was reached at a concentration of 70 mM ^{3}H-6-hydroxydopamine. Neither an increase in the initial concentration nor the addition of further doses of ^{3}H-6-hydroxydopamine after the binding plateau had been reached could achieve any further increase in the quantity of covalently bound radioactivity. The fact that both the rate of oxidation and the covalent binding of ^{3}H-6-hydroxydopamine to bovine albumin are pH-dependent suggests that oxidation of 6-hydroxydopamine is a prerequisite for the subsequent covalent binding to the protein molecule. This is further supported by the fact that the anti-oxidant $Na_2S_2O_5$ almost completely abolished the binding of radioactivity to albumin under experimental conditions (pH 7.4, 38° C) that otherwise favor this covalent binding (Saner and Thoenen, 1971b).

If we are correct in our working hypothesis that nucleophilic groups of macromolecules are involved in covalent binding of 6-hydroxydopamine, acetylation of bovine albumin should drastically reduce the binding of radioactivity. This is indeed the case, as shown by experiments reported in detail elsewhere (Saner and Thoenen, 1971b). To exclude the possibility that denaturation of bovine albumin, resulting from acetylation, is responsible as such for the reduced binding of radioactivity, we studied the effect of heat-denaturation. In contrast to acetylation, heat-denaturation reduced only immaterially the binding of radioactivity.

The results of the *in vivo* and *in vitro* experiments with ^{3}H-6-hydroxydopamine are compatible with the hypothesis that the destruction of adrenergic neurons by 6-hydroxydopamine results from covalent binding of oxidation products of this amine to biological macromolecules, that this reaction is nonspecific, and that the degree to which and selectivity with which adrenergic neurons are damaged depend on the efficiency of the 6-hydroxydopamine transport by the neuronal membrane pump.

Concluding Remarks

Surgical sympathectomy is still the method of choice for the denervation of organs which are supplied by a single, easily accessible ganglion. However, for general sympathectomy or denervation of organs with a more complex innervation, the surgical procedure is too cumbrous and time-consuming, especially for experiments that require a large number of animals. In such cases, immunological or chemical sympathectomy is preferable.

The fact that 6-hydroxydopamine destroys only nerve terminals if given to adult animals, and ganglionic cell bodies if given to newborn animals, makes it possible to achieve a "permanent chemical sympathectomy" by treatment of newborn animals and a "reversible chemical sympathectomy" by treatment of adult animals.

Although both immunological and chemical sympathectomy involve the whole sympathetic nervous system, these two methods also have their limitations, and there are considerable differences in the effectiveness with which single organs are denervated. It is worthy of note that there is a very close correlation between the susceptibility of ganglia of newborn animals to nerve growth factor antiserum and to 6-hydroxydopamine. The question arises, therefore, whether there is a parallel development (and disappearance) of the susceptibility to nerve growth factor antiserum and the transport mechanism for phenethylamines, since the accumulation of 6-hydroxydopamine is a prerequisite for its destructive effect.

In adult animals, the organ differences in the degree of denervation most probably result from differences in blood supply, both with respect to organ mass and, in particular, with respect to the norepinephrine content, which is a measure for the density of the adrenergic innervation. The denser the adrenergic innervation of an organ, the smaller is the share of 6-hydroxydopamine delivered by the bloodstream to a single nerve ending.

Since 6-hydroxydopamine does not cross the blood-brain barrier, the central adrenergic neurons are not affected by systemic administration of 6-hydroxydopamine. However, intraventricular or intracerebral injection of 6-hydroxydopamine leads to a selective destruction of adrenergic neurons. As is the case in the periphery, the nerve terminals are predominantly affected and there are also considerable differences in the extent of destruction between the different brain regions. Attempts to destroy adrenergic neurons by systemic administration of 6-hydroxy-DOPA have been disappointing, and there is no evidence that the modest reduction in cerebral norepinephrine content results from a destruction of adrenergic neurons, there being no corresponding reduction in tyrosine hydroxylase.

As to the mechanism of action of 6-hydroxydopamine, it has been shown that the transport of 6-hydroxydopamine into the adrenergic neuron is a prerequisite for the destructive effect, whereas the accumulation in the storage vesicles is not necessary. *In vivo* and *in vitro* experiments with ³H-6-hydroxydopamine have provided strong evidence that oxidation products of 6-hydroxydopamine are covalently bound to nucleophilic groups of biological macromolecules, that this reaction is nonspecific, and that the high degree of selectivity of damage to adrenergic neurons (nerve terminals only in adults; cell bodies in newborn animals) depends on the efficiency with which 6-hydroxydopamine is accumulated by the neuronal membrane pump.

References

Angeletti, P. U., and Levi-Montalcini, R. 1970. *Proc. Nat. Acad. Sci.* U.S. 65: 114-21.

Axelrod, J., Hertting, G., and Potter, L. 1962. *Nature* (Lond.) 194:297.

Bartholini, G., and Pletscher, A. 1967. *J. Pharmacol. Exp. Ther.* 161:14-20.

Bartholini, G., Richards, J. G., and Pletscher, A. 1970. *Experientia* 26:142-44.

Bartholini, G., Thoenen, H., and Pletscher, A. 1971. In *6-Hydroxydopamine and Catecholamine Neurons*, T. Malmfors and H. Thoenen (Eds.), North Holland, Amsterdam. pp. 163-70.

Bennett, T., Burnstock, G., Cobb, J. L. S., and Malmfors, T. 1970. *Brit. J. Pharmacol.* 37:802-9.

Berkowitz, B. A., Spector, S., Brossi, A., Focella, A., and Teitel, S. 1970. *Experientia* 26:982.

Bloom, F. E. 1971. In *6-Hydroxydopamine and Catecholamine Neurons*, T. Malmfors and H. Thoenen (Eds.), North Holland, Amsterdam. pp. 135-50.

Bloom, F. E., Algeri, S., Groppetti, A., Revuelta, A., and Costa, E. 1969. *Science* 166:1284-86.

Burkard, W. P., Jalfre, M., and Blum, J. 1969. *Experientia* 25:1295-96.

Cobb, J. L. S., and Bennett, T. 1971. In *6-Hydroxydopamine and Catecholamine Neurons*, T. Malmfors and H. Thoenen (Eds.), North Holland, Amsterdam. pp. 33-46.

Corrodi, H., Clark, W. G., and Masnoka, D. I. 1971. In *6-Hydroxydopamine and Catecholamine Neurons*, T. Malmfors and H. Thoenen (Eds.), North Holland, Amsterdam. pp. 187-92.

Dahlström, A., and Fuxe, K. 1964. *Acta Physiol. Scand.* 62 suppl. 232:1.

Evetts, K. D., and Iversen, L. L. 1970. *J. Pharm. Pharmac.* 22:540-43.

Evetts, K. D., Kretsky, N. J., Iversen, L. L., and Iversen, S. D. 1970. *Nature* (Lond.) 225:961.

Finch, L., and Leach, G. D. H. 1970. *J. Pharm. Pharmac.* 22:354-60.

Furness, J. B., Campbell, G. R., Gillard, S. M., Malmfors, T., Cobb, J. L. S., and Burnstock, G. 1970. *J. Pharmacol. Exp. Ther.* 174:111-22.

Fuxe, K., and Sedvall, G. 1965. *Acta Physiol. Scand.* 64:75-86.

Geffen, L. B., and Ostberg, A. 1969. *J. Physiol.* (Lond.) 204:583-92.

Gillespie, J. S., and Muir, T. C. 1967. *Brit. J. Pharmacol.* 30:78-87.

Glassmann, E., and Wilson, J. E. 1970. *Brain Res.* 21:157-68.

Hamberger, B., and Malmfors, T. 1967. *Acta Physiol. Scand.* 70:412-18.

Häusler, G. 1971. In *6-Hydroxydopamine and Catecholamine Neurons,* T. Malmfors and H. Thoenen (Eds.), North Holland, Amsterdam. pp. 193-204.

Häusler, G., Haefely, W., and Hürlimann, A. 1969. *Symp. on the Physiol. and the Pharmacol. of Vascular Neuroeffector Systems,* Interlaken (in press).

Häusler, G., Haefely, W., and Thoenen, H. 1969. *J. Pharmacol. Exp. Ther.* 170: 50-61.

Häusler, G., Thoenen, H., Haefely, W., and Hürlimann, A. 1968. *Naunyn-Schmiedeberg's Arch. Exp. Path. Pharmak.* 261:398-411.

Hertting, G., Axelrod, J., and Whitby, L. G. 1961. *J. Pharmacol. Exp. Ther.* 134:146-53.

Hertting, G., and Peskar, B. 1971. In *6-Hydroxydopamine and Catecholamine Neurons,* T. Malmfors and H. Thoenen (Eds.), North Holland, Amsterdam. pp. 279-290.

Hertting, G., and Schiefthaler, T. 1964. *Int. J. Neuropharmacol.* 3:65-69.

Iversen, L. L. 1965. In *Advances in Drug Research 2* N. J. Harper and A. B. Simmonds (Eds.), Academic Press, London, pp. 1-46.

Iversen, L. L., and Uretsky, N. J. 1971. In *6-Hydroxydopamine and Catecholamine Neurons,* T. Malmfors and H. Thoenen (Eds.), North Holland, Amsterdam. pp. 171-186.

Jalfre, M., and Haefely, W. 1971. In *6-Hydroxydopamine and Catecholamine Neurons,* T. Malmfors and H. Thoenen (Eds.), North Holland, Amsterdam. pp. 333-346.

Jonsson, G. 1971. In *6-Hydroxydopamine and Catecholamine Neurons,* T. Malmfors and H. Thoenen (Eds.), North Holland, Amsterdam. pp. 87-100.

Jonsson, G., and Sachs, C. 1970. *Europ. J. Pharmacol.* 9:141-55.

Kapeller, K., and Mayor, D. 1967. *Proc. Roy. Soc. B* 167:282-92.

Kapeller, K., and Mayor, D. 1969. *Proc. Roy. Soc. B* 172:39-51.

Langer, S. Z. 1966. *J. Pharmacol. Exp. Ther.* 151:66-72.

Langer, S. Z., Draskoczy, P. R., and Trendelenburg, U. 1967. *J. Pharmacol. Exp. Ther.* 157:255-73.

Laverty, R., Sharman, D. F., and Vogt, M. 1965. *Brit. J. Pharmacol.* 24:549-60.

Lever, J. D., and Esterhuizen, A. C. 1961. *Nature* (Lond.) 192:566-67.

Levi-Montalcini, R., and Angeletti, P. U. 1966. *Pharmacol. Rev.* 18:619-28.

Levi-Montalcini, R., and Angeletti, P. U. 1968. *Physiol. Rev.* 48:534-69.

Lightman, S. L., and Iversen, L. L. 1969. *Brit. J. Pharmacol.* 37:638-49.

Lindmar, R., Loeffelholz, K., and Muscholl, E. 1967. *Experientia* 23:933-34.

Lotti, V. J., and Porter, C. C. 1970. *J. Pharmacol. Exp. Ther.* 172:406.

Malmfors, T. 1971. In *6-Hydroxydopamine and Catecholamine Neurons,* T. Malmfors and H. Thoenen (Eds.), North Holland, Amsterdam. pp. 47-58.

Malmfors, T., and Sachs, C. 1968. *Europ. J. Pharmacol.* 3:89-92.

Molinoff, P. B., Weinshilboum, and Axelrod, J. 1970. *Fed. Proc.* 29:278.

Mueller, R. A. 1971. In *6-Hydroxydopamine and Catecholamine Neurons*, T. Malmfors and H. Thoenen (Eds.) North Holland, Amsterdam. pp. 291-302.

Mueller, R. A., Thoenen, H., and Axelrod, J. 1969a. *Science* 163:468-69.

Mueller, R. A., Thoenen, H., and Axelrod, J. 1969b. *J. Pharmacol. Exp. Ther.* 169: 74-79.

Ong, H. H., Creveling, C. R., and Daly, J. W. 1969. *J. Med. Chem.* 12:458.

Porter, C. C., Totaro, J. A., and Stone, C. A. 1963. *J. Pharmacol. Exp. Ther.* 140: 308-16.

Porter, C. C., Totaro, J. A., and Burcin, A. 1965. *J. Pharmacol. Exp. Ther.* 150: 17-22.

Richards, J. G. 1971. In *6-Hydroxydopamine and Catecholamine Neurons*, T. Malmfors and H. Thoenen (Eds.), North Holland, Amsterdam. pp. 151-62.

Saner, A., and Thoenen, H. 1971a. In *6-Hydroxydopamine and Catecholamine Neurons*, T. Malmfors and H. Thoenen (Eds.), North Holland, Amsterdam. pp. 265-276.

Saner, A., and Thoenen, H. 1971b. *J. Mol. Pharmacol.* (in press).

Sedvall, G. C., and Kopin, I. J. 1967. *Biochem. Pharmacol.* 16:39-46.

Senoh, S., Creveling, C. R., Udenfriend, S., and Witkop, B. 1959a. *J. Amer. Chem. Soc.* 81:6236-40.

Senoh, S., and Witkop, B. 1959b. *J. Amer. Chem. Soc.* 81:6222-31.

Senoh, S., Witkop, B., Creveling, C. R., and Udenfriend, S. 1959c. *J. Amer. Chem. Soc.* 81:1768-69.

Smith, C. B. 1963. *J. Pharmacol. Exp. Ther.* 142:343.

Smith, C. B., Trendelenburg, U., Langer, S. Z., and Tsai, T. H. 1966. *J. Pharmacol. Exp. Ther.* 51:87-94.

Stein, L. 1964. *Fed. Proc.* 23:836.

Stone, C. A., Porter, C. C., Stavorski, J. M., Ludden, C. T., and Totaro, J. A. 1964. *J. Pharmacol. Exp. Ther.* 144:196-204.

Stone, C. A., Stavorski, J. M., Ludden, C. T., Wenger, H. C., Ross, C. A., Totaro, J. A., and Porter, C. C. 1963. *J. Pharmacol. Exp. Ther.* 142:147-56.

Thoenen, H. 1970. *Nature* (Lond.) 228:861-62.

Thoenen, H. 1971a. In *Handbook of Experimental Pharmacology*, "Catecholamines," Springer, Berlin-Heidelberg-New York.

Thoenen, H. 1971b. In *6-Hydroxydogamine and Catecholamine Neurons*, T. Malmfors and H. Thoenen (Eds.), North Holland, Amsterdam. pp. 75-86.

Thoenen, H., Haefely, W., Gey, K. F., and Hürlimann, A. 1967. *Naunyn-Schmiedeberg's Arch. Exp. Pharmak. Path.* 259:17-33.

Thoenen, H., Mueller, R. A., and Axelrod, J. 1969a. *J. Pharmacol. Exp. Ther.* 169:249-54.

Thoenen, H., Hürlimann, A., and Haefely, W. 1969b. *Europ. J. Pharmacol.* 6:29-37.

Thoenen, H., and Tranzer, J. P. 1968. *Naunyn-Schmiedeberg's Arch. Exp. Path. Pharmak.* 261:271-88.

Thoenen, H., Tranzer, J. P., and Häusler, G. 1970. In *New Aspects of Storage and Release Mechanisms of Catecholamines*, Springer, Berlin-Heidelberg-New York.

Tranzer, J. P., and Richards, J. G. 1971. In *6-Hydroxydopamine and Catecholamine*

Neurons, T. Malmfors and H. Thoenen (Eds.), North Holland, Amsterdam. pp. 15-32.

Tranzer, J. P., und Thoenen, H. 1967a. *Naunyn-Schmiedeberg's Arch. Exp. Path. Pharmak.* 257:343-44.

Tranzer, J. P., und Thoenen, H. 1967b. *Experientia* 23:743-45.

Tranzer, J. P., and Thoenen, H. 1968. *Experientia* 24:155-56.

Tranzer, J. P., Thoenen, H., Snipes, R. L., and Richards, J. G. 1969. *Recent Prog. Brain Res.* 31:33-46.

Trendelenburg, U. 1971. In *Handbook of Experimental Pharmacology,* "Catecholamines," Springer, Berlin-Heidelberg-New York.

Trendelenburg, U., and Wagner, K. 1971. In *6-Hydroxydopamine and Catecholamine Neurons,* T. Malmfors and H. Thoenen (Eds.), North Holland, Amsterdam. pp. 215-24.

Ungerstedt, U. 1968. *Europ. J. Pharmacol.* 5:107-10.

Ungerstedt, U. 1971. In *6-Hydroxydopamine and Catecholamine Neurons,* T. Malmfors and H. Thoenen (Eds.), North Holland, Amsterdam. pp. 315-32.

Uretsky, N. J., and Iversen, L. L. 1969. *Nature* (Lond.) 221;557-59.

Uretsky, N. J., and Iversen, L. L. 1970. *J. Neurochem.* 17:269-78.

Van Orden III, L. S., Bensch, K. G., Langer, S. Z., and Trendelenburg, U. 1967. *J. Pharmacol. Exp. Ther.* 157:274-83.

Weissman, A., Koe, B. K., and Tenen, S. S. 1966. *J. Pharmacol. Exp. Ther.* 151:339.

Wolinsky, H., and Glagov, S. 1967. *Circulat. Res.* 20:409-21.

11

False Aminergic Transmitters

IRWIN J. KOPIN

It was once widely accepted that a neuron releases only one transmitter substance; but during the last several years it has been shown that the mechanisms for synthesis, storage, and release of neurochemical transmitters are not absolutely specific. More than one compound may be present in nerve endings and may be released, particularly after drug treatment. Furthermore, even under physiologic circumstances more than one substance may be released from a nerve ending in response to nerve stimulation.

Origin of the Concept of "False" Transmitters

The concept that a physiological transmitter may be replaced by an inactive nonphysiological analogue was first proposed when Burgen et al. (1956) found that triethylcholine was acetylated by the choline acetylase of brain tissue almost as effectively as choline. They speculated that triethylcholine might be converted *in vivo* to a physiologically inert neurohumor. Bowman and Rand (1961) subsequently found that triethylcholine markedly reduced muscular contraction in response to nerve stimulation without interfering with conduction of the nerve action potential or blocking the response of muscle to acetylcholine. They suggested that triethylcholine interferes with synthesis of acetylcholine and cited the possibility that triethylacetylcholine may have been formed and functioned as an inactive "false" transmitter. Bull and Hemsworth (1963) demonstrated

339

that triethylcholine inhibits synthesis of acetylcholine by inhibiting uptake of choline but were unable to show the occurrence of triethylacetylcholine *in vivo*. The possibility that false transmitter formation explained the actions of triethylcholine was subsequently discarded.

Nonspecificity of Synthesis, Storage, and Release of Amines

Nonspecificity of the processes for synthesis, storage, and release of amine neurochemical transmitters allows for the substitution of other amines for the physiologic transmitter. Such false neurotransmitters are usually less active than the amines for which they substitute and produce a decrease in the efficiency of transmission at nerve endings in which they accumulate.

Norepinephrine is formed from tyrosine by the sequential action of three enzymes. Tyrosine hydroxylase converts tyrosine to DOPA, and this step is considered to be rate-limiting (Levitt et al., 1965) in formation of dopamine or norepinephrine. The enzyme is relatively specific but does act on α-methyltyrosine to produce small amounts of α-methyl-DOPA (Maitre, 1965).

Decarboxylation of dopa is carried out by L-aromatic amino acid decarboxylase (Lovenberg et al., 1962). It is a relatively nonspecific enzyme present in serotonergic (converting 5-hydroxytryptophan to serotonin) and adrenergic neurons and in other tissues (liver, kidney), which can catalyze the decarboxylation of α-methylamino acids as well as its natural substrates. Its specificity appears to vary, depending on its source (Hagen, 1962), so that the decarboxylase isolated from the adrenal medulla does not decarboxylate p-tyrosine, histidine, or tryptophan. The decarboxylase in brain, however, can decarboxylate α-methyl analogues of DOPA, m-tyrosine, etc, to produce the corresponding amines (Carlsson and Lindqvist, 1962). Presumably the decarboxylase present in serotonergic neurons which converts 5-hydroxytryptophan to serotonin is also able to decarboxylate L-DOPA. Similarly the enzyme in dopaminergic and noradrenergic neurons can decarboxylate exogenous 5-hydroxytryptophan to form serotonin.

Dopamine-β-hydroxylase is relatively nonspecific and will convert a variety of phenylethylamines to phenylethanolamine derivatives (Creveling et al., 1962). It is localized in synaptic vesicles, and transport of dopamine (or other amines) into the vesicles must precede β-hydroxylation. The transport process at the vesicular membrane is also nonspecific, and many amines may compete with dopamine for entry into the vesicles.

The nonspecificity of the enzymes involved in conversion of tyrosine to norepinephrine results in the conversion of a number of nonphysiological compounds to analogues of norepinephrine. Thus after administration of α-methyl-m-tyrosine or α-methyl-DOPA, Carlsson and Lindqvist (1962) found α-methyl-m-hydroxyphenylethanolamine (metaraminol) or α-methylnorepinephrine in brain.

Musacchio et al. (1965a, 1965b) found that the β-hydroxyl derivatives formed from a number of phenylethylamine derivatives are retained in the same subcellular structure as is norepinephrine, the synaptic vesicles. Phenylethylamines which had only one hydroxyl group were not retained in the particulate fractions. They concluded that compounds having the phenylethylamine structure and which contain either a catechol- or a β-hydroxyl group can occupy the site at which norepinephrine is bound.

It is believed that release of neurotransmitters from nerve endings results from extrusion of the contents of the synaptic vesicles by exocytosis. Neurophysiological studies provided the first evidence that discrete quanta of acetylcholine are resealed at neuromuscular junctions. The evidence supporting the view that storage vesicles serve as the coin of quantal release of acetylcholine has been reviewed by Katz (1962). A similar mechanism has been suggested for the release of epinephrine from the granules of the adrenal medulla. Douglas and Poisner (1966) found stoichiometric release of adenine nucleotides and catecholamines, and a number of investigators have found that chromagranin (the protein associated with bound catecholamines) and dopamine-β-hydroxylase (which is also present in the storage granules) are released with catecholamines from the adrenal medulla (Kirshner et al., 1966; Schneider et al., 1967; Viveros et al., 1969).

A similar mechanism is thought to function at sympathetic nerve endings. Release of dopamine-β-hydroxylase (Gewirtz and Kopin, 1970b) and chromagranin (De Potter et al., 1969) with norepinephrine is not, however, stoichiometric. It may be a consequence of binding of most of the vesicular enzyme to the membrane. Recent studies in our laboratory (Weinshilboum, Thoa, Johnson, Axelrod, and Kopin, 1971) indicate that there is a stoichiometric relationship between norepinephrine and dopamine-β-hydroxylase released from the guinea pig vas deferens. The ratio of released catecholamine to released dopamine-β-hydroxylase is similar to that found in the soluble contents of the synaptic vesicles. Because other amines which are retained by norepinephrine storage particles are also released, the site from which release occurs appears to have properties which are very similar to the vesicles (Kopin, 1968).

Shortly after Carlsson and Lindqvist (1962) demonstrated formation of α-methylnorepinephrine and metaraminol from administered amines and their precursors, it was found that they are released from the heart by sympathetic nerve stimulation (Muscholl and Maitre, 1963; Crout et al., 1964). The number of verified false transmitters rapidly increased, and they have been used as pharmacological tools to study the physical processes of storage, release, and uptake at sympathetic nerve endings.

Octopamine, the β-hydroxylated derivative of tyramine, is of particular interest. It can be formed after the decarboxylation of tyrosine and its metabolite, p-hydroxymandelic acid, is normally present in urine of human subjects on a glucose diet (von Studnitz et al., 1964). After administration of a monoamine oxidase inhibitor (MAO), octopamine accumulates in the tissues (Kakimoto and Armstrong, 1962). Since it does not accumulate in sympathetically denervated organs (Kopin et al., 1965), it is likely that the sympathetic nerves are the site of amine retention. Furthermore, labelled octopamine (formed from administered radioactive tyramine) can be released by sympathetic nerve stimulation.

The recent development of a sensitive and specific method for assay of endogenous octopamine (Molinoff et al., 1969) has permitted demonstration of octopamine release from sympathetic nerves without monoamine oxidase inhibition. Thus both octopamine and norepinephrine are released from the isolated perfused cat spleen during stimulation (Gewirtz, Molinoff, and Kopin, in preparation). Normally, sympathetic nerve endings contain much more norepinephrine than octopamine; but after inhibition of monoamine oxidase, octopamine increases markedly and partially displaces norepinephrine. Displacement of norepinephrine by octopamine has been suggested as the mechanism through which monoamine oxidase inhibitors may interfere with sympathetic neuronal function (Kopin et al., 1965).

Selective Release of Newly Synthesized Neurotransmitters

When release of norepinephrine is evoked by stimulation of sympathetic nerves, synthesis of the catecholamine is accelerated and the levels of transmitter in the tissues remain relatively constant (see review by Weiner, 1970). Inhibition of synthesis of norepinephrine by blocking tyrosine hydroxylation with α-methyltyrosine reduces the amount of norepinephrine released by nerve stimulation (Thoenen et al., 1966; Kopin et al., 1968). If ^{3}H-norepinephrine has been administered to the animal 24 hours before perfusion of its spleen, the specific activity of the catecholamine released during constant stimulation is lower than that found in the spleen unless synthesis is inhibited with α-methyltyrosine (Kopin et al., 1968).

The interpretation that newly formed unlabelled norepinephrine is released with the stored labelled amine is supported by the observation that norepinephrine released by nerve stimulation from a spleen perfused with radioactively labelled tyrosine has a higher specific activity than the catecholamine formed in the spleen (Kopin et al., 1968). The relative enrichment of released catecholamine by newly synthesized transmitter appears to vary with the interval and rate of stimulation (Gewirtz and Kopin, 1970a). Selective release of newly formed labelled norepinephrine has been found in the perfused rabbit heart (Stjärne and Weirnmalm, 1970) and in the guinea pig vas deferens (Thoa et al., 1971). Thierry et al. (1970) have obtained evidence for selective utilization of newly formed norepinephrine in brain during stress of electrical shocks. Thus it appears that amines released from the synaptic vesicles at the nerve ending are replaced to a significant extent by newly synthesized transmitter.

Selective utilization of newly formed transmitter may be important in explaining the effects of false transmitters and their precursors in altering the release of the physiological transmitter. Andén and Magnusson (1964) depleted a large portion of the norepinephrine content of the heart, brain, and other tissues by combined treatment with α-methyl-m-tyrosine (400 mg/kg, i.p. daily for 2 days) and metaraminol (0.2 mg/kg 4 hours before) and found little if any impairment of sympathetic neuronal function. Haefely et al. (1966, 1967) were able to demonstrate some impairment of the effect of sympathetic nerve stimulation on the nictitating membrane of cats pretreated with α-methyl-m-tyrosine, but the heart rate and blood pressure of the animals were not greatly altered.

Crout et al. (1964) found that although levels of cardiac metaraminol were similar 2 hours or 17 to 20 hours after administration of the amine, more metaraminol could be released by sympathetic nerve stimulation at the earlier time. They suggested that the metaraminol taken up had shifted from an "available" to a "less readily available" pool. The apparent lack of relationship between the endogenous norepinephrine content and the amount released by nerve stimulation as well as the decrease in availability and effectiveness of previously taken-up or endogenously formed false transmitters may be explained by the role of synthesis in replacing the released amines.

Shortly after administration of a nonphysiologic amine or its precursor, norepinephrine at the sites from which the amine is released by nerve stimulation is displaced to about the same extent as the catecholamine in the less available stores. After release of the amines from the more available sites, the amines which replace the released substances are derived from new synthesis as well as from mobilization. If only precursors of norepinephrine are available, then the physiologic catecholamine replaces the released amines. Function of the neuron is not impaired when the amine available for release is active, even when the less available stores may have been replaced by inactive compounds. However, if precursors of false transmitters are present in concentrations sufficiently high to compete with dopamine for entry into the synaptic vesicles and subsequent conversion to norepinephrine, then both the false and physiologic amines replace the released amines. This may result in diminished release of the active transmitter even when reserve stores have not been greatly depleted.

Serotonin Storage in Catecholaminergic Neurons

The parenchymal cells of the pineal gland, which contain high concentrations of serotonin, are innervated by sympathetic nerve fibers. A considerable portion of the serotonin synthesized in these cells appears to be released, transported across the neuronal membrane of the sympathetic nerves, and stored in norepinephrine-containing vesicles (Owman, 1965). Carlsson et al. (1963) have previously shown that serotonin is taken up by catecholamine storage granules isolated from the adrenal medulla. Taxi and Droz (1966) found by radioautography that after injection of ^{14}C-5-hydroxytryptophan, radioactivity presumably due to ^{14}C-serotonin accumulated in the guinea pig vas deferens. Subsequently Thoa et al. (1969) showed that labelled serotonin can be taken up by the guinea pig vas deferens after incubation with the amine *in vitro* and that the uptake could be blocked by drugs such as cocaine, imipramine, and ouabain, which interfere with sympathetic neuronal uptake of norepinephrine. Furthermore drugs which deplete catecholamines from vas deferens also release the labelled serotonin accumulated during incubation *in vitro*.

Uptake and retention of serotonin by catecholaminergic neurons in the central nervous system were demonstrated by Lichtensteiger et al. (1967). Mice were pretreated with reserpine (to deplete amines) and nialamide (to prevent destruction of accumulated amines), after which serotonin or 5-hydroxytryptophan was administered. Exposure of the tissue to formaldehyde vapor using the techniques developed by Falck, Hillarp, et al. (1962) for histological demonstration of biogenic amines revealed fluorescence typical of serotonin in the tubero-infundibular neurons which normally contain dopamine. Thus in the brain as well as in peripheral adrenergic neurons the uptake and storage mechanisms for catecholamines may be sufficiently nonspecific to allow accumulation of indoleamine and phenylethylamine derivatives. It is likely that accumulated indoleamines may also be released by nerve stimulation and meet the criteria for false adrenergic transmitters.

Catecholamines in Serotonin Storage Sites

Serotonin is present in the argentaffin cells of the gastrointestinal tract, mast cells, platelets, and neurons of the central nervous system. The ready availability of human blood platelets has made it an attractive tissue for the study of amine storage. It has been hoped that the mechanism of amine binding in platelet organelles and in neurons is sufficiently similar to allow valid extrapolation of observations in platelets to events in brain. DePrada and Pletscher (1969) found that platelets accumulate a number of amines and speculated that if the platelet storage mechanism is similar to that of neurons which contain serotonin, then a similar situation might occur in brain.

There is some evidence that after administration of large doses of L-DOPA, dopamine formed by aromatic amino acid decarboxylase in serotonergic neurons will replace serotonin from its storage sites and act as a false serotonergic transmitter. Butcher et al. (1970) have presented histological evidence that dopamine formed from exogenous L-DOPA can accumulate in serotonergic neurons. Large doses of L-DOPA reduce levels of serotonin and transiently increase the cerebral level of 5-hydroxyindoleacetic acid (Bartholini et al., 1968; Butcher and Engel, 1969). In brain slices and synaptosomes (Ng et al., 1970; Ng et al., 1971a), L-DOPA markedly increases the efflux of labelled dopamine and serotonin. The releasing action of L-DOPA is blocked by decarboxylase inhibitors so that dopamine formation appears to be necessary.

Since pretreatment with 6-hydroxydopamine (which destroys catechol-aminergic neurons) (see chapter by Thoenen) markedly reduces the DOPA-induced release of dopamine but does not alter release of serotonin, dopamine appears to release serotonin from the serotonergic neurons. In brain slices from rats pretreated with 6-hydroxydopamine, synthesis and electrical stimulation-induced release of radioactive dopamine formed from ^{14}C-tyrosine or tracer doses of ^{3}H-DOPA are markedly reduced (Ng et al., 1971b). When high concentrations of L-DOPA are used, how-ever, 6-hydroxydopamine pretreatment reduces only slightly the electrical stimulation-induced release of dopamine. High doses of L-DOPA thus ap-pear to form dopamine in noncatecholaminergic cells from which the amine can be released by electrical stimulation. Presumably dopamine is formed in other aminergic neurons which contain a decarboxylase. It has already been shown that dopamine formed from L-DOPA releases sero-tonin and accumulates in serotonergic neurons. It appears likely, therefore, that when high concentrations of L-DOPA are available, serotonergic neurons are the source of the dopamine released from brain slices by electrical depolarization. Thus serotonergic neurons appear to form, store, and release dopamine as well as serotonin, provided large amounts of dopa are available.

The role of dopamine as a false serotonergic transmitter in the brains of patients treated with L-DOPA is not known, but its formation in cells where it is not normally present may be partially responsible for the pro-duction of toxic side effects or therapeutic benefits.

Conclusion

The concept that functional alterations in synaptic efficacy may result from substitution of the physiologic transmitter by a false inactive com-pound has been fruitful. It has provided a molecular basis to explain the actions of several drugs which are precursors for, or are themselves, false transmitters. Furthermore it may partially explain the effects of other drugs which alter metabolism of endogenous substances to result in the accumulation of amines. In the future it is likely that more examples of neurotransmitter and humoral substitutes will be found which may explain, on a molecular level, pathological as well as pharmacological alterations in functions.

References

Andén, N.-E., and Magnusson, T. 1964. In *Symposium on Cholinergic and Adrenergic Transmission,* A. Carlsson, G. B. Koelle, and W. W. Douglas (Eds.), Pergamon Press, London-New York, pp. 319-28.
Bartholini, G., DePrada, M., and Pletscher, A. 1968. *J. Pharm. Pharmacol.* 20:228.
Bowman, W. C., and Rand, M. J. 1961. *Brit. J. Pharmacol.* 17:176.
Bull, G., and Hemsworth, B. A. 1963. *Nature* (Lond.) 199:487.
Burgen, A. S. V., Burke, G., and Desborats-Shonbaum, M. 1956. *Brit. J. Pharmacol.* 11:308.
Butcher, L. L., and Engel, J. 1969. *Brain Res.* 15:223.
Butcher, L. L., Engel, J., and Fuxe, K. 1970. *J. Pharm. Pharmacol.* 22:313.
Carlsson, A., Hillarp, N.-Å., and Waldeck, B. 1963. *Acta Physiol. Scand.* 59 suppl. 215:1.
Carlsson, A., and Lindqvist, M. 1962. *Acta Physiol. Scand.* 54:87.
Creveling, C. R., Daly, J. W., Witkop, B., and Udenfriend, S. 1962. *Biochim. Biophys. Acta* 64:125.
Crout, J. R., Alpers, H. S., Tatum, E. L., and Shore, P. A. 1964. *Science* 145:828.
DePrada, M., and Pletscher, A. 1969. *Europ. J. Pharmacol.* 7:45.
DePotter, W. P., Schaeporyver, A. F., Muerman, E. J., and Smith, A. D. 1969. *J. Physiol.* (Lond.) 204:102.
Douglas, W. W., and Poisner, A. A. 1966. *J. Physiol.* (Lond.) 183:236.
Everett, G. M., and Wiegard, R. G. 1962. *Proc. Int. Pharmacol. Meet.* 8:85.
Falck, B., Hillarp, N.-Å., Thieme, G., and Thorp, A. 1962. *J. Histochem. Cytochem.* 10:348.
Gewirtz, G. P., and Kopin, I. J. 1970a. *J. Pharmacol. Exp. Ther.* 175:514.
Gewirtz, R. P., and Kopin, I. J. 1970b. *Nature* (Lond.) 227:406.
Haefely, W., Huerlimann, A., and Thoenen, H. 1966. *Brit. J. Pharmacol.* 26:172.
Haefely, W., Huerlimann, A., and Thoenen, H. 1967. *Brit. J. Pharmacol.* 31:105.
Hagen, P. 1962. *Brit. J. Pharmacol.* 18:175.
Kakimoto, Y., and Armstrong, M. D. 1962. *J. Biol. Chem.* 237:422.
Katz, B. 1962. *Proc. Roy. Soc. B* 155:455.
Kirschner, N., Sage, N. J., Smith, W. J., and Kirshner, A. G. 1966. *Science* 154:529.
Kopin, I. J. 1968. *Ann. Rev. Pharmacol.* 8:377.
Kopin, I. J., Breese, G. R., Krauss, K. R., and Weise, V. K. 1968. *J. Pharmacol. Exp. Ther.* 161:271.
Kopin, I. J., Fischer, J. E., Musacchio, J. M., Horst, W. D., and Weise, V. K. 1965. *J. Pharmacol. Exp. Ther.* 147:186.
Levitt, M., Spector, S., Sjoerdsma, A., and Udenfriend, S. 1965. *J. Pharmacol. Exp. Ther.* 148:1.

Lichtensteiger, W., Mutzner, V., and Langeman, N. 1967. *J. Neurochem.* 14:489.

Lovenberg, W., Weissbach, H., and Udenfriend, S. 1962. *J. Biol. Chem.* 237:89.

Maitre, L. 1965. *Life Sci.* 4:2249.

Molinoff, P. B., Landsberg, L., and Axelrod, J. 1969. *J. Pharmacol. Exp. Ther.* 170:253.

Musacchio, J. M., Kopin, I. J., and Weise, V. K. 1965a. *J. Pharmacol. Exp. Ther.* 148:22.

Musacchio, J. M., Weise, V. K., and Kopin, I. J. 1965b. *Nature* (Lond.) 205:606.

Muscholl, E., and Maitre, L. 1963. *Experientia* 19:658.

Ng, K.-Y., Chase, T. N., Colburn, R. W., and Kopin, I. J. 1970. *Science* 170:76.

Ng, K.-Y., Chase, T. N., Colburn, R. W., and Kopin, I. J. 1971a. *Science* 172:487.

Ng, K.-Y., Colburn, R. W., and Kopin, I. J. 1971b. *Nature* (Lond.) 230:331.

Owman, C. 1965. *Recent Prog. Brain Res.* 10:423.

Schneider, F. M., Smith, S. D., and Winkler, H. 1967. *Brit. J. Pharmacol.* 31:94.

Stjärne, L., and Weirnmalm, Å. 1970. *Acta Physiol. Scand.* 80:428.

Taxi, J., and Droz, B. 1966. *C.R. Hebd. Séances Acad. Sci.* (D) (Paris) 263:1237.

Thierry, A.-M., Blanc, G., and Glowinski, J. 1970. *Europ. J. Pharmacol.* 10:139.

Thoa, N. B., Eccleston, D., and Axelrod, J. 1969. *J. Pharmacol. Exp. Ther.* 196:68.

Thoa, N. B., Johnson, D. G., and Kopin, I. J. *Europ. J. Pharmacol.* (in press).

Thoenen, H., Haefely, W., Gey, K. F., and Huerlimann, A. 1966. *Life Sci.* 5:723.

Viveros, O. H., Arqueros, L., and Kirshner, N. 1969. *Science* 165:911.

Weiner, N. 1970. *Ann. Rev. Pharmacol.* 10:273.

Weinshilbaum, R., Thoa, N. B., Johnson, D. G., Axelrod, J., and Kopin, I. J. 1971. *Science* (in press).

12
Some New Facts About Synthesis, Storage, and Release Processes of Monoamines in the Central Nervous System

J. GLOWINSKI

Introduction

In 1966, after two fascinating years spent with Dr. J. Axelrod at the NIMH, I was fortunate enough to get together a research group in order to carry on studies on the metabolism and functions of transmitter substances in the central nervous system. I would like to review and discuss the main biochemical results obtained in our laboratory during the last few years. Most of our work has been dedicated to the study of central monoaminergic neurons.

We were first interested in applying some of the techniques and concepts developed in Dr. Axelrod's laboratory to studies of the turnover of central norepinephrine (NE) in various physiological or pharmacological states. The first experiments, with Dr. S. S. Kety, on the effect of "foot shock" stress on the activity of central noradrenergic neurons, have been extended. This stress situation has been successfully used as an experimental tool to study the properties of the various intraneuronal forms of NE storage in noradrenergic neurons.

Many factors have contributed to the development of our researches on the nigro-striatal system of dopaminergic neurons. Stimulated by the early finding of Carlsson and his coworkers (1958), who first detected very high

Most of the results described in this review article were obtained during the last five years, with my colleagues of the group N B: M. J. Besson, G. Blanc, A. Chéramy, M. Hamon, F. Héry, F. Javoy, M. Lopez, and A. M. Thierry. We should like also to mention the names of visiting scientists who have contributed largely to some of the studies reported: Drs. S. S. Kety, J. Macon, J. Musacchio, and L. Sokoloff (U.S.A.); M. Fekete (Hungary); P. Feltz, L. Julou, Y. Morot-Gaudry, B. Scatton, and J. F. Pujol (France).

levels of dopamine (DA) in the caudate nuclei, I started my own work in this field at the Pasteur Institute, studying the qualitative metabolism of labelled DA, in the rat brain after its intraventricular injection (Milhaud and Glowinski, 1962). Moreover, from our work with Dr. L. L. Iversen on the regional metabolism of catecholamines, we knew that dopaminergic terminals in the striatum could be easily and heavily labelled (Glowinski and Iversen, 1966a). Therefore, there was some hope of success in studying *in vivo* the release of DA. Finally, this project was also stimulated by the neurophysiological studies of Professor D. A. Fessard on this important pathway, her great interest in the problems linked to Parkinson's disease, and her strong motivation to combine electrophysiological and biochemical approaches in a fundamental research.

Curiously, it was Dr. Axelrod who, in 1966, introduced me to Professor Jouvet. As soon as we met, there was no doubt that we would be involved in research on serotonin (5-HT) metabolism. Dr. Pujol, one of his assistants, came to our laboratory and immediately started to work on the variations of 5-HT metabolism in sleep processes. Our work on the metabolism of 5-HT in central serotoninergic neurons was also, later on, markedly motivated by Dr. C. Kordon's interest in the role of serotoninergic neurons in ovulation processes. After neuropharmacological experiments which helped us demonstrate the involvement of serotoninergic terminals localized in the median eminence (Kordon *et al.*, 1968; Hamon *et al.*, 1970) in the control of LH release, we decided to explore more thoroughly the various biochemical problems involved in 5-HT metabolism.

In conclusion, we will present various data related to the estimation, intra- and interneuronal regulation of synthesis, to the intraneuronal storage or compartmentalization, and finally to the release and inactivation of NE, DA, and 5-HT. It is interesting to note that basic problems about the processes of central amine metabolism have very often risen in the course of physiological studies.

Noradrenergic Neurons

Three main steps can be distinguished in our research on central noradrenergic neurons—attempts to appreciate changes in their activity in various situations, particularly acute or chronic stressful states; attempts to demonstrate and to study the characteristics of the various forms of NE storage as well as their respective roles under different levels of neuronal activity; attempts to understand the role of the various steps of NE formation in the regulation of the amine synthesis. Some methodological problems will be discussed first, since in many experiments noradrenergic neurons have been labelled with tritiated NE injected intracisternally to study the amine turnover or utilization.

Methodological Problems

It is now well established that central catecholaminergic neurons can be labelled specifically with tracer quantities of ^{3}H-catecholamines (CA) injected into the cerebrospinal fluid. This enables the study of various aspects of the metabolism of these amines in central noradrenergic and dopaminergic neurons. The main experiments, which have shown the specificity of the ^{3}H-CA uptake in the various catecholaminergic neurons, as well as the similarity of the disposition of the exogenous and endogenous amines, were mostly performed from 1964 to 1966 in Dr. Axelrod's laboratory, with my colleagues Drs. Iversen, Snyder, and Reivich. They have been extensively reviewed: in Glowinski and Axelrod, 1966; Glowinski and Baldessarini, 1966; Glowinski, 1967a. The original technique to circumvent the blood-brain barrier was to inject the labelled amine stereotaxically in the lateral ventricle. Noble et al. (1967) later on simplified this method: a very short needle introduced directly into the lateral ventricle through a small hole precisely localized on the surface of the parietal bone, using superficial coordinates delimited from the junction of frontal and parietal bones. This method is quite similar to that described for the intraventricular injection in newborn and young rats of different ages (Glowinski, 1967b). Another injection site was chosen by Schanberg et al. (1967), who used the intracisternal route. This method is very fast, it requires only light anesthesia and avoids the simultaneous labelling of dopaminergic terminals of the striatum; this is particularly convenient for studies on noradrenergic neurons. Both the intraventricular and intracisternal methods have been widely used to label noradrenergic neurons in examining central NE turnover modifications in various experimental conditions. These techniques present advantages and limitations as do other methods available to estimate central NE turnover. Some criticisms have been recently put forth by Costa and Neff (1970), but as it will be seen they do not always appear pertinent. It is known that D- and

L-norepinephrine have some slight differences in their central metabolism, as previously discussed (Glowinski *et al.,* 1965; Iversen and Glowinski, 1966a); the minor error brought by the use of D-L-^{3}H-NE may be eliminated by injecting L ^{3}H-NE, now readily available. Generally, ^{3}H-epinephrine formed in tissues from injected ^{3}H-NE is not separated in chemical ^{3}H-NE determinations. The small quantities of ^{3}H-epinephrine accumulated in tissues (McGeer and McGeer, 1964), compared to ^{3}H-NE, indicates that epinephrine-containing neurons are minor relative to the numerous systems of noradrenergic neurons. Consequently, the error introduced by the combined estimation of the two amines is also very limited. More serious is the inconvenience linked to the geographical heterogeneous labelling of catecholaminergic neurons. Undoubtedly, the neurons which lie near the site of injection or the subarachnoidal space take up more ^{3}H-NE than those localized in deeper structures. Furthermore, after intraventricular injection of ^{3}H-NE the striatal dopaminergic neurons take up and store important quantities of the labelled amine. However, autoradiographic studies (Aghajanian and Bloom, 1967; Reivich and Glowinski, 1697; Descarries and Droz, 1970) with labelled NE have shown that most of the central catecholaminergic neurons are labelled. The error which could be attributed to the simultaneous labelling of dopaminergic and noradrenergic neurons or to the regional differences in the initial specific activity of NE in noradrenergic neurons can be greatly minimized. The intracisternal route may be used instead of the intraventricular approach, and NE turnover may be measured in well-defined structures and not in the whole brain. By taking into account these few remarks, valid information about modifications of NE turnover in various areas of the brain may be obtained by following the temporal changes of NE specific activity, up to six hours after the initial labelling of noradrenergic neurons. This was originally demonstrated in studies on the regional turnover of NE using this method as well as ^{3}H-NE precursors or α methyl-para-tyrosine (α.MpT) (Iversen and Glowinski, 1966b). Comparable results were obtained with the three procedures mentioned; in all cases the NE turnover was much more rapid in the cortex, the cerebellum, and the hippocampus than in other structures of the brain. The differences in NE turnover observed in this earlier study, may be explained by recent combined histochemical and lesion experiments. These experiments indicate that the three structures previously mentioned are mainly innervated by a dorsal noradrenergic pathway originating in the locus coeruleus (Ungerstedt, 1971). This pathway is quite distinct from a ventral noradrenergic pathway which originates in various cell groups of the lower brain stem and innervates the medulla and the pons, the mesencephalon, the hypothalamus, and the septal area (Ungerstedt, 1971).

Despite its limitations, the method of estimation of central NE turnover, based on the direct labelling of noradrenergic neurons with tritiated NE, was preferred for various reasons to the other methods available when we decided, in 1966 with Dr. S. Kety, to determine changes in noradrenergic neuron activity in various physiological or pharmacological states. Inhibition of synthesis with α.MpT was avoided to eliminate the possible alterations in functions of both peripheral and central catecholaminergic neurons occurring immediately after the inhibitor injection. It is, in fact, now well established that animal behavior and important physiological functions are disturbed after α.MpT treatment. Central noradrenergic neurons were not labelled by injecting labelled tyrosine intravenously since the estimation of the radioactive NE utilization for several hours in discrete brain regions requires the administration of large amounts of the precursor. Furthermore, the separation of labelled NE from its precursors and their metabolites is not as fast and easy as the estimation of ^{3}H-NE accumulated in tissues after direct labelling with the exogenous amine.

Effect of Various Experimental States on the Activity of Central Noradrenergic Neurons

In our earlier investigations the changes in NE specific activity occurring from a half-hour or one hour to four or six hours after the intracisternal ^{3}H-NE administration were taken as an index of NE turnover. During this period ^{3}H-NE disappears in a single exponential phase in all structures of the rat brain. It was thus assumed, for simplification, that the amine was localized in a single compartment in noradrenergic neurons, and that endogenous amine levels were reasonably stable. In these conditions, the rate of NE utilization reflects its rate of synthesis. We know now, from various recent experiments, that NE synthesis is always largely underestimated when calculated on this basis. Therefore, the single compartment model can no longer be used to estimate the synthesis rate of the amine. Nevertheless, valid comparative information can be obtained with this approach about NE turnover modifications in different experimental situations and consequently about changes in noradrenergic neuron activity.

First, we observed an acceleration of central NE turnover under stress. The stressful situation was produced by series of electrical shocks delivered to the paws of rats housed in individual boxes; the shocks were applied for six periods of 10 minutes each, alternating with rest periods of 20 minutes. The over-all stress session lasted for three hours. Under these conditions, when the stress was given two hours after the intracisternal ^{3}H-NE injection, the NE specific activity was always markedly reduced at the end of the stress in the various structures of the brain and in the spinal cord, indicating a general activation of the central noradrenergic neurons (Thierry *et al.,* 1968a). Higher current intensities of the shocks further enhanced the acceleration of NE turnover and increased markedly the ^{3}H-normetanephrine accumulation in tissues. This suggests that large amounts of ^{3}H-NE are released from nerve terminals under these experimental conditions. Similar indications about the increased activity of noradrenergic neurons with this stress were obtained with the other methods available for the estimation of NE turnover: i.e., measuring the disappearance rate of labelled NE endogenously synthesized from its labelled precursor (Thierry *et al.,* 1968a) and estimating the decline of endogenous NE after α.MpT administration (Thierry, 1968). Increased NE synthesis could also be demonstrated *in vitro* by measuring the ^{3}H-CA formed from ^{3}H-tyrosine in brain-stem slices of stressed animals (Thierry *et al.,* 1971a).

A second application of the NE turnover studies by direct labelling of the noradrenergic neurons with ^{3}H-NE (direct labelling method) was made in sleep studies. Since lesion and pharmacological studies implicated noradrenergic neurons in sleep processes (see review Jouvet, 1969), we sought to measure noradrenergic neuronal activity during suppression or rebound of paradoxical sleep (PS). Rats, placed on small supports surrounded by water for 91 hours, were selectively deprived of PS and exhibited a marked PS rebound for five hours following the deprivation period (Mouret *et al.,* 1969). During these five hours NE turnover was markedly accelerated in various parts of the brain and spinal cord of animals allowed to rest and thus to exhibit PS rebound, as compared with animals left in the deprived situation (Pujol *et al.,* 1968). This effect was observed even after a shorter period (24 hours) of PS deprivation (Héry and Lopez, unpublished observations). NE turnover was even more accelerated in the telencephalon-diencephalon during the PS rebound periods than in the brain stem-mesencephalon, of rats previously deprived for 91 hours. This may be mainly related to the innervation of higher brain structures by the dorsal noradrenergic pathway which plays a major role in PS. Indeed, the destruction of the locus coeruleus abolishes PS (Jouvet, 1969). Increased synthesis of ^{3}H-CA from ^{3}H-tyrosine was found in brain-stem slices of rats allowed for five hours to have a rebound of PS, as compared with animals continuously deprived of PS (Héry and Lopez, unpublished observations). The decrease of O_2 atmospheric pressure induced by high altitude may be also used to deprive rats of PS. Turnover of NE in brains of rats placed in high altitude was reduced as compared with that of animals returned to normal O_2 atmospheric pressure after a 24-hour period in high altitude (Klein and Héry, in preparation).

Modifications of endocrinological functions were also shown to affect the activity of central NE neurons. NE turnover in the brain stem of rats was accelerated a few days after adrenalectomy (Javoy et al., 1968a).

The effects of psychotropic drugs on NE turnover in the brain were examined with the method of direct labelling of noradrenergic neurons. The complex action of D-amphetamine on NE turnover is particularly interesting. High doses of the drug given acutely (20 mg/kg i.p.) or smaller doses given chronically (5 mg/kg once a day for 4 days s.c.; or 0.5 mg/kg once a day for 15 days s.c.) had no effect on NE turnover. Acceleration of NE turnover was detected only in the brain stem-mesencephalon and not in the telencephalon-diencephalon after the acute injection of 5 mg/kg (i.p.) of the drug. This dose of D-amphetamine also potentiated markedly the effect of the "electric foot shock" stress on noradrenergic neurons localized in lower parts of the brain. The specific activity of NE in the brain stem of these animals was less than 50 per cent that of animals submitted to only the three-hour stress session previously described (Javoy et al., 1968b). These results were confirmed by in vitro studies; pretreatment of animals with a single intraperitoneal injection of 5 mg/kg of D-amphetamine enhanced the total accumulation of ^{3}H-CA formed from ^{3}H-tyrosine in brain-stem slices and released in the incubating medium (Besson et al., 1969c).

In most of the studies reported, we have indicated that results on NE turnover obtained with the "direct labelling method" were confirmed by other approaches and particularly by the in vitro determination of CA synthesis. This good correlation, seen in different experimental conditions, clearly demonstrates that valid information on alterations of central NE turnover may be obtained with the "direct labelling method." Therefore, the statements of Costa and Neff (1970) and Persson (1970), who proposed to reject definitively this very easy and quick method of turnover estimation, are rather surprising and difficult to explain. Moreover, to my knowledge, no data inconsistent with the results on turnover studies previously described with this method by other authors have been reported. Interesting observations about the involvement of central noradrenergic neurons in various physiological or pharmacological states have been obtained with this method. For example, Bliss *et al.* (1968) and Taylor and Laverty (1969) have also observed an acceleration of NE turnover under stressful conditions; changes in central noradrenergic neuron activity were detected during experimental hypertension (Nakamura *et al.*, 1971). Increases in NE turnover were also observed selectively in the hypothalamus after modification of the environmental temperature (Simmonds and Iversen, 1969), and chronic treatment with desmethylimipramine (DMI) over a few days' period was shown to activate central noradrenergic neurons (Schildkraut *et al.*, 1970).

In our earlier investigations, we sought to elicit sustained changes in the activity of noradrenergic neurons. Central NE turnover was accelerated much more in animals given the stress of three-hour "electric foot shock" session once a day for four days than in animals submitted to a single stress session (Thierry *et al.*, 1968a). Curiously, the chronic stress situation particularly enhanced the turnover of NE in the telencephalon-diencephalon, suggesting a preferential sustained activation of the noradrenergic dorsal pathway. Similar observations were made after the application of electroshock twice a day for a 10-day period. Twenty-four hours after the last electroshock session, NE turnover was still markedly accelerated in various parts of the brain. The effect was again more pronounced in the telencephalon-diencephalon than in the brain stem-mesencephalon (Kety *et al.*, 1967). This sustained activation of NE turnover was linked to or associated with an increase of tyrosine hydroxylase activity in various parts of the brain (Musacchio *et al.*, 1969).

Various Forms of NE Storage in Central
Noradrenergic Neurons

In the course of our investigations on central NE metabolism new data were obtained supporting the existence of different forms of NE storage in noradrenergic terminals. First, we observed that ^{3}H-NE newly taken up disappeared very rapidly over a short period immediately after a three-hour "electric foot shock" session. The diminished accumulation of ^{3}H-NE in tissues 30 minutes after its intracisternal administration could have been attributed to an inhibition of the uptake process. However, this interpreta-tion was rejected because we did not detect changes in NE uptake in brain-stem slices of stressed animals (Thierry et al., 1971a). It thus appeared that ^{3}H-NE newly taken up in neurons could be mobilized very rapidly for extraneuronal utilization. Second, we were surprised to see in other experi-ments that desmethylimipramine (DMI), given acutely in small doses, did not accelerate NE turnover estimated by the "direct labelling method," as-suming a single compartment for NE storage. ^{3}H-NE did not disappear more rapidly one hour after its injection, and the endogenous amine levels were not affected. Unlike the amphetamine effect, DMI did not enhance the stress effect on NE turnover. These results were not expected for vari-ous reasons: DMI, a potent inhibitor of NE uptake, had been shown before to accelerate the utilization of ^{3}H-NE newly formed from ^{3}H-DA in various structures of the brain (Glowinski et al., 1966); a similar DMI treatment increased the synthesis of ^{2}H-CA from ^{3}H-tyrosine in brain-stem slices (Besson et al., 1969c). Third, Sedvall et al. (1968) reported that the rate of NE synthesis, calculated on the basis of ^{14}C-amine formation from ^{14}C-tyrosine injected intravenously, was higher than NE synthesis rate esti-mated from different turnover studies made on the assumption of a single compartment for NE storage. All this information led us to reexamine more seriously the problem of NE storage in central noradrenergic neurons.

We knew from experiments made in 1965 with Drs. Kopin and Axelrod that ^{3}H-NE taken up in catecholaminergic neurons of the rat brain disap-peared in three major phases over a 48-hour period (Glowinski et al., 1965). Similar observations were made in various structures of the brain (Iversen and Glowinski, 1966a). The initial short and rapid phase of ^{3}H-NE disappearance is followed by two other phases lasting for several hours. The half-life of ^{3}H-NE disappearance is successively about 1, 3, and 17 hours in these three phases. This may correspond to the distribution of the amine in three main "pools," possibly visualized as intraneuronal com-partments, in which the amine is utilized at different rates. Therefore, var-ious experiments were carried on by Drs. Thierry and Blanc to explore further the respective properties of the different phases of the amine utili-zation. They particularly studied the first phase, neglected in our early studies which favored the second phase. Electric foot-paw shock was used as a stressor to examine changes in NE mobilization from various storage forms. The main results may be summarized as follows: (1) A mild stress,

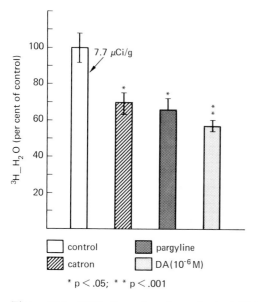

Figure 12-1   Utilization of newly synthesized ^{3}H-NE under stress in the brain stem of the rat. Eight groups of rats received 23 μCi of L-3-5-^{3}H-tyrosine (27 Ci/m mole) intracisternally. Rats of four groups received electric foot shock for 15 minutes, 2, 5, 20, or 180 minutes after the ^{3}H-amino acid injection; stressed and control rats were killed 17, 20, 35, and 195 minutes after ^{3}H-tyrosine injection. ^{3}H-NE was estimated in the brain stem. Results are expressed as per cent of controls $\pm$ S.E.M. (From Thierry, *et al.*, 1970)

lasting for only 15 minutes, markedly accelerated the utilization of newly taken up ^{3}H-NE, or of ^{3}H-NE newly synthesized from ^{3}H-DA or ^{3}H-tyrosine in the brain stem of the rat (Fig. 12.1): ^{3}H-NE levels were decreased by 20 to 27 per cent during this short period. This stress had no significant effect on endogenous NE levels. (2) This mild stress, of short duration, had no effect on exogenous or endogenously synthesized ^{3}H-NE still stored in tissue three hours after its initial accumulation or formation from ^{3}H-DA or ^{3}H-tyrosine injected intracisternally. (3) Only a long stress (the three-hour electric shock session previously described) could accelerate significantly the utilization of ^{3}H-NE, still bound in tissues two or three hours after its injection. The ^{3}H-amine, affected by this stress, is localized in a compartment in which its half-life is about three hours. In these conditions, the endogenous amine levels were always decreased by about 20 to 25 per cent. (4) The "three-hour stress" was less effective on ^{3}H-NE still in tissues 20 hours after its intracisternal administration; nevertheless, this later form of ^{3}H-NE was also utilized at a faster rate (Thierry *et al.*, 1970, 1971a). In conclusion, these results indicate that NE newly taken up or newly synthesized in central noradrenergic terminals is mainly localized in a compartment (A) from which the amine is preferentially utilized for release under activation of neurons. This compartment can thus be regarded as a "functional compartment." The exogenous or endogenously synthesized amine stored for a longer period is predominantly localized in a compartment (B), which may represent a "main storage compartment." This compartment (B), where NE half-life is about two to three hours, may act as a reservoir for compartment A. Turnover studies described changes in utilization of NE localized in this compartment. A third compartment (C), containing an amine form utilized at a much slower rate (half-life: 17 hours), may have also a "reservoir" role. Slight activation of central noradrenergic neurons induced in physiological or pharmacological states will affect only the NE localized in compartment A. Changes in the rate of utilization of NE in compartment B or C will occur in acute emergency situations or in long-term activation of noradrenergic neurons. These changes are likely to be seen when the amine content of compartment A has been reduced to a minimal level, despite the existence of the regulatory process provided by the rapid enhancement of the amine synthesis. Therefore, the various methods of turnover estimation based on the assumption of a single compartment for the amine storage cannot be used to demonstrate rapid and mild changes in the activity of noradrenergic neurons particularly seen in behavioral or physiological states (Glowinski *et al.*, 1971a). Much more attention should be given to the disposition of the newly taken up or newly synthesized transmitter.

Some New Aspects on NE Synthesis and Its Regulation

Further evidence about the existence of various forms of NE storage, exhibiting differences in their rates of utilization, were obtained with the help of the synthesis inhibitors α.MpT (Spector *et al.*, 1965) and FLA 63 (Svensson and Waldeck, 1969; Florvall and Corrodi, 1970). These inhibitors act, respectively, at the first and last step of NE synthesis. From these studies preliminary indications were obtained about the main characteristics of compartments A and B previously described and about the rate of NE synthesis in noradrenergic neurons (Thierry *et al.*, 1971b). Finally, the differences observed in the effects of FLA 63 and α.MpT on NE metabolism on the one hand, and in the effects of α.MpT on DA and NE disposition in noradrenergic terminals on the other, revealed the important role of the last step of NE formation in the regulation of its synthesis (Thierry *et al.*, 1971c).

1). The early effects of both inhibitors on NE levels were examined carefully in the cortex, a structure which until now has been shown to contain mainly noradrenergic and not dopaminergic terminals (Ungerstedt, 1971). The amine did not decline monophasically, as generally described: two phases of NE disappearance could be detected in the first four to six hours after the administration of both inhibitors. This indicates again the existence of a form of NE utilized at a much faster rate than that reported for NE still stored in tissues one hour after NE synthesis inhibition (Thierry *et al.*, 1971a). After the injection of FLA 63, a very rapid acting inhibitor of the DA-NE conversion, NE levels decreased immediately and very rapidly during the first five minutes, then, by a still unexplained process, returned rapidly to almost control levels, and, finally, declined with a half-life of about two hours for several hours. After α.MpT administration, a completely different picture was seen: surprisingly, NE levels increased during the first five minutes, then declined in two successive phases, a short and rapid one lasting for about 45 minutes followed by a much longer one (Fig. 12-2). In this second phase the rate of NE disappearance was significantly slower (half-life: 3 hours) than that observed after FLA 63 (Thierry *et al.*, 1971b,c). The differences observed after FLA 63 and α.MpT are very likely linked to the regulatory role of the last step of NE synthesis which, as it will be discussed below, still operates after α.MpT administration. In any case these results confirmed the data obtained with isotopic methods: the first rapid and short-lasting phase of NE decline both after FLA 63 and α.MpT may correspond to the rapid utilization of NE localized in the "functional compartment" (A) and the slower phase of NE decline to the amine utilization in the "main storage compartment" (B).

2. The heterogeneous storage, seen for cortical NE, raised some questions about the real rate of NE synthesis in the brain. It is probable that previous estimations based on the existence of a single compartment have largely underestimated the rate of the amine synthesis. Synthesis rates of NE in the cortex of the rat were thus found to be about 0.4 to 0.6 μg/g/hr when calculated from the initial rise of cortical NE levels occurring in the first 10 minutes after the administration of pargyline (Glowinski *et al.*,

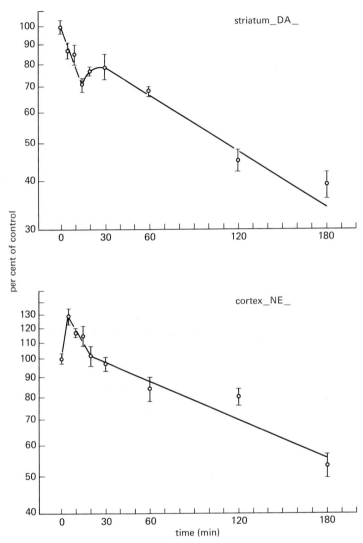

Figure 12-2   Effects of α-methyl-p-tyrosine on striatal DA and cerebral cortical NE levels in the rat. Groups of rats received α.MpT (200 mg/kg i.p.) and were killed at various times intervals after treatment with this inhibitor of catecholamine synthesis. DA was estimated in pooled striata, and NE in the cerebral cortex. The absolute DA and NE levels in control animals were 10 μg/g and 0.3 μg/g respectively. Results are the mean ± S.E.M. of groups of eight animals. (Experiments by Javoy, Thierry, and Blanc)

1971b; Thierry *et al.,* 1971c). These values of NE synthesis rates are about five to seven times higher than previous estimations based on the monophasic NE decline observed from one to six hours after α.MpT (Iversen and Glowinski, 1966a; Ho *et al.,* 1970). However, this very high synthesis rate of cortical NE obtained with the MAO inhibitor method may result partly from the increased availability of its precursor DA. Neglecting the period during which NE levels return to normal levels, possibly corresponding to the flow of NE still present in axons, we have calculated, from the curve of NE decline obtained after FLA 63 administration, approximate characteristics of the "functional" and "main storage" compartments (Fig. 12-3) (Thierry *et al.,* 1971b; Thierry, Blanc, and Glowinski, in preparation). The size of the "functional compartment" was obtained by subtracting the quantity of NE disappearing in the "main storage compartment" in the initial five minutes after FLA 63 injection, from the total amount of NE which disappeared during this initial period. It represents about 20 per cent of the total cortical NE content. The NE half-life in the "functional compartment" was approximately 5 to 10 minutes, and thus, is much more rapid than the rate of NE utilization in the "main storage compartment." Assuming a steady state situation and calculating independently the NE turnover rate in each compartment, NE turnover in the "functional compartment" was estimated to be about seven times that of the "main storage compartment." The total rate of NE turnover, which in these conditions equals the rate of NE synthesis, was found to be about 0.6 μg/g/hr in this structure of the brain, a value much higher than previous estimations. These evaluations, similar to those obtained with MAO inhibitors, further demonstrate the importance of the "functional compartment" in cortical noradrenergic neurons. Similar preliminary observations could be made for other structures of the brain.

3. Endogenous levels of CA in noradrenergic neurons seem to regulate the amine synthesis by a mechanism of end-product inhibition occurring at the first step of synthesis. This was originally proposed by Costa and Neff (1966) and Spector *et al.* (1967), who demonstrated in *in vivo* studies an inhibition of NE synthesis and turnover after acute or chronic treatment with an MAO inhibitor. Drs. Thierry and Blanc were able to confirm these results *in vitro:* in the cortex slices of rats injected with pargyline, one hour before death, the rate of formation of tritiated water formed during the conversion of 3.5-ditritiotyrosine to ^{3}H-DOPA was significantly decreased, as compared to control animals (Thierry, and Blanc, unpublished

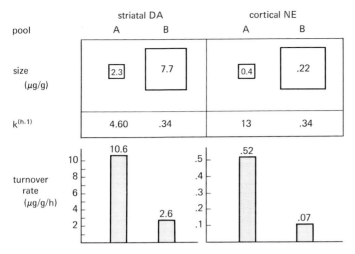

Figure 12-3   Evaluations of the rate constant and turnover rate of DA and NE, in the "functional" and "main storage" compartments of striatal dopaminergic and cerebral cortical noradrenergic terminals. Rate constants k (fraction of the pool turned over per unit of time) and turnover rates were calculated on the basis of the experimental curves on the time course of striatal DA decline after α.MpT administration (200 mg/kg i.p.) and of cerebral cortical NE decline after FLA 63 administration (40 mg/kg i.p.). The sizes of the compartments were also approximately evaluated, from experimental curves, by subtracting the quantities of amine disappearing in the "main storage compartment" during the initial rapid amine decline, which followed α.MpT or FLA 63 injection, from the total amount of DA or NE which disappeared during this period; the sizes of DA and NE "main storage" compartments were obtained by subtracting the size of the "functional" compartment from the total amine level in control animals. The small rising phase of DA and NE occurring between the two phases of amine decline after α.MpT and FLA 63 respectively in the striatum and in the cortex was neglected for the calculations; a steady state situation was assumed for each compartment and their turnover rates were calculated independently. (Experiments made by Javoy, Thierry, and Blanc)

observations). The last step of NE synthesis seems also to play an important role in the regulation of NE synthesis; this was particularly observed in α.MpT-treated animals. The availability of stored DA to be converted into NE for a long time after inhibition of the first step of synthesis is suggested by various experiments mainly made on the cortex of the rat, a structure innervated by the dorsal noradrenergic pathway.

The following observations were made: (a) NE disappeared much more rapidly after inhibition of the DA-NE conversion with FLA 63 than after inhibition of the tyrosine-DOPA step with α.MpT. Similar data have been obtained on the whole brain of the rat with FLA 63 (Persson and Waldeck, 1970) or with other inhibitors of the last step of NE synthesis, disulfiram (Goldstein and Nakajima, 1967), or α-α'-dydypiridil (Bapna et al., 1970). It is unlikely that this effect can be attributed to the lack of the activating effect of dopaminergic neurons on the noradrenergic neurons as a consequence of α.MpT treatment, as suggested by Persson and Waldeck (1970), since these authors have found a similar half-life for ^{3}H-NE synthesized from ^{3}H-tyrosine in control or α.MpT-treated rats. (b) NE levels were not changed 30 minutes after the α.MpT administration (Thierry et al., 1971c) despite the complete inhibition of NE synthesis observed a few minutes after the drug injection as shown by the immediate decrease of DA levels in the cortex or in the striatum, a dopaminergic structure. (c) The NE/DA ratio increased very rapidly, and then more slowly as a function of time, in the cortex after α.MpT treatment. More important changes in this NE/DA ratio, which mainly result from a faster DA decline, are seen after activation of noradrenergic neurons with thioproperazine, a potent neuroleptic (Thierry et al., 1971c), or under stress (Thierry, Blanc, and Glowinski, in preparation) in α.MpT-treated animals.

Other data seem also to indicate that the last step of NE synthesis modulates independently the NE formation in situations other than α.MpT treatment. (a) Marked changes in the NE/DA ratio level occur also in the rat cortex after inhibition of MAO with pargyline. A simultaneous increase of both amines is rapidly followed by a rapid and selective decrease of DA levels leading to an increase of the NE/DA ratio (Thierry, Blanc, and Glowinski, in preparation). (b) As with NE, newly synthesized or newly taken up DA is utilized preferentially and at a faster rate in the brain stem of stressed rats (Thierry et al., 1971a); this may be explained not only by the simultaneous enhanced release of DA and NE from noradrenergic terminals but also by the acceleration of the conversion of DA to NE under activation of noradrenergic neurons. (c) Finally, NE appears to be synthesized at a much slower rate than its precursor DA in noradrenergic neurons. The maximal accumulation of ^{3}H-NE in the brain stem of rats was delayed as compared to ^{3}H-DA after the intracisternal administration of ^{3}H-tyrosine (Thierry et al., 1971a). Similarly, ^{3}H-DA appeared much more rapidly than ^{3}H-NE in brain-stem or cortical slices of rats incubated for various times with ^{3}H-tyrosine (Thierry and Blanc, unpublished observations).

Dopaminergic Neurons

The very well-defined nigro-striatal dopaminergic system represents a relatively simple and unique model for biochemical studies on transmitter substances. This system of neurons has many advantages as compared to systems of noradrenergic neurons for studying the process of release, or the problems linked to the regulation of the transmitter biosynthesis. First, in the cat or in the rat, the numerous dopaminergic terminals are mainly localized in the caudate nucleus or in the striatum structures which contain very high quantities of DA. Second, the cell bodies of the dopaminergic neurons are all grouped in the pars compacta of the substantia nigra, which in both species can be easily stimulated or destroyed by stereotaxic techniques. Finally, DA is synthesized from tyrosine in only two steps, and labelled DA can be easily and rapidly separated from its precursors or metabolites; there is only one rate-limiting step, which does not seem to be the case in noradrenergic neurons. Our researches on this system of neurons, mainly made by Drs. Besson, Chéramy, and Javoy, have followed since 1967 two main complementary directions: attempts to understand the processes of regulation of DA synthesis in terminals and also in cell bodies; attempts to study the release of DA from dopaminergic terminals under direct or indirect activation of the nigro-striatal dopaminergic system.

Synthesis of DA and Its Regulation

Two approaches have been generally used in all our studies to appreciate changes in DA synthesis in the striatum of the rat.

1. A method was developed to measure in tissue slices the rate of conversion of 3-5 ditritiotyrosine into DOPA, the first and rate-limiting step of the amine synthesis (Besson *et al.*, 1971e). This *in vitro* method is based on the estimation of radioactive water formed during the reaction. Various experiments were first set up to test the specificity of this method: ^{3}H-DA accumulated in rat striatal slices and their incubating medium was measured simultaneously to ^{3}H-H$_2$O. Both ^{3}H-DA and ^{3}H-H$_2$O levels increased linearly as a function of time during a 30-minute incubation of the striatal slices with ^{3}H-tyrosine. Both ^{3}H-DA and ^{3}H-H$_2$O levels were reduced to less than 90 per cent of control values shortly after treatment of

the animals with α.MpT, the inhibitor of tyrosine hydroxylase. Finally both ^{3}H-DA and ^{3}H-H$_2$O levels were parallelly affected by drugs or ions such as K$^+$, which act on synthesis without interfering with the metabolic inactivation of the amine (Besson *et al.,* 1971e).

In the course of these preliminary studies we also observed that the total quantities of ^{3}H-DA accumulated in tissues, and released in the incubating medium, were almost identical to the quantities of ^{3}H-H$_2$O. This indicates that *in vitro* ^{3}H-DA newly synthesized is well protected from enzymatic inactivation by MAO or COMT. Similar observations could be made after inhibition of DA reuptake with amphetamine or acceleration of DA synthesis with thioproperazine (Besson *et al.,* 1971e) or amantadine (Scatton *et al.,* 1971), a drug used in Parkinson treatment. This may be related to the marked reduction of the release of DA, very likely induced by the lack of normal nerve impulses, as suggested by the relatively small quantities of ^{3}H-DA accumulated in the medium as compared to those found in tissues, and to the rapid *in vivo* inactivation of ^{3}H-DA newly synthesized from ^{3}H-tyrosine (Javoy and Glowinski, in preparation). However, different findings were made on cortical slices in comparable *in vitro* experiments on NE synthesis (Thierry and Blanc, unpublished observations): ^{3}H-CA levels were found much lower than those of ^{3}H-H$_2$O, indicating a rapid *in vitro* inactivation of the amines. The differences observed between dopaminergic and noradrenergic neurons may be related to slight differences in the inactivating properties of MAO or COMT in these respective neuronal systems.

2. The *in vivo* estimation of DA synthesis has been generally made by injecting ^{3}H-tyrosine intravenously or intraventricularly and by measuring the ^{3}H-DA levels and the tyrosine specific activity at short time intervals after the labelled amino acid injection. However, we will report results obtained with another new approach originally developed to measure synthesis of amines in very discrete areas or nuclei of the brain. This method consists in injecting 0.05 to 0.2 μl of a ^{3}H-tyrosine solution with the help of a glass microneedle, and in estimating ^{3}H-DA levels in the brain or in the area injected shortly after the labelled amino acid administration. This local stereotaxic micro-injection technique allows the selective labelling of about 1 mm^3 of tissue: more than 95 per cent of the total ^{3}H-DA or ^{3}H-CA accumulated in the whole brain was found in the striatum or in the ventromedial nucleus of the hypothalamus, 15 minutes after the micro-injection of ^{3}H-tyrosine (Javoy *et al.,* 1970). This new technique may be

used to estimate changes in the initial accumulation of ^{3}H-DA occurring in various experimental situations in the group of dopaminergic cell bodies which lie in the pars compacta of the substantia nigra or in structures containing small quantities of catecholaminergic terminals. It is still difficult to appreciate the local tyrosine specific activity in tissues and even more in the dopaminergic neurons, although this information is necessary to calculate the absolute rate of DA synthesis. About 50 to 60 per cent of the newly synthesized ^{3}H-DA is inactivated by MAO during the 15 minutes which follow the micro-injection of the amino acid. This was indicated by the differences observed in the accumulation of ^{3}H-DA and ^{3}H-methoxy-dopamine in control rats and in animals pretreated with a MAO inhibitor 5 or 10 minutes before ^{3}H-tyrosine injection (Javoy and Glowinski, in preparation). Therefore, the initial accumulation of the newly synthesized catecholamines underestimates the absolute synthesis of the transmitters and can be only used as an index of synthesis in comparative studies. Despite these limitations, valid information may be obtained about changes in aminergic neuron activity in small structures or discrete areas of the brain. This was indicated by the comparable results obtained with the *in vivo* and *in vitro* methods just described, in studies on the effect of psychotropic drugs on DA synthesis in the striatum of the rat.

Effects of Some Psychotropic Drugs on DA Synthesis. The accumulation of ^{3}H-DA found in tissues 15 minutes after the *in vivo* micro-injection of ^{3}H-tyrosine has been generally compared to the total accumulation of ^{3}H-DA or ^{3}H-H$_2$O at the end of a 15-minute incubation period, both in striatal slices and their incubating medium. The effects of reserpine and thioproperazine, representing two different types of neuroleptics, were first analyzed with these methods. Twenty-four hours after reserpine treatment (2 or 5 mg/kg i.p.), both the *in vivo* and *in vitro* accumulations of ^{3}H-DA were, as expected, decreased markedly. This drug affects the storage capacity of this amine in vesicles and therefore enhances the intraneuronal catabolic inactivation of the transmitter; thus ^{3}H-H$_2$O levels did not decrease as much as ^{3}H-DA levels in the *in vitro* studies, nevertheless they were significantly reduced as compared to those of control animals. Reserpine not only affects the amine storage but also decreases the amine synthesis (Besson *et al.,* 1971e). This effect on DA synthesis was not associated with changes in tyrosine hydroxylase activity (Table 12-1). Similarly chronic treatment with reserpine did not affect the enzyme activity in the striatum (Chéramy et al., 1971; Besson et al., 1971d). Since tyrosine hydroxylase activity in the brain stem was increased after acute (Mueller et al., 1969) or chronic treatment with reserpine (Besson et al., 1971d), differences may exist between the characteristics of regulation of dopaminergic and noradrenergic neurons under reserpine treatment. The storage capacity of dopaminergic neurons for newly synthesized DA reappeared very rapidly a few days after reserpine treatment as shown by the recovery, as a function of time, of the normal in vivo and in vitro accumulation of ^{3}H-DA formed from ^{3}H-tyrosine (Chéramy, Javoy, and Besson, unpublished observations). This very likely corresponds to the arrival of newly formed DA-containing granules in dopaminergic terminals, as suggested by Häggendal and Dhalström's (1971) experiments on peripheral noradrenergic neurons of reserpinized rats.

Various workers have shown that neuroleptics of the butyrophenone or the phenothiazine type accelerate the synthesis and turnover of DA in the striatum (Anden et al., 1964b; Roos, 1965; Scharman, 1966; Da Prada and Pletscher, 1966; Corrodi et al., 1967a; Nybäck and Sedvall, 1969). Comparable results were obtained with our in vivo and in vitro methods using thioproperazine, a potent neuroleptic of the phenothiazine type (Table 12-1). Small doses of this drug (5 mg/kg i.p.) rapidly increased both the in vivo (Javoy et al., 1970) and in vitro (Chéramy et al., 1970; Besson et al., 1971e) accumulation of ^{3}H-DA as well as the in vitro formation of radioactive water (Besson et al., 1971e). The in vitro results imply that the indirect activation of DA neurons, linked to the blockade of DA receptors as originally proposed by Corrodi et al. (1967a), rapidly, induces sustained changes in DA synthesis. Moreover, this effect can be still detected in slices although the tyrosine hydroxylase activity is not affected (Chéramy et al., 1971). The acceleration of DA synthesis detected in vitro only after the previous in vivo injection of the drug can also be seen when thioproperazine is given after amphetamine, a drug which inhibits DA synthesis 90 minutes after its intraperitoneal injection (Besson et al., 1971e). Indeed DA synthesis recovered almost to normal level immediately after the administration of thioproperazine; this biochemical effect associated with the blockade of the pharmacological effects of amphetamine further suggests an interneuronal activation of dopaminergic neurons under neuroleptic treatment (Chéramy et al., 1970). Thioproperazine seems to activate DA synthesis rapidly both in dopaminergic terminals and cell bodies as indicated by the simultaneous increased initial

TREATMENT	SCHEDULE	In vitro DA synthesis $^3H-H_2O$ $\mu Ci/g$ ①			In vivo DA synthesis ^3H-DA $\mu Ci/g$ ②			Tyrosine hydroxylase activity $\mu moles$ $^3H-H_2O/g/hr$ ③		
		CONTROL	TREATED	PER CENT CHANGE	CONTROL	TREATED	PER CENT CHANGE	CONTROL	TREATED	PER CENT CHANGE
Thioproperazine	5 mg/kg (3 hr)	12.0	20.3	+69	21.0	46.0	+120	1.13	1.18	N.S.
Reserpine	2 mg/kg (24 hr)	13.5	8.7	−36	11.9	5.9	−46	1.24	1.25	N.S.
Amphetamine	5 mg/kg (90 min)	12.0	1.1	−40	23,0	11.5	−50	0.77	0.78	N.S.
Pargyline	75 mg/kg (2 hr)	7.6	4.1	−46	*46.1	30.6	−27	—	—	—

Table 12-1   Effects of acute treatment with psychotropic drugs on DA synthesis and tyrosine hydroxylase activity in the striatum of the rat. All drugs were injected intraperitoneally. In vitro ^3H-DA synthesis was estimated on striatal slices by measuring the ^3H-H_2O formed during the conversion of L-3-5-ditritiotyrosine into DOPA during a 15-minute incubation. In vivo DA synthesis was estimated by measuring the accumulation of ^3H-DA in the striatum 15 minutes after the micro-injection of ^3H-tyrosine. Tyrosine hydroxylase activity was estimated on a semi-purified enzyme preparation obtained from striatal homogenates by measuring the ^3H-H_2O formed during the conversion of ^3H-tyrosine into ^3H-DOPA. All results obtained on DA in in vivo accumulation or in vitro synthesis were statistically significant. Under all drug treatments tyrosine specific activity estimated in the in vitro experiments was not significantly affected. Results are the mean of data obtained on 8 striata (in vitro DA synthesis, tyrosine hydroxylase activity) or groups of 8 to 10 animals (in vivo DA synthesis).* Control animals in the in vivo striatal DA synthesis estimation of pargyline pretreated animals were animals injected with ^3H-tyrosine 3 minutes after a single injection of pargyline (75 mg/kg i.p.). Therefore the differences mentioned correspond to ^3H-DA 15 minute accumulation at a shorter time (3 minutes) or a longer time (120 minutes) after pargyline treatment. (Experiments made by Besson, Chéramy, Mussachio, Gauchy: 1, 3, and Javoy 2)

accumulation of ^3H-DA observed in the striatum and in the substantia nigra after local micro-injection of ^3H-tyrosine (Javoy et al., 1970). The increase in the fluorescence of dopaminergic cell bodies observed by Andén et al. (1966) after treatment with a neuroleptic is thus, very likely, related to the activation of DA synthesis. This general rapid acceleration of DA synthesis in dopaminergic neurons is probably induced by the enhanced release of the transmitter shown both in vitro in the rat (Chéramy et al., 1970) and in vivo in the cat (Besson, Chéramy, and Gauchy, unpublished observation) after the acute administration of thioproperazine. However, recent data obtained with the in vitro technique reveal that the neuroleptic mechanism of action on dopaminergic or noradrenergic neurons is much more complex than suggested by the observations made in acute treatment of the drugs. Chronic treatment with small doses of thioproperazine over eight days or more had an opposite effect on DA synthe-

sis than did acute treatment: namely, a significant reduction of the transmitter synthesis (Scatton, Garett, and Julou, personal communication).
This effect has as yet not been related to changes in tyrosine hydroxylase
activity in the striatum, although a decrease in the enzyme activity was
found in the brain stem and in the cortex (Besson *et al.*, 1971d). This long-
term effect of this neuroleptic on the activity of dopaminergic neurons
cannot be adequately explained with our present knowledge, but it suggests complex temporal interneuronal regulation of dopaminergic neurons.
This biochemical change may be of great importance for the understanding
of the potent clinical effect of the drug, only acting after chronic administration to patients. During their extensive study on the action of thioproperazine on striatal DA synthesis Julou, Garett, and Scatton have detected another interesting point: an inverse relationship between the effect
of the drug on DA synthesis and that on endogenous DA levels. The rate
of DA synthesis, estimated with the *in vitro* "tritiated water method," increased as a function of time during the first three hours following acute
thioproperazine treatment (2 mg/kg s.c.); it then returned to normal levels
in a few hours. The maximal level of DA synthesis was correlated with
the maximal decrease of the endogenous DA content which never exceeded
25 per cent of control levels under the various doses tested. This reduction
of DA levels may correspond to the complete utilization of the amine
localized in the "functional compartment" of dopaminergic terminals.
This compartment has been found to contain approximately 25 per cent of
the total amine content of striatal dopaminergic terminals (Javoy and
Glowinski, 1971a). It is therefore tempting to suggest that the intensity of
DA synthesis is directly related to the changes in the DA content in the
"functional compartment"; the rapid increase in DA synthesis could correspond to an immediate regulating process in order to overcome the faster
utilization of the newly synthesized transmitter.

Amphetamine affects various processes of DA metabolism in the dopaminergic neurons of the nigro-striatal system. This drug is a potent inhibitor of the DA uptake process (Coyle and Snyder, 1969a). Both D- and
L-amphetamine treatments enhance the release of newly synthesized DA,
as indicated by the increased quantities of ^{3}H-DA released into the incubating medium of rat striatal slices (Besson *et al.*, 1969c), and by the increased output of newly synthesized ^{3}H-DA during continuous superfusion
of the cat caudate nucleus with ^{3}H-tyrosine. This effect, also detected after
direct application of the drug on dopaminergic terminals, may be related

to the direct releasing effect of the drug and to the inhibition of the re-
uptake process. Surprisingly, this enhanced extraneuronal utilization of
DA newly synthesized was not, as expected, associated with a compensatory increase in DA synthesis, although DA endogenous levels were not
decreased but even slightly increased. A reduction of about 40 to 50 per
cent of the initial accumulation of ^{3}H-DA formed from ^{3}H-tyrosine in
dopaminergic terminals was detected with the *in vivo* micro-injection technique, 90 minutes after amphetamine treatment (5 mg/kg i.p.) (Javoy
et al., 1970). Similar data were obtained for the *in vitro* accumulation of
both ^{3}H-DA and ^{3}H-H_2O formed from ^{3}H-tyrosine in striatal slices of amphetamine-pretreated animals (Besson *et al.*, 1971e). (Table 12-1). The
extent of DA synthesis inhibition was identical with increasing doses of
D-amphetamine from 1 mg/kg to 10 mg/kg; moreover this effect was also
seen after addition of small concentrations (10^{-7} M) of the drug in the
incubating medium of control striatal slices, indicating its direct effect on
the biosynthetic process. Finally, the specific activity of tyrosine in slices
was not affected by the amphetamine pretreatment (Besson *et al.*, 1971e).
Both these *in vivo* and *in vitro* results clearly demonstrate that D-amphetamine inhibits DA synthesis at its first and rate-limiting step. Kinetic analysis of the DA synthesis could be made by incubating striatal slices with
increasing concentrations of ^{3}H-tyrosine: in a concentration range in which
the tyrosine uptake was a linear function of the amino acid concentration
in the incubating medium, initial rates of DA synthesis in slices could be
measured and K_m and V_{max} for DA synthesis in slices could be calculated,
following the Lineweaver and Burk method of analysis, assuming that ^{3}H-
tyrosine newly taken up in slices is preferentially used for DA synthesis.
In these conditions V_{max} values for DA synthesis were 18.2 and 13.3
mμmole/g/hr in striatal slices of normal and amphetamine-pretreated rats,
respectively. Moreover amphetamine was found to inhibit DA synthesis
from tyrosine by a noncompetitive mechanism for tyrosine. As tyrosine
hydroxylase activity was not changed after amphetamine treatment (Chéramy *et al.*, 1971), the drug may inhibit DA synthesis by enhancing cytoplasmic DA levels. These play a critical role in the regulation of the
tyrosine-DOPA conversion, probably by competing with the cofactors
involved in the first-rate limiting step of DA synthesis, as previously suggested by experiments on peripheral noradrenergic neurons (Ikeda *et al.*,
1966).

Various remarks are prompted by the inhibitory effect of amphetamine on DA synthesis. (1) As already mentioned striatal DA endogenous levels were not decreased after amphetamine treatment despite the marked decrease in the amine synthesis and the potent effect of the drug on the amine release. These results are difficult to explain according to the hypothesis of a single compartment model for DA storage; they favor the idea of the existence of various forms of DA in dopaminergic terminals differently affected by the drug. (2) As suggested by the enhanced initial accumulation of ^{3}H-DA seen in dopaminergic cell bodies after local ^{3}H-tyrosine micro-injection in the substantia nigra (Javoy *et al.*, 1970), DA synthesis may be increased in cell bodies after amphetamine treatment despite the inhibitory effect of the drug on dopaminergic terminals. This may imply that a drug could act differently on cell bodies and on terminals. (3) An acute amphetamine treatment similar to that used in the previous experiments on dopaminergic neurons had been shown to increase NE turnover (Javoy *et al.*, 1968b) and ^{3}H-CA synthesis from ^{3}H-tyrosine in the brain stem (Besson, *et al.*, 1969c). D-amphetamine, which affects the uptake of CA in both dopaminergic and noradrenergic neurons (Coyle and Snyder, 1969a) and stimulates the liberation of these transmitters (Besson *et al.*, 1969a, c) acts differently on the synthesis regulation of the amines in the noradenergic and dopaminergic terminals.

Regulation of DA Synthesis in DA Terminals. The synthesis of DA in dopaminergic terminals seems to be modulated by a mechanism of negative feedback control: increased intraneuronal levels of DA in dopaminergic terminals appear to inhibit DA synthesis at its first and rate-limiting step. These conclusions could be made from *in vivo* and *in vitro* experiments in which DA synthesis was estimated with the two methods previously described.

(a) In a first group of experiments, DA synthesis was estimated as a function of time after inhibition of MAO with pargyline (75 mg/kg i.p.) by measuring the *in vivo* accumulation of ^{3}H-DA fifteen minutes after the microinjection of ^{3}H-tyrosine in the striatum. As a result of the protection from MAO inactivation, ^{3}H-DA levels were markedly increased (60 per cent), as compared to control animals, when the labelled amino acid was injected almost immediately (3 minutes) after pargyline administration. However, ^{3}H-DA levels were significantly reduced in groups of animals treated for a longer time period (> 30 minutes) (Table 12-1) or chronically (3 days) with pargyline as compared to those found in animals injected with ^{3}H-tyrosine shortly (3 minutes) after the drug administration. The formation of DA appears to be inhibited as soon as 30 minutes after MAO inhibition when DA levels have already reached about 160 per cent of control levels (Javoy and Glowinski, 1971b; Javoy and Glowinski, in preparation).

(b) In a second group of experiments, DA synthesis was estimated *in vitro* in striatal slices by measuring ^{3}H-H_2O formed during the conversion of L-3,5-^{3}H-tyrosine to DOPA and accumulated over a 15 minute period. The formation of tritiated water was reduced by 30 to 40 per cent as compared with control rats 60 minutes after pargyline or pheniprazine (Fig. 12-4). This effect was not related to changes in tyrosine specific

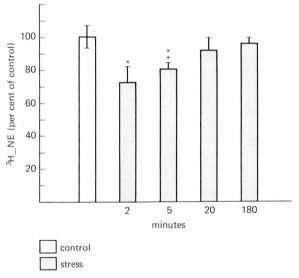

Figure 12-4   Effect of increased DA levels on *in vitro* ^{3}H-DA synthesis, from ^{3}H-tyrosine, in dopaminergic terminals of the rat. ^{3}H-DA synthesis was estimated by incubating, for 20 minutes, striatal slices with 25 μCi/ml of L-3,4-ditritiotyrosine (40 Ci/mmole). ^{3}H-H_2O formed during the conversion of ^{3}H-tyrosine to ^{3}H-DOPA was used as an index of the first step of ^{3}H-DA synthesis. Endogenous DA levels were increased either by pretreatment of rats with pargyline (75 mg/kg i.p.) or pheniprazine (Catron) (5 mg/kg i.p.) given 60 minutes before death, or by preincubating slices for 10 minutes with DA (10^{-6}M) added in the incubating medium. ^{3}H-H_2O formed in control slices was 7.7 μCi/g. Endogenous tyrosine levels were unchanged at the time of ^{3}H-DA synthesis estimation. Results, expressed in per cent of control values, are the mean $\pm$ S.E.M. of data obtained on 7 or 8 striata. (Experiments made by Javoy)

activity since tyrosine endogenous levels or ³H-tyrosine accumulation in slices were not modified by these treatments. A similar inhibition of DA synthesis was observed at longer intervals after pargyline treatment or in rats treated chronically with the MAO inhibitor (Javoy and Glowinski, 1971b; Javoy and Glowinski, in preparation). This reduction of DA synthesis was not related to changes in tyrosine hydroxylase activity since the enzyme activity was identical to that of control animals after chronic treatment with pargyline (one injection of 40 mg/kg, s.c. once a day over 13 days) (Besson et al., 1971d). The effect of increased intraneuronal DA levels on the amine synthesis was finally demonstrated directly by incubating striatal slices with a small concentration of nonlabelled DA (10^{-6}M): DA synthesis was markedly reduced as observed one hour after MAO inhibition (Fig. 12-4). Moreover, the effect of the exogenous DA on ³H-DA synthesis could be prevented with benztropine, an inhibitor of DA uptake (Javoy and Glowinski, in preparation). In conclusion, small changes in intraneuronal DA levels induce rapidly sustained modifications of the DA synthesis easily detected *in vitro*.

DA Synthesis and Multistorage Forms of DA. As previously mentioned, the maximal velocity of DA synthesis in striatal slices can be calculated following the Lineweaver and Burk method by measuring the initial rates of DA synthesis under various concentration ranges of tyrosine with the help of the "tritiated water method" (Besson et al., 1971e). Under these conditions the maximal rate of DA synthesis in intact striatal slices was 18.2 mμmol/g/hr. This rate of DA synthesis is much lower than that of tyrosine hydroxylase activity estimated on a partly purified enzyme preparation and with an excess of substrate and cofactors, about 496 mμmol/g/hr in the striatum (Musacchio et al., 1970). This *in vitro* DA synthesis rate in striatal slices is similar to that calculated from *in vivo* turnover studies made on the basis of a single compartment model for DA storage. From the curve of DA disappearance obtained one hour after α.MpT treatment, Costa and Neff (1966) have calculated that the rate of DA synthesis was 18.6 mμmol/g/hr in the caudate nucleus of the rabbit. With the same methodology and assumptions for DA storage, we found a rate of synthesis of about 17 mμmol/g/hr in the striatum of the rat (Javoy and Glowinski, 1971a). However, the maximal rate of DA synthesis obtained *in vitro* is probably underestimated when compared to that occurring *in vivo* since the amine synthesis rate may be dependent on nerve impulse activity, as it has been shown in peripheral noradrenergic neurons (see review Weiner, 1970). In this case, the synthesis rate of DA calculated from the *in vivo* turnover study based on a single compartment model is also underestimated since it is comparable to that obtained in *in vitro* studies. In fact, we found various data suggesting the existence of more than one form of DA storage in dopaminergic terminals, indicating therefore that the assumption of a single compartment model for DA storage cannot be retained to calculate the *in vivo* rate of DA synthesis. First, newly synthesized ^{3}H-DA from ^{3}H-tyrosine seems to be preferentially released from DA terminals as shown in *in vivo* studies on the cat caudate nucleus (Besson *et al.*, 1971b, Besson *et al.*, 1971c). Second, DA levels in the rat striatum do not decline monophasically after inhibition of DA synthesis with α.MpT as previously assumed, but in two distinct and separated phases: an initial and rapid one, lasting for 15 minutes, and a much slower one, starting 30 minutes after the drug injection and lasting for a few hours (Javoy and Glowinski, 1971a) Fig. 12-2). These two phases are separated by a period during which DA levels return to almost normal levels as observed for NE after administration of FLA 63. The two successive phases of DA decline may correspond in the main to the utilization of DA in a "functional" compartment and in a "main storage" compartment. The characteristics of these two compartments have been approximated from the experimental curves, neglecting the raising phase of DA levels, possibly related to DA axonal flow, and assuming that DA is used simultaneously in the two compartments. The sizes of the two compartments in dopaminergic terminals were found to be, respectively, 2.3 and 7.7 μg, the half-lives of DA utilization 9 and 124 minutes, and the turnover rate of DA 10.6 and 2.6 μg/g/hr in the "functional" and "main storage" compartments. Consequently, the total rate of DA synthesis was found to be not less than 13.2 μg/g/hr ($\neq$ 65 mμmol/g/hr), assuming that both compartments were in a steady state situation. According to these estimations, the turnover of DA in the "functional" compartment was about four times that of the "main storage" compartment (Javoy and Glowinski, 1971a) (Fig. 12-3). Further evidence of the very high *in vivo* rate of DA synthesis was obtained by measuring the 10- to 15-minute initial rate of DA accumulation after MAO inhibition. In these conditions the DA synthesis was estimated to be about 20 to 25 μg/g/hr (Javoy and Glowinski, 1971b). As various forms of storage of DA coexist in dopaminergic terminals exhibiting different characteristics, new methods should be developed to measure more precisely the absolute rate of DA synthesis in *in vivo* conditions.

Release of Dopamine

The experiments on DA release carried on in our laboratory during the last few years, mainly by Drs. Besson and Chéramy, have been based on the labelling of dopaminergic terminals with ^{3}H-DA synthesized endogenously from L-^{3}H-tyrosine, its original precursor. A labelled amino acid of very high specific activity was used to detect very small quantities of ^{3}H-DA released. This approach has been chosen for two main reasons: (1) The spectrofluorimetric methods available were not sensitive enough to measure accurately quantities of DA lower than 3 to 5 ng. Despite the original successful experiments of McLennan (1964-65), the use of microspectrofluorimetric methods seems hazardous since Portig and Vogt (1966-68) failed to obtain consistent data under pharmacological or electrical activation of dopaminergic neurons and also did not detect a spontaneous release of the amine. (2) Direct labelling of dopaminergic terminals with ^{3}H-DA was avoided to eliminate possible artifacts linked to the release of small quantities of ^{3}H-DA not stored in dopaminergic terminals. In contrast, direct labelling of dopaminergic terminals with ^{3}H-tyrosine provides great security about the specificity of the ^{3}H-DA release, since tyrosine hydroxylase is localized only in dopaminergic neurons (Goldstein *et al.*, 1967). It allows the study of the relationship between synthesis and release processes. Furthermore, this technique is about a thousand times more sensitive than the DA spectrofluorimetric method since the minimal amounts of ^{3}H-DA detectable are about 5 to 10 pg.

However, technical precautions must be taken. First, since the ^{3}H-tyrosine should be as pure as possible in order to get low blank of ^{3}H-tyrosine and to eliminate the ^{3}H-DOPA contamination, the labelled amino acid is purified just before each experiment. Second, ^{3}H-DA must be well separated from ^{3}H-tyrosine if very small quantities of ^{3}H-DA in medium particularly rich in ^{3}H-tyrosine are to be detected. Microtechniques based on alumina adsorption and ion-exchange chromatography on amberlite CG.50 used, allow the reproducible extraction and separation of about one mole of ^{3}H-DA in medium containing 10^5 moles of the labelled amino acid. Finally, the identity of ^{3}H-DA extracted from superfusing or incubating medium has been checked by cochromatography after acetylation of the amine.

Our researches were made successively *in vitro* on the rat striatum and *in vivo* on the caudate nucleus of the cat. In both cases release of ^{3}H-DA endogenously synthesized was successively examined after previous labelling of dopaminergic terminals with ^{3}H-tyrosine for short periods (acute labelling) or during simultaneous and constant labelling of the dopaminergic terminals with the labelled amino acid (continuous labelling). The *in vitro* studies were designed and carried out as a simplified model for the development of the *in vivo* studies. In preliminary studies to detect the release of the transmitter, "acute labelling" was used both *in vitro* and *in vivo;* this procedure was quickly abandoned for "continuous labelling" as more important release of DA was seen when the transmitter had been newly synthesized.

In vitro Studies. Acute labelling experiments were made on the isolated striatum of the rat which was first incubated for 45 to 60 minutes with L-^{3}H-tyrosine (15.6 μCi of 28.2 Ci/mmole) and then superfused with a physiological medium. Superfusates were collected in serial 15-minute fractions over a two-hour period. The spontaneous release of ^{3}H-DA from dopaminergic terminals as well as the release of the transmitter induced by drugs, other transmitters, or depolarizing procedures could be easily demonstrated (Besson *et al.,* 1969a). The main results obtained can be summarized briefly: (a) the curve of ^{3}H-DA decline in the successive collected fractions was characteristic and different from the curve of disappearance of inert substances such as ^{14}C-urea and ^{3}H-inulin or ^{3}H-tyrosine the precursor of ^{3}H-DA. Two distinct phases of DA decline, suggesting the existence of two forms of DA with different dynamic characteristics of utilization, could be seen. Moreover, the ^{3}H-DA decline as a function of time was different from that observed for ^{3}H-5-HT formed from ^{3}H-tryptophan in the isolated striatum (Besson *et al.,* 1969b) or for ^{3}H-NE formed from ^{3}H-tyrosine in the isolated brain stem (Glowinski, 1970). (b) The release of ^{3}H-DA was markedly stimulated by increased concentrations of K$^+$ in the superfusing medium, or by electrical field stimulation. (c) D-amphetamine and phenyprazine (Catron), an MAO inhibitor structurally related to amphetamine, markedly enhanced the output of ^{3}H-DA when introduced in low concentrations (10^{-6}M) for 15 minutes in the superfusing medium (Besson *et al.,* 1969a). These effects seem specific since amphetamine concentrations a hundred times higher had almost no effect on the release of ^{3}H-5-HT previously synthesized from ^{3}H-tryptophan (Glowinski, 1970). (d) Acetylcholine (5.10^{-5}M) and 5-HT (5.10^{-5}M), two substances found in high concentrations in the striatum, very likely acting as transmitters, increase the release of ^{3}H-DA. Their effect, however, was not as pronounced as that seen after amphetamine but seemed quite specific since no change could be seen in the output of total radioactivity, represented mainly by ^{3}H-tyrosine. Furthermore, acetylcholine had absolutely no effect on the release of substances mainly localized in the extraneuronal space such as ^{3}H-inulin or ^{14}C-urea.

More ^{3}H-DA was released in collected fractions relative to the ^{3}H-DA content in tissues immediately after the end of the synthesis period with ^{3}H-tyrosine than later on. It suggested that DA newly synthesized was preferentially released spontaneously. This, however, could not be fully demonstrated in these experiments since DA specific activity could not be estimated in superfusates. Nevertheless, these observations led us to develop the "continuous labelling" method to estimate preferentially the release of the newly synthesized transmitter. Slices of striatum were thus incubated with ^{3}H-tyrosine for 15 to 30 minutes, and the ^{3}H-DA released in the incubating medium as well as the ^{3}H-amine contained in tissues were measured at the end of the incubating period. As already mentioned, this technique also gives information about synthesis, since total ^{3}H-DA accumulated in tissues and incubating medium can be estimated. This approach is particularly appropriate for simultaneous study of the effects of psychotropic drugs or ions on release and synthesis processes. The drugs may be administered *in vivo* to the animals, or in some cases added to the incubating medium when they act directly on aminergic neurons. Enhanced quantities of transmitter in the incubating medium may be linked to enhanced release, or to inhibition of reuptake, or to both processes. Complementary experiments should be performed to distinguish these two effects. Enhanced release of ^{3}H-DA newly synthesized was demonstrated under various conditions: increased K^+ concentrations in the medium, pretreatment of animals with a neuroleptic such as thioproperazine (Chéramy et al., 1969) or anti-parkinson drugs such as amantadine (Scatton, et al., 1971), all situations in which an acceleration of the transmitter synthesis has been seen. Pronounced release of newly synthesized ^{3}H-DA could be also detected when synthesis was inhibited, as after pretreatment of animals with amphetamine or after addition of this drug to the incubating medium (Besson *et al.*, 1969c). Reduction of ^{3}H-DA release was seen 5 or 24 hours after reserpine treatment, which also inhibits DA synthesis. However, rapid recovery of normal release could be seen in the two following days despite the low content of endogenous DA levels still seen in dopaminergic terminals (Chéramy and Besson, unpublished observations). As previously discussed, this may be linked to the arrival or formation of new DA-containing vesicles in dopaminergic terminals; they could thus represent the "functional compartment" of the amine already described. Therefore changes in the release of DA induced by direct or indirect activation of dopaminergic neurons can be easily detected with this very sensitive approach which is particularly suitable for the study of effects of very small doses of psychotropic drugs.

In vivo Studies. The *in vivo* studies on DA release in the cat were made with the "cup technique" originally used by Mitchell (1966) to study the release of acetylcholine from the cortex surface. This method was adapted to our problem. Briefly, a specially designed cup is applied stereotaxically on the ventricular dorsal surface of the caudate nucleus, previously exposed by removal of overlying tissue. Small tubes fixed to the cup allow the continuous superfusion of the surface of the caudate nucleus as well as its continuous oxygenation. Superfusates can be continuously collected at a rate of about 6 ml per hour (Besson *et al.,* 1971a). This new approach has some advantages over the other two methods available: first, the number of dopaminergic terminals superfused is much larger than that obtained with the push-pull cannulae method used by McLennan (1964-65) and more recently by McKenzie and Szerb (1968), Riddell and Szerb (1971), and Voigtlander and Moore (1971); second, only catecholaminergic neurons of the caudate nucleus are superfused; this may not be the case with the ventricular perfusing technique used by Portig and Vogt (1969). Furthermore, the cup technique eliminates the artifacts which may be produced with the push-pull cannulae method. As previously discussed by Vogt (1969), local increase of leakage of substances present in tissues as a result of unspecific changes in permeability or blood supply caused by an inflow of impulses may occur. The physiological integrity of the tissue lying under the cup is maintained for a long period. This is indicated by the usual changes in the electrical activities of cells normally recorded following the stimulation of the substantia nigra (Besson *et al.*, 1971a) and by the constant increase in ^{3}H-DA content of the caudate nucleus seen over a few hours during continuous labelling of dopaminergic terminals with ^{3}H-tyrosine (Besson, Chéramy, and Gauchy, in preparation). Finally it should also be mentioned that most of the radioactivity found in tissues is concentrated into a very thin tissue layer localized just under the cup.

Both the spontaneous and evoked release of ^{3}H-DA could be demonstrated under "acute" or "continuous" labelling of the dopaminergic terminals in the unanesthetized cat immobilized with flaxedil. The best results were obtained with the continuous labelling method by superfusing ^{3}H-tyrosine (30 to 50 μCi/ml, 52 Ci/m mole) at a rate of 6 ml/hr and by collecting fractions of 5 to 10 minutes' duration. This method which is very reproducible, provides very rapidly an almost constant release of ^{3}H-DA for many hours. Therefore, this allows the comparison of results obtained by repeated administrations of drugs or electrical stimulations on the same animal. In fact, ^{3}H-DA was detected almost immediately after the onset of superfusion, its release increasing rapidly during the first hour and thereafter much more slowly. Despite the formation of small quantities of ^{3}H-NE in the caudate nucleus detected only a few hours after the onset of superfusion, ^{3}H-DA was the only ^{3}H-CA identified in superfusates (Besson et al., 1971a).

The main results already obtained can be summarized as follows: (a) quantities of ^{3}H-DA representing about 5 to 10 pg of the labelled amine were collected in a 10-minute fraction during spontaneous release; (b) depolarization of dopaminergic terminals with K$^+$ induced a marked and short-lasting release of the transmitter, about ten times the amount of DA spontaneously released; depolarization with a local stimulation was surprisingly much less effective, although the mechanical stimulation produced by the introduction of the electrode in the tissue under the cup caused an abrupt and important rise of ^{3}H-DA release; (c) pronounced reduction of ^{3}H-DA spontaneous release (about 65 per cent) was seen after the abolition of nerve impulses in neurons with tetrodotoxin introduced into the cup; (d) various drugs were shown to increase the output of newly synthesized ^{3}H-DA: benztropine, an inhibitor of the DA uptake process (Besson, Chéramy, Gauchy, and Glowinski, in preparation); pargyline, an irreversible MAO inhibitor which induced a small but constant rise in ^{3}H-DA output; D- and L-amphetamine which when introduced into the cup or given intravenously (Fig. 5), increased (probably because of their direct releasing properties) more markedly the release of the transmitter than did benztropine (Besson et al., 1971a); phenyprazine, which had a rapid

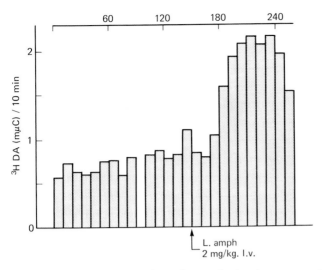

Figure 12-5   Effect of l-amphetamine on the *in vivo* release of ^{3}H-DA, newly synthesized from ^{3}H-tyrosine, from dopaminergic terminals of the cat caudate nucleus. L-3-5-^{3}H-tyrosine (40 Ci/mmole) was continuously superfused (30 μCi/ml/10 min) in a cup on the ventricular surface of the caudate nucleus of an anaesthetized cat. The figure illustrates the effect of an intravenous injection of l-amphetamine (2 mg/kg) on the release of ^{3}H-DA. Superfusates were collected in serial fractions of 10 minutes, and ^{3}H-DA was estimated in each fraction. (Experiment by Besson and Chéramy)

and pronounced effect on DA release (five to seven times the DA spontaneous release), much more comparable to the amphetamine effect than to that of pargyline (Besson, Chéramy, Gauchy, and Glowinski, in preparation); and finally thioproperazine, a potent neuroleptic, which induced a small but persistent rise in ^{3}H-DA release after its intravenous administration; (e) small concentrations of 5-HT introduced into the cup markedly increased the release of newly synthesized ^{3}H-DA for short periods; the effect was much more pronounced than that observed *in vitro* on the isolated striatum; changes in ^{3}H-DA release were also seen after acetylcholine addition in presence of eserine, but the effects were less pronounced and not so reproducible (Besson, Chéramy, Gauchy, and Glowinski, in preparation).

In further experiments, attempts have also been made to study the evoked release of DA induced by electrical stimulation of the substantia nigra, which contains the DA cell bodies (Andén *et al.*, 1964a; Poirier and Sourkes, 1965; Bedard *et al.*, 1969). Other workers have done similar experiments with the cat, but all have not obtained identical results. This may be related to the difficulty of the experiments as well as the diversity of the methodology used.

With the push-pull cannulae method, McLennan (1964) was not able to detect the release of DA under stimulation of the substantia nigra; positive results were obtained only during the stimulation of the nucleus centro medianus. More recently, with a similar method, and under labelling of dopaminergic terminals with ^{14}C-tyrosine, Riddell and Szerb (1971) observed a release of ^{14}C-DA. They obtained successful results in only a few experiments during long-term and intense stimulation of the rostral portion of the substantia nigra, but consistent data were seen after stimulation of the medial forebrain bundle. Portig and Vogt (1966-68) have also attempted to measure the release of DA from the caudate nucleus with the ventricular perfusing method. They reported that the amine was sometimes released but inconsistently, and in very small quantities, and that furthermore the latent period between stimulation and emergence of the amine was variable. However, increases of homovanillic acid output in perfusates were seen in most of the experiments, during short or long stimulation of the substantia nigra. Sizable increase in homovanillic acid content in the superfusates was detected after short stimulation periods, this was attributed to the slow diffusion of the acid and not to the prolonged activation of dopaminergic neurons (Portig and Vogt, 1969). With the same method and after previous labelling of dopaminergic terminals with ^{3}H-DA, von Voigtlander and Moore (1971) have detected in a few experiments a very small increase of ^{3}H-DA release during short stimulation periods. The effect was slightly more apparent just after the end of the stimulation.

Surprisingly, in our preliminary experiments on about 25 cats, we were not able to detect an average significant increase in the release of ^{3}H-DA newly synthesized, in the 10-minute fraction corresponding to the stimulation period, under various conditions of stimulation of the substantia nigra. However, ^{3}H-DA release was found to be significantly enhanced in the immediately following fraction. These results suggest that complex events may occur during stimulation; they may be related to the effects of the stimulation on cells localized in or near the pars compacta of the substantia nigra and in relation with dopaminergic neurons. It should also be mentioned that significant enhanced release of ^{3}H-DA could be seen in some experiments during stimulation of other mesencephalic structures of the brain (Besson, Chéramy, Gauchy, Glowinski, and Albe Fessard, in preparation).

Complementary information may be obtained with "acute labelling experiments" as observed in the *in vitro* experiments. The acute labelling experiments were mainly carried out in cat preparation in order to study the role of various forms of DA storage in release processes. First, as observed with the isolated striatum of the rat, ^{3}H-DA declined in two distinct phases in the fractions collected successively just after the acute labelling with ^{3}H-tyrosine. In the two phases, the half-life of ^{3}H-DA was about 18 and 60 minutes (Besson *et al.*, 1971a). The initial rapid phase may reflect the fast utilization of ^{3}H-DA newly synthesized and localized in the "functional compartment." It should be noted that the duration of the first phase and the ^{3}H-DA initial half-life are quite comparable to those observed in the early DA disappearance seen in the rat striatum immediately after α.MpT treatment (Javoy and Glowinski, 1971a). The effects of drugs on ^{3}H-DA stored in tissues for a long time were examined under acute labelling and compared with those obtained with continuous labelling experiments. Amphetamine, and phenyprazine (Catron) (Besson, *et al.*, 1971a) evoked the ^{3}H-DA release much more markedly during continuous labelling with the ^{3}H-amino acid than in acute labelling experiments in which the drugs were added to the cup at long intervals after the end of ^{3}H-DA synthesis. These observations, as well as the rapid and pronounced decrease in ^{3}H-DA release, detected in continuous labelling experiments after intravenous injection of α.MpT (Besson, Chéramy, Gauchy, and Glowinski, 1971c), strongly suggest that newly synthesized DA is more available for extraneuronal release than DA stored in tissues for longer periods.

Serotoninergic Neurons

The study of 5-HT metabolism in central serotoninergic neurons is relatively more difficult than in catecholaminergic neurons. Central serotoninergic neurons cannot be directly labelled with exogenous radioactive 5-HT since the amine may be partly taken up in catecholaminergic neurons (Shaskan and Snyder, 1970). Moreover, the exogenous amine does not appear to behave quite like endogenous 5-HT (Sanders-Bush and Sulzer, 1969). Parachlorophenylalanine (PCPA) has been generally used to inhibit 5-HT synthesis selectively (Koe and Weissman, 1966), but this drug also slightly affects the metabolism of CA and does not inhibit completely the *in vivo* formation of 5-HT (Diaz *et al.,* 1968). Recently, as will be discussed, MAO inhibitors (MAOI), as well as probenecid, have been found to affect the metabolism of centrol tryptophan (Tagliamonte *et al.,* 1971; Glowinski *et al.,* 1971b). Therefore, their use is not particularly appropriate for the estimation of 5-HT turnover according to methods previously described (Tozer *et al.,* 1966; Neff *et al.,* 1967). The best approach yet available to detect changes in synthesis or utilization of 5-HT in the brain is to label central 5-HT neurons with radioactive tryptophan, the original precursor of 5-HT. As in our studies on central catecholaminergic neurons, combined *in vivo* and in *vitro* methods have been used in most experiments. Our researches have been limited to two main directions: (1) attempts to detect changes in activity of central 5-HT neurons induced by modifications of environment or physiological states and by psychotropic drugs; (2) attempts to demonstrate the regulatory processes of 5-HT synthesis.

Changes in Serotoninergic Neuron Activity

The activity of central serotoninergic neurons has been examined in most of our earlier studies on stress and sleep, parallel to the activity of central catecholaminergic neurons. Pronounced increases in the activity of serotoninergic neurons were found in situations representing severe physical modifications of the environment. More recently, very important changes of 5-HT metabolism were also detected after examination of the activity of serotoninergic neurons at various times of the day (they may have more important physiological significance). The results obtained as well as those gained in a few drugs studies made to examine specific problems of 5-HT metabolism confirm and extend our knowledge of the metabolic characteristics of central serotoninergic neurons.

1) *Effects of Stress and Sleep Deprivation.* As previously mentioned, two types of acute stress were used in our studies: a long stress session corresponding to repetitive periods of application of electrical shock to paws of rats over 180 minutes, and a short stress session corresponding to a single 15-minute application of electrical shock. The changes in 5-HT

turnover were estimated in the brain stem of rats by measuring the temporal changes of 5-HT specific activity after previous labelling of serotoninergic neurons with L-³H-tryptophan injected intracisternally. Acceleration of 5-HT turnover was only seen during long stress experiments (Thierry et al., 1968b); no effect could be detected with the short stress session, which is quite different from that observed on noradrenergic neurons (Thierry et al., 1971a). The change of 5-HT utilization seen under the 180-minute stress was associated with a pronounced increase of 5-HT synthesis as indicated by the direct estimation of ³H-5-HT formation and initial accumulation in brain tissues after intravenous injection of ³H-tryptophan. In contrast to the observations made on noradrenergic neurons, the increase in 5-HT synthesis was not potentiated by a chronic stress treatment (Thierry et al., 1968b), suggesting a short duration of the stress effect. Pain or increased temperature related to the intense muscular exercise induced by the long stress, may be responsible for the serotoninergic neuron activation. In fact, high environmental temperature has been shown to accelerate 5-HT turnover (Reid et al., 1968; Corrodi et al., 1967; Tagliamonte et al., 1971). On the other hand, PCPA, the inhibitor of tryptophan hydroxylase, and lesions of the midbrain raphé in rats, both of which markedly reduced the 5-HT brain levels, have been shown to block the analgesic effect of morphine (Tenen, 1968; Samanin et al., 1970).

Various lesion and pharmacological studies support the hypothesis of a functional role of central serotoninergic neurons in sleep processes (Jouvet, 1969). This led us to investigate the effects of physical modifications of sleep states on the central metabolism of 5-HT, using an approach similar to that of our studies on the effects of PS deprivation on central noradrenergic neurons (Pujol et al., 1968). As already described, p. 000), rats were selectively deprived of PS for 91 hours by putting them on small supports surrounded by water; 5-HT synthesis and utilization were estimated in various structures of the brain at the end of this deprivation period. The following main observations could be made: (1) a markedly increased accumulation of ³H-5-HT was observed in all brain tissues of PS-deprived animals as compared to control rats 45 minutes after the intracisternal injection of ³H-tryptophan. The specific activity of 5-HT was increased significantly (about 50 per cent) in the telencephalon-diencephalon, the brain stem-mesencephalon, and in the spinal cord. These effects were associated with parallel increases in the tryptophan specific activity of the various structures and resulted from an enhanced

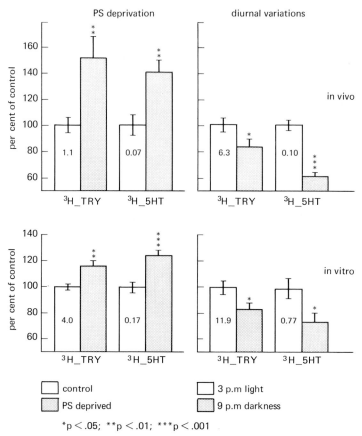

Figure 12-6 Effect of paradoxical sleep (PS) deprivation and diurnal variations on
³H-5-HT formation from ³H-tryptophan in the brain stem of the rat. ³H-5-HT
formation from ³H (G)-tryptophan (5.4 Ci/mmole) was estimated *in vivo* (upper
part) and *in vitro* (bottom part). In the experiments on PS deprivation (1) (left
part), rats were deprived of PS for 91 hours by putting them on small supports surrounded by water, and ³H-5-HT formation was estimated just at the end of the PS
deprivation period in the brain stem-mesencephalon. In the experiments on 5-HT
diurnal variations (II) (right part), rats were subjected to alternate cycles of 12
hours of light and darkness (light from 7 a.m. to 7 p.m. and darkness from 7 p.m. to
7 a.m.) for three weeks, and ³H-5-HT formation in the brain stem was estimated in the
middle of two successive light and dark periods. In the experiments (1) control and
PS-deprived rats were injected intracisternally with 25 μCi of ³H-tyrptophan under
light ether anaesthesia and killed 45 minutes later. Brain stem-mesencephalon slices of
control and PS-deprived rats were incubated for 30 minutes with 10 μCi of ³H-tyrptophan. Endogenous levels of 5-HT and tryptophan were unchanged at the time of estimation of ³H-HT formation (Héry *et al.*, 1971). In the experiments (II) rats kept in

accumulation of the labelled amino acid (Fig. 12-6). (2) Synthesis of 5-HT was also estimated *in vitro* on brain-stem slices of PS-deprived animals. Specific activities of 5-HT and tryptophan were estimated in tissues at the end of a 30-minute incubation with ^{3}H-tryptophan. As in the *in vivo* experiments, the 5-HT specific activity was markedly increased in tissues of PS-deprived animals; ^{3}H-tryptophan accumulation was less, but significantly enhanced, and tryptophan specific activity was not affected. (3) No effect could be seen *in vivo* or *in vitro* experiments when ^{3}H-5 hydroxy-tryptophan was substituted for ^{3}H-tryptophan. (4) The effect of PS deprivation on the utilization of 5-HT could be estimated by labeling central serotoninergic neurons of PS-deprived animals with the help of ^{3}H-tryptophan injected intracisternally. ^{3}H-5-HT levels in tissues of rats allowed to rest for 90 minutes after the injection of the amino acid were compared with those of rats put back on small support surrounded by water for 45 minutes, 45 minutes after the injection of ^{3}H-tryptophan. The ^{3}H-5-HT levels in the brain stem-mesencephalon of the second group of animals were reduced significantly (about 30 per cent), indicating a faster utilization of the newly synthesized ^{3}H-5-HT during PS deprivation (Héry *et al.,* 1970).

There is little doubt that the experimental situation used to deprive animals of PS markedly accelerates the synthesis and utilization of 5-HT in various brain structures. This effect is, very likely, in great part the result of PS deprivation; however, the stressful procedure used may affect not only sleep processes. The marked activation of central serotoninergic neurons seen in PS-deprived animals may be explained by the impossibility of triggering PS; serotoninergic neurons are probably involved in this process since the reduction of 5-HT levels produced by lesions or drugs was associated with a diminution of PS (Jouvet, 1969; Jouvet *et al.,* 1966; Mouret *et al.,* 1968). The biochemical results obtained, suggest that the tryptophan transport is specifically facilitated during activation of 5-HT

---

light or darkness were injected with 50 μCi of ^{3}H-tryptophan under light anaesthesia and killed 15 minutes later. Brain-stem slices were incubated for 30 minutes with 25 μCi of ^{3}H-tryptophan. Endogenous levels of 5-HT and tryptophan were respectively 0.64 μg/g, 4.19 μg/g and 0.53 μg/g, 3.71 μg/g in the brain stem of rats kept in light and darkness. (Experiments made by Héry and Lopez) ^{3}H-5-HT and ^{3}H-tryptophan were estimated in tissues in *in vivo* as well *as in vitro* studies. Results, expressed as per cent of respective controls (1) or of values obtained in animals kept in light (II), are the mean $\pm$ S.E.M. of groups of 8 to 10 animals. Numbers correspond to the absolute values of ^{3}H-tryptophan and ^{3}H-5-HT (expressed in μCi/gr.) in control animals.

synthesis. The increased accumulation of ^{3}H-tryptophan in tissues observed *in vivo* but also in the *in vitro* experiments supports this statement. However, the activation of the ^{3}H-tryptophan-^{3}H-5-hydroxytryptophan conversion may also be involved in the activation of 5-HT synthesis, as suggested by the increased ratio of the 5-HT and tryptophan-specific activities detected in brain-stem slices of PS-deprived animals. The differences in the results obtained with ^{3}H-tryptophan and ^{3}H-5-hydroxytryptophan indicate the major role of the first step of synthesis in the regulation of 5-HT formation.

Diurnal Variations of 5-HT Metabolism. Diurnal variations in 5-HT levels of the rat brain have been noted by various workers (Quay, 1968; Montanaro and Graziani, 1966; Scheving *et al.,* 1968); they suggest marked changes in the activity of central serotoninergic neurons. Recent experiments made by Dr. Héry in our laboratory indicate that the study of serotoninergic neuron activity at various times of the day provides an interesting experimental physiological model for understanding the regulatory processes of central 5-HT metabolism (Héry, Lopez, and Glowinski, in preparation). Groups of rats placed in special boxes, in constant temperature and noise environment, were submitted to regular alternative cycles of 12 hours of light and 12 hours of darkness for at least three weeks. First, we decided to estimate 5-HT synthesis and turnover in various brain structures during a 12-hour period corresponding to 6 hours of light followed by 6 hours of darkness. The synthesis of 5-HT was examined every two hours by injecting L-^{3}H-tryptophan intracisternally in different groups of rats. Labelled and endogenous 5-HT and tryptophan were estimated in the hypothalamus, cortex, and brain stem of animals 15 minutes after the labelled amino acid injection. Marked changes in 5-HT metabolism occur between light and dark periods: (1) 5-HT levels were significantly higher (about 20 per cent) in the various brain structures during the light period; (2) ^{3}H-5-HT accumulation as well as 5-HT specific activity in the three structures were also markedly increased (about 50 per cent) during these first 6 hours; these effects were associated with a parallel increase in ^{3}-H-tryptophan specific activity, resulting almost entirely from an increased accumulation of the labelled amino acid in tissues (Fig. 12-6); (3) relatively more ^{3}H-5-hydroxyindole acetic acid (^{3}H-5-HIAA), as compared to ^{3}H-5-HT levels in tissues, was found in all groups of animals killed in the middle of the dark period. In a second experiment the synthesis of 5-HT was estimated *in vitro:* brain stem slices from groups of rats killed in the middle of the light and dark periods were incubated with ^{3}H-tryptophan for 30 minutes, 5-HT specific activity was found higher (35 per cent) in slices of animals killed during the light period than in those of animals sacrificed during darkness. This effect was again associated with a parallel increase in ^{3}H-tryptophan accumulation (30 per cent) and ^{3}H-tryptophan specific activity. The total formation of ^{3}H-5-HT and of its main metabolite, accumulated both in slices and incubating medium, was also markedly enhanced during light, demonstrating the acceleration of ^{3}H-5-HT synthesis during this environmental situation. On the other hand, much more ^{3}H-5-HIAA was formed during darkness than during light; moreover, as in the *in vivo* experiments, the ^{3}H-5-HIAA/^{3}H-5-HT ratio increased significantly during darkness.

The *in vivo* and *in vitro* experiments indicate clearly that 5-HT synthesis and turnover are markedly accelerated during the light period as compared to the dark period. If small changes could be seen between the various groups of rats within each 6-hour period, they were not at all comparable to the striking biochemical changes occurring as soon as the animals were put in darkness (Héry, Lopez, and Glowinski, in preparation). The well-known behavioral differences seen in rats between the light and dark periods of the day may be related to the changes in serotoninergic neuron activity. The turnover of 5-HT appears maximal when the animals exhibit minimal activity. Schwartz and Aghajanian (1969) have already reported similar diurnal changes in serotoninergic neuron activity. They obtained significant results only with animals kept in a quiet environment. A control of 5-HT synthesis at the level of the tryptophan transport across the neuronal membrane appears clearly in these experiments: the increased 5-HT synthesis was closely associated with an activation of the initial accumulation of ^{3}H-tryptophan in the *in vivo* and also in the *in vitro* experiments. The observations made in previous stress and sleep studies are thus confirmed. In fact, such an hypothesis had been suggested a few years ago (Graham-Smith, 1968), and various studies have indicated that the rate of 5-HT synthesis depends on tryptophan availability (Ashcroft *et al.,* 1965; Consolo *et al.,* 1965; Gal and Drewes, 1962; Green *et al.,* 1962). The relatively high K_m of tryptophan hydroxylase for tryptophan provides the likely explanation of these results (Jequier *et al.,* 1967; McGeer *et al.,* 1968). Moreover, Tagliamonte *et al.* (1971) have recently reported that various treatments which stimulate 5-HT synthesis also produce a marked increase in brain tryptophan. The acceleration of the amine synthesis is thus very likely related to the increased levels of the amino acid which probably resulted from the activation of the tryptophan transport into neurons, as indicated by our experiments. These authors also mentioned that the increase in brain tryptophan could be dissociated from changes in plasma tryptophan: in the various pharmacological or environmental situations used to stimulate 5-HT synthesis, the increase in brain tryptophan levels occurs with or without changes in plasmatic tryptophan levels. This observation also agrees with our own findings since the enhanced initial accumulation of ^{3}H-tryptophan in tissues could be seen after intracisternal administration of the amino acid and, even more convincing, in *in vitro* studies on brain tissue slices. As our effects were detected in experimental situations in which no psychotropic drugs were used, changes in the regulation of tryptophan uptake may be directly related to the rate of 5-HT utilization and/or synthesis. The activation of 5-HT turnover in brain is very often associated with a small increase in endogenous 5-HT levels, as observed in our different experiments; this effect may be more or less pronounced according to the structure examined. Increased 5-HIAA levels are often seen but not always (Tagliamonte et al., 1971), possibly indicating a direct relationship between the acceleration of 5-HT synthesis and the 5-HT utilization as generally assumed. However, this is not always the case; 5-HT newly synthesized may be utilized at a faster rate when 5-HT synthesis is at its minimal level. The relatively enhanced ^{3}H-5-HIAA levels found in tissues of animals in dark environment, as compared with those of ^{3}H-5-HT, support this hypothesis. Therefore, apparently, changes in 5-HT utilization and synthesis processes may not be simultaneously and closely related in physiological states.

Effects of MAO Inhibitors and Imipramine on 5-HT Metabolism. In our earlier studies on 5-HT metabolism, the disappearance of labelled 5-HT in the rat brain was followed, for many hours, after the intracisternal injection of ^{3}H-tryptophan (Thierry *et al.,* 1968). If the initial amine decline appeared rapid for a short period, the labelled amine as well as the 5-HT specific activity decayed monoexponentially for at least 6 hours, one hour after the injection of the labelled amino acid. During this period the ^{3}H-amine half-life was about 2 hours. From this exponential curve of 5-HT utilization, the turnover rate of 5-HT was calculated, with the assumption that the amine was localized in a single homogenous pool. Our estimation, 0.18 μg/g/hr, was smaller than those obtained by various workers with other methods (Neff et al., 1967: 0.37 μg/g/hr; Giacalone et al., 1968: 0.22 and 0.29 μg/g/hr). Continuous ^{3}H-5-HT synthesis from small quantities of ^{3}H-tryptophan still available in tissues a few hours after its intracisternal administration may be only partly responsible for the relatively slow decay of the labelled amine. The discrepancy between the 5-HT turnover rate estimations may be just explained by differences in 5-HT metabolism possibly seen in various strains of rats. Another possibility, which cannot be excluded, is the existence of more than one storage form of 5-HT in serotoninergic neurons, as observed in catecholaminergic neurons. This led us to undertake a few experiments to test this last hypothesis.

In a first group of experiments, 5-HT synthesis was estimated by measuring the initial rate of 5-HT accumulation after the inhibition of MAO with pargyline or phenyprazine, in order to compare the results obtained with estimations based on previous turnover studies. To our surprise, 5-HT levels did not increase linearly as a function of time, during the first one or two hours, as generally reported (Costa and Neff, 1970). In the various structures of the rat brain examined, or in the whole mouse brain, two successive rises of amine levels were seen, but they were separated by a phase of short duration during which 5-HT levels remained constant or even declined. From the initial rapid rise lasting for 10 to 15 minutes, values of about 1.7 μg/g/hr to 3.3 μg/g/hr were obtained for the rate of 5-HT synthesis in mouse brain, according to the experiments and the MAOI used. Similar observations could be made in specific structures of the rat brain. For example, from the initial 5-minute rise of 5-HT levels in the cortex, synthesis rates of about 1 μg/g/hr to 2.5 μg/g/hr were found with pargyline and phenyprazine respectively (Hamon et al., 1971; Glowinski et al., 1971). All these estimations are three to six times greater than those previously described for the mouse brain (Valzelli and Garattini, 1968; Rosecrans, 1970) and the rat cortex (Ho et al., 1970). Despite these large differences in the rates of 5-HT synthesis obtained, as compared to previous studies with MAOI or other methods available, we could not absolutely conclude that the true rate of 5-HT synthesis had been largely underestimated. Tryptophan levels were found to parallel closely the initial complex evolution of 5-HT levels in the first 30 minutes after MAO inhibition, although the effect was less pronounced (Morot-Gaudry, Hamon, Bourgoin, and Glowinski, in preparation). Similar observations of enhanced

tryptophan levels in brain have been seen after treatment of rats with phen-
elzine, another MAOI (Tagliamonte *et al.*, 1971). Therefore, MAOI may
also stimulate temporary 5-HT synthesis.

In a second group of experiments, control and MAOI-treated mice
(pargyline 75 mg/kg i.p., was given one minute before ^{3}H-tryptophan injection) were killed 10 minutes after the intravenous injection of ^{3}H-tryp-
tophan to examine the early disposition of brain ^{3}H-5-HT. ^{3}H-5-HIAA
levels in tissues of control animals were about 30 per cent those of ^{3}H-5-
HT, and the total ^{3}H-5-HIAA and ^{3}H-5-HT content was comparable to
that of ^{3}H-5-HT of MAOI-treated mice in which the acid metabolite was
almost undetectable (Hamon *et al.*, 1971). Therefore, about 25 per cent
of the ^{3}H-5-HT formed in the first 10 minutes had been inactivated in normal animals, suggesting a very rapid half-life (about 15 to 20 minutes) of
the newly synthesized transmitter. Another indirect indication of the rapid
utilization of the newly formed ^{3}H-5-HT was obtained in studies on the
effects of imipramine on ^{3}H-5-HT synthesis from ^{3}H-tryptophan. As have
other workers (Schubert *et al.*, 1970), we observed an inhibition of ^{3}H-5-
HT synthesis from ^{3}H-tryptophan with large doses of the drug (20 mg/kg
i.p.); this was seen *in vivo* by measuring the ^{3}H-5-HT accumulation in the
hypothalamus of rats at short intervals (7 and 15 minutes) after the intracisternal injection of ^{3}H-tryptophan, and *in vitro* by measuring the ^{3}H-5-
HT accumulation in tissues and incubating medium of hypothalamic slices
at the end of a 30-minute incubation with the labelled amino acid. However, different results were obtained with smaller doses of the drug. In the
in vivo experiments the ^{3}H-5-HT accumulation was significantly decreased
by 30 per cent, 15 minutes after ^{3}H-tryptophan injection, but was comparable to that of normal animals at an earlier time (7 minutes). Therefore, relatively small doses of the drug did not seem to affect ^{3}H-5-HT synthesis, but only the reuptake process of the amine. This was confirmed in
in vitro experiments: ^{3}H-5-HT levels were increased in incubating medium
of hypothalamic slices of imipramine-pretreated animals, and total ^{3}H-5-
HT levels accumulated in slices and medium were not reduced, as compared to those of control animals, at the end of the incubation with
^{3}H-tryptophan. Therefore, the *in vivo* reduced accumulation observed in
imipramine-treated animals, 15 minutes after ^{3}H-tryptophan administration, suggests that important quantities of newly synthesized ^{3}H-5-HT are
rapidly released extraneuronally and inactivated by MAO. These preliminary results are in favor of a multicompartmental model for the intraneu-

ronal storage of 5-HT (Hamon *et al.*, 1971). However, further convincing experimental proofs should be obtained if this hypothesis is to be accepted.

Regulation of 5-HT Synthesis

Preliminary information suggesting the existence of a control of 5-HT synthesis by end-product inhibition was obtained in our study on the effects of stress on cerebral 5-HT metabolism. Electric shock applied to rat paws during a 180-minute session according to a protocol previously described (p .000: noradrenergic neurons) induced only a slight and not significant increase in 5-HT levels (20 per cent). In contrast, the 5-HT brain content could be doubled by the stress situation when the endogenous amine levels had been previously lowered with a long-term PCPA treatment (350 mg/kg, i.p., 42 hours before the stress session). The activation of 5-HT synthesis appeared thus facilitated by the low intraneuronal levels of the transmitter (Thierry *et al.*, 1968b). Further information about the role of intraneuronal levels of 5-HT in the regulation of the transmitter synthesis has been obtained in more recent *in vivo* and *in vitro* studies in which 5-HT levels were increased with MAOI administered *in vivo* or with exogenous 5-HT added in the incubating medium of brain tissue slices.

In a first group of experiments, the initial (15-minute) accumulation of ^{3}H-5-HT synthesized from intracisternally injected L-^{3}H-tryptophan was examined in the brain stem of rats at various times after the administration of phenyprazine or pargyline. Short and long treatments were used to compare 5-HT synthesis in situations in which 5-HT endogenous levels were markedly different. Furthermore, as MAO activity was inhibited in all cases, the 5-HT accumulation represented a good index of 5-HT synthesis. The 15-minute ^{3}H-5-HT accumulation was markedly increased (175 to 200 per cent) 20, 35, or 75 minutes after phenyprazine treatment (5 mg/kg i.p.) as compared with control animals. This very likely resulted from the protection of newly synthesized ^{3}H-5-HT from rapid MAO inactivation. However, the 15-minute initial accumulation of ^{3}H-5-HT formed from ^{3}H-tryptophan was significantly reduced (30 to 40 per cent) 180 minutes after MAOI treatment, as compared with all shorter treatments used (20, 35, or 75 minutes). Similar results were obtained when animals were treated with pargyline instead of phenyprazine. The diminished accumulation of ^{3}H-5-HT observed between the long (180 minutes) and short ($\leqslant$ 75 minutes) treatments with MAOI was attributed to an inhibition of 5-HT synthesis, induced by the rise in intraneuronal 5-HT levels occurring between the short and long MAOI treatments (5-HT levels were respectively 150 and 300 per cent of control levels, 35 and 180 minutes after phenyprazine injection) (Macon et al., 1971). However, Millard and Gal (1971) have recently made one observation about the interpretation of our data: they have attributed the increased accumulation of ^{3}H-5-HT formed from ^{3}H-tryptophan, shortly after MAOI treatment, to a stimulation of 5-HT synthesis related to the initial temporary rise of corticoids in plasma induced by the drug. However, they have neglected the role of MAOI towards the protection of newly synthesized 5-HT. If stimulation of 5-HT synthesis is involved, this will be only for a short time period since increases in tryptophan levels in brain tissues have been observed only in the first 15 to 20 minutes after MAO inhibition. Therefore, the reduction of ^{3}H-5-HT formation observed 180 minutes after MAO inhibition, as compared with the effects seen 75 minutes after, seems to be mainly attributable to the increase in 5-HT levels. This statement may be reinforced by the differences in 5-HT synthesis found between acute long-term treatment (3 hours) and chronic treatment (48, 24, and 3 hours before death) with phenyprazine (10 mg/kg i.p.). The chronic treatment with the MAOI further enhanced the steady state level of endogenous 5-HT and produced a corresponding decrease in ^{3}H-5-HT synthesized from ^{3}H-tryptophan, as compared to the acute long-term treatment (3 hours) in the whole brain of the rat. In summary, we have observed a direct relationship between the increase in 5-HT tissues levels and the reduction of ^{3}H-5-HT synthesis from ^{3}H-tryptophan. The long-term inhibiting effect of MAOI on ^{3}H-5-HT synthesis, observed as soon as 5-HT levels were about twice normal levels, was not linked to a decrease of tryptophan specific activity in tissues. In contrast, a slight increase in ^{3}H-tryptophan accumulation was detected when ^{3}H-5-HT synthesis was inhibited, suggesting a decreased uptake or utilization of ^{3}H-tryptophan in serotoninergic neurons. Finally, the long-term effect of MAOI on 5-HT synthesis is related to processes occurring at the first and rate-limiting step of the amine synthesis, since no differences could be seen in the ^{3}H-5-HT formation from ^{3}H-5-hydroxy-tryptophan between short- and long-term treatments with MAOI (Macon et al., 1971).

More recently, in a second group of experiments, Drs. Hamon, Bourgoin, and Morot-Gaudry have estimated the in vitro ^{3}H-5-HT synthesis from ^{3}H-tryptophan by measuring both the ^{3}H-5-HT and the ^{3}H-5-HIAA accumulated in striatal slices and their incubating medium, 15 or 30 minutes after the beginning of the incubation. The following observations were made: (1) The formation of ^{3}H-5-HT was markedly reduced (about 30 per cent) in striatal slices of animals treated 3 hours before with phenyprazine (10 mg/kg) or pargyline (75 mg/kg), as compared to control untreated animals. The effect was even more striking when the total formation of ^{3}H-5-HT and ^{3}H-5-HIAA was compared in striatal slices of control and MAOI-treated rats (Fig. 12-7). As no changes in tryptophan specific activity could be detected in slices after MAOI treatment, results obtained indicate that these long-term drug treatments have induced an inhibition

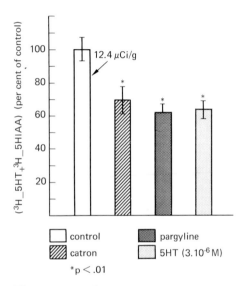

Figure 12-7   Effect of increased 5-HT levels on *in vitro* ^{3}H-5-HT synthesis, from ^{3}H-tryptophan, in serotoninergic terminals of the rat brain. ^{3}H-5-HT synthesis was estimated by incubating, for 30 minutes, striatal slices with 4 μCi/ml of ^{3}H (G) tryptophan (4.4 Ci/m mole). Total ^{3}H-5-HT and ^{3}H-5-HIAA formed and accumulated in slices and their incubating medium were used as an index of ^{3}H-5-HT synthesis. Endogenous 5-HT levels were increased either by pretreatment of rats with pargyline (75 mg/kg i.p.) or pheniprazine (Catron) (10 mg/kg i.p.) given 180 minutes before death, or by pre-incubating slices for 10 minutes with 5-HT (3.10^{-6}M) added to the incubating medium. Total ^{3}H-5-HT and ^{3}H-5-HIAA formed in controls amounted to 2.4 μCi/g. Endogenous tryptophan levels were unchanged at the time of ^{3}H-5-HT synthesis estimation. Results, expressed in per cent of control values, are the mean ± S.E.M. of data obtained on 10 striata. (Experiments by Hamon and Morot-Gaudry)

of ^{3}H-5-HT synthesis from ^{3}H-tryptophan. (2) Similar inhibition of ^{3}H-5-HT synthesis was seen after pre-incubation of striatal slices of control animals with exogenous 5-HT (3.10^{-6}M). The increased intraneuronal levels of the amine induced a 30 to 50 per cent reduction of the total accumulation of ^{3}H-5-HT and its metabolite ^{3}H-5-HIAA in tissues and their incubating medium, as compared to control slices. Moreover, the inhibiting effect of exogenous 5-HT on ^{3}H-5-HT synthesis could be prevented by chlorimipramine, an inhibitor of the amine uptake process at the neuronal membrane level (Hamon, Bourgoin, Morot-Gaudry, and Glowinski, in preparation; Glowinski *et al.,* 1971).

The existence of a mechanism of negative feedback control for 5-HT synthesis by end-product inhibition was already suggested a few years ago by Eiduson (1966); however, this hypothesis has been rejected by Lin *et al.* (1969), Millard and Gal (1971), and Meek and Fuxe (1971) only on the basis of *in vivo* experiments with MAOI. To the contrary, our *in vivo* and *in vitro* studies give good arguments in favor of this hypothesis. The reduction of the amine synthesis does not seem to be related to a change of tryptophan hydroxylase activity as suggested by the very rapid effect of the rise in intraneuronal 5-HT levels on the *in vitro* ^{3}H-5-HT synthesis. The best working hypothesis is that 5-HT levels control in some way the tryptophan transport into serotoninergic neurons, which, as previously discussed, plays an important role in the regulation of 5-HT synthesis. The recent observations of Aghajanian and Graham (1970), who detected decreased electrical activity in serotoninergic cell bodies of the rat midbrain raphé nuclei after treatment with MAOI, are in agreement with our biochemical results and further support the concept of an end-product inhibition control of 5-HT synthesis in central serotoninergic neurons.

Conclusion

During the last five years we have learned a lot about the specific properties of the central dopaminergic, noradrenergic, and serotoninergic neurons, particularly concerning their anatomical distribution and morphological aspect at the ultramicroscopic level on the one hand, and their role in important functions of the CNS and their sensitivity to various psychotropic drugs on the other. Specific properties of their metabolism have also been discovered and have stimulated new researches. Some examples, described in this review, are particularly relevant: as in dopaminergic neurons, the first step of synthesis in central noradrenergic neurons plays a major role in the regulation of the amine formation; however, the last step of NE synthesis may also contribute efficiently to the modulation of NE formation. The regulatory role of the DA-NE conversion is very likely of great importance not only in pharmacological but also in physiological states. If it is sound to suspect the contribution of the tyrosine transport process for its possible regulatory role in DOPA formation in catecholaminergic neurons, so far very little evidence of this has been obtained. However, new information has been gained about the importance of the process of tryptophan transport in the regulation of 5-HT synthesis. As already discussed, it seems of prime importance to bear in mind that changes in tryptophan uptake into neurons seen under various pharmacological treatments, and also during PS deprivation or diurnal variations of serotoninergic neuron activity, are independent of tryptophan plasmatic levels. Another interesting point has been noted about the possible differences between noradrenergic and dopaminergic neurons in the regulatory processes of amine biosynthesis. It concerns the changes in tyrosine-hydroxylase activity: apparently, tyrosine-hydroxylase activity is much more easily affected in noradrenergic than in dopaminergic neurons. Nevertheless, more experiments are needed to verify further the validity of our preliminary observations. It is likely that other major differences will be discovered, especially concerning the storage and release processes of these three amines in their respective neurons. For example, recent stress studies and estimations of amine release in slices suggest that, as peripheral neurons, the central noradrenergic neurons can particularly release two substances, DA and NE, both of which may act as transmitters. However, despite the progress made in *in vivo* studies on DA release, we have still relatively little informaton about the *in vivo* release of NE and 5-HT in the CNS for making fruitful comparisons. In contrast, the development of kinetic studies on slices of isolated brain structures has markedly extended our knowledge about the specific properties of the amines' uptake process in their respective neurons (Snyder, 1970). In other respects, we should also be aware of the possible differences in the dynamic characteristics of the distinct systems of neurons acting with an identical transmitter substance. As underlined in a few occasions in this article, the dorsal and ventral noradrenergic pathways seem to differ considerably: we knew from earlier work that NE subcellular distribution was quite different in the cortex or the cerebellum than in other brain structures (Glowinski and Iversen, 1966b), and that NE turnover was much more rapid in these two higher structures; we have recently seen also that these two main systems of noradrenergic neurons appear to react differently under long-term activating stimuli.

Besides their specific properties the various types of central aminergic neurons exhibit major resemblances which have been much discussed. Among the general observations made, we can first point out that the rate of the amines' synthesis, in their respective neuronal systems, is much more important than has been reported during the past years. The sophisticated mathematical models used have no doubt been oversimplified. High rates of synthesis, about five to ten times the previous estimations, have already been noted for DA and NE, respectively, in striatal dopaminergic and noradrenergic terminals. Some preliminary data, although less conclusive, suggest that the rate of 5-HT synthesis is also more important than generally reported. Furthermore, in catecholaminergic neurons, as well as in serotoninergic neurons, the synthesis of amines is, in all cases, controlled by a negative feedback acting by end-product inhibition. As has been directly shown in *in vitro* studies, this regulatory process is operating at the first step of synthesis. However, further work is required to determine precisely on exactly which biochemical process the intraneuronal amines are acting. There seem to be some slight differences in the sensitivity of these regulatory processes: smaller variations in the intraneuronal amine levels may be required in terminals of catecholaminergic and particularly dopaminergic neurons than in those of serotoninergic neurons to detect inhibiting effect on the amine synthesis. Isotopic studies, as well as experiments wtih synthesis inhibitors, have shown the existence of various forms of amine storage in both noradrenergic and dopaminergic terminals. Numerous data have thus been obtained in favor of the simplified "two compartments model" for the disposition of the amines in their respective terminals. Preliminary information suggests that this concept is also a valid working hypothesis for further studies on 5-HT storage in central serotoninergic neurons. The biochemical demonstration of the existence of a "functional compartment" in catecholaminergic neurons confirms and supports previous observations made in pharmacological (Weissman *et al*, 1966; Rech *et al.*, 1968) and endocrinological studies (Kordon and Glowinski, 1969). It is particularly interesting to note that the half-lives of the amines in this compartment have been evaluated as never exceeding 20 minutes. Furthermore, as revealed by preliminary and approximative estimations made on catecholaminergic neurons, the quantities of amine turning over per unit of time in the "functional compartment," which contains about 20 to 25 per cent of the stored amine, are in the order of five to ten times those of the "main storage compartment." Finally, there is strong evidence that most of the newly synthesized transmitter, localized in the "functional compartment," is used for extraneuronal release. All these observations indicate our progress in detecting subtle changes in the activity of aminergic neurons in physiological states. Therefore, they emphasize the current possibility of obtaining close correlations between biochemical changes in neurotransmitter metabolism and behavioral or psychopharmacological effects.

The first observations suggesting the main role of newly synthesized transmitter in release processes prompt us to develop new biochemical and methodological approaches in order to follow more precisely the rapid metabolic changes occurring in central aminergic neurons. In general, as it has been described, the aminergic neurons have been labelled with the help of ^{3}H-tyrosine or ^{3}H-tryptophan, the original amine precursors. Attempts have been made to compare, as much as possible, results obtained by *in vitro* studies on slices of isolated structures and *in vivo* studies on localized area of the brain. The development of the "radioactive water method" for the estimation of the rate of the first rate-limiting step of CA synthesis in slices and the use of microstereotaxic techniques to appreciate local *in vivo* changes in synthesis give an idea of our progress. These new techniques have already been particularly useful for examining the effects of various psychotropic drugs on biosynthesis processes. The use of radioactive amino acids has been also fruitful for the *in vitro* studies on ^{3}H-CA or ^{3}H-5-HT release processes. It seems important to recall that rapid changes in neuronal activity induced by drugs or modifications of the environment may evoke sustained biochemical changes on synthesis and release of the amines detectable *in vitro*. Finally, the successful experiments obtained on the spontaneous and the evoked release of newly synthesized ^{3}H-DA during continuous labelling, with ^{3}H-tyrosine, of the superficial dopaminergic terminals of the cat caudate nucleus, indicate that important progress can now be rapidly made in the understanding of release processes. Moreover, this *in vivo* methodology, undoubtedly applied in the near future to the study of NE and 5-HT release processes, will be of great help for further research into the role and relationships of central aminergic neurons.

References

Aghajanian, G. K., and Bloom, F. E. 1967. *J. Pharmacol. Exptl. Therap.* 156:407.

Aghajanian, G. K., and Graham, A. 1970. *Fed. Proc.* 29:251, Abs. 26.

Andén, N. E., Carlsson, A., Dahlström, A., Fuxe, K., Hillarp, N. Å., and Larsson, K. 1964a. *Life Sci.* 3:523.

Andén, N. E., Roos, B. E., and Werdinius, B. 1964b. *Life Sci.* 3:149.

Andén, N. E., Dahlström, A., Fuxe, K., and Hökfelt, T. 1966. *Acta. Physiol. Scand.* 68:419.

Ashcroft, G. W., Eccleston, D., and Crawford, T. B. B. 1965. *J. Neurochem.* 12:483.

Bapna, J., Neff, N. H., and Costa, E. 1970. *Neuropharmacology* 9:333.

Bedard, P., Larochelle, L., Parent, A., and Poirier, L. J. 1969. *Exp. Neur.* 25:365.

Besson, M. J., Chéramy, A., Feltz, P., and Glowinski, J. 1969a. *P.N.A.S.* (U.S.A.) 62:741.

Besson, M. J., Chéramy, A., Feltz, P., and Glowinski, J. 1969b. *J. Physiol.* (Paris) 61:90.

Besson, M. J., Chéramy, A., and Glowinski, J. 1969c. *Eur. J. Pharmacol.* 7:111.

Besson, M. J., Chéramy, A., Feltz, P., and Glowinski, J. 1971a. *Brain Research* 32: 407.

Besson, M. J., Chéramy, A., Feltz, P., and Glowinski, J. 1971b. *Proc. Int. Uni. Physiol. Sci.* 9:60, n°168.

Besson, M. J., Chéramy, A., Gauchy, C., and Glowinski, J. 1971c. *J. Physiol.* (Paris) in press.

Besson, M., J., Chéramy, A., Gauchy, C., and Musacchio, J. M. 1971d. *Europ. J. Pharmacol.* in press.

Besson, M. J., Chéramy, A., and Glowinski, J. 1971e. *J. Pharmacol. Exptl. Therap.* 177:196.

Bliss, E. L., Ailion, J., and Zwanziger, J. 1968. *J. Pharmacol. Exptl. Therap.* 154: 493.

Carlsson, A., Lindqvist, M., Magnusson, T., and Waldeck, B. 1958. *Science* 127:471.

Chéramy, A., Besson, M. J., and Glowinski, J. 1970. *Europ. J. Pharmacol.* 10:206.

Chéramy, A., Besson, M. J., and Musacchio, J. M. 1971. *J. Pharmacol.* (Paris) 1:23.

Consolo, S., Garattini, S., Ghielmetti, R., Morselli, P., and Valzelli, L. 1965. *Life Sci.* 4:625.

Corrodi, H., Fuxe, K., and Hökfelt, T. 1967a. *Life Sci.* 6:767.

Corrodi, H., Fuxe, K., and Hökfelt, T. 1967b. *Acta Physiol. Scand.* 71:224.

Costa, E., and Neff, N. H. 1966. In E. Costa, L. Côte, and M. Yahr (Eds.), *Biochemistry and Pharmacology of the Basal Ganglia* (Raven Press, Hewlett: New York), p. 141.

Costa, E., and Neff, N. H. 1970. In A. Lajtha (Ed.), *Handbook of Neurochemistry* (Plenum Press: New York-London), 4:p. 45.

Coyle, J. T., and Snyder, S. H. 1969a. *J. Pharmacol. Exptl. Therap.* 170:221.

Coyle, J. T., and Snyder, S. H. 1969b. *Science* 166:899.

Da Prada, M., and Pletscher, A. 1966. *Experientia* 22:465.

Descarries, L., and Droz, B. 1970. *J. Cell. Biol.* 44:385.

Diaz, P. M., Ngai, S. H., and Costa, E. 1968. *Adv. in Pharmacology* 6 B:75.

Eiduson, S. 1966. *J. Neurochem.* 13:923.

Florvall, L., and Corrodi, H. 1970. *Acta Pharmaceutica suecica* 7:7.

Gal, E. M., and Drewes, P. A. 1962. *Proc. Soci. Exp. Biol.* 110:368.

Giacalone, E., Tansella, M., Valzelli, L., and Garattini, S. 1968. *Biochem. Pharmacol.* 17:1315.

Glowinski, J. 1967a. *Actualités Pharmacol.* (Paris) 20:29.

Glowinski, J. 1967b. Thèse de Doctorat ès sciences (Paris). Metabolisme des catécholamines dans le cerveau du rat.

Glowinski, J. 1970. In H. J. Schümann and G. Kroneberg (Eds.), *New Aspects of Storage and Release Mechanisms of Catecholamines* (Springer-Verlag: Berlin-Heidelberg-New York), p. 237.

Glowinski, J., Kopin, I., and Axelrod, J. 1965. *J. Neurochem.* 12:25.

Glowinski, J., and Axelrod, J. 1966. *Pharmacol. Rev.* 18:775.

Glowinski, J., and Baldessarini, R. 1966. *Pharmacol. Rev.* 18:1201.

Glowinski, J., and Iversen, L. 1966a. *J. Neurochem.* 13:665.

Glowinski, J., and Iversen, L. 1966b. *Biochem. Pharmacol.* 15:977.

Glowinski, J., Alexrod, J., and Iversen, L. 1966. *J. Pharmacol. Exptl. Therap.* 153: 30.

Glowinski, J., Besson, M. J., Chéramy, A., and Thierry, A. M. 1971a. In E. Costa and L. L. Iversen (Eds.), *Advances in Biochemical Psychopharmacology* (in press). Studies in neurotransmitters at the synaptic level.

Glowinski, J., Hamon, M., Javoy, F., and Morot-Gaudry, Y. 1971b. In E. Costa and M. Sandler (Eds.), *Advances in Biochemical Psychopharmacology* (in press). Monoamine oxydases: new vistas (Sardinia).

Goldstein, M., and Nakajima, K. J. 1967. *Pharmacol. Exptl. Therap.* 157:96.

Goldstein, M., Anagnoste, B., Owen, W. S., and Battista, A. F. 1967. *Brain Research.* 4:298.

Graham-Smith, D. G. 1968. *Adv. Pharmacol.* 6 A:37.

Green, H., Greebarg, S. M., Erickson, R. W., Sawyer, J. L., and Ellison R. J. 1962. *J. Pharmacol. Exptl. Therap.* 136:174.

Häggendal, J., and Dahlström, A. 1971. *J. Pharm. Pharmacol.* 23:81.

Hamon, M., Javoy, F., Kordon, C., and Glowinski, J. 1970. *Life Sci.* 9:167.

Hamon, M., Morot-Gaudry, Y., Javoy, F., and Glowinski, J. 1971. In J. Domonkos, A. Fonyo, I. Huszak, and J. Szentagothai (Eds.), Third meeting of the Int. Soc. for Neurochem. (Akadémiai Kiado: Budapest), p. 325.

Héry, F., Pujol, J. F., Lopez, M., Macon, J., and Glowinski, J. 1970. *Brain Research* 21:391.

Ho, A. K. S., Loh, H. H., Craves, F., Hitzemann, R. J., and Gershon, S. 1970. *Europ. J. Pharmacol.* 10:72.

Ikeda, M., Fahien, L. A., and Udenfriend, S. 1966. *J. Biol. Chem.* 241:4452.

Iversen, L. L., and Glowinski, J. 1966a. *Neurochem.* 13:671.

Iversen, L. L., and Glowinski, J. 1966b. *Nature* (London) 210:1006.

Javoy, F., Glowinski, J., and Kordon, C. 1968a. *Europ. J. Pharmacol.* 4:103.

Javoy, F., Thierry, A. M., Kety, S. S., and Glowinski, J. 1968b. *Commun. Behav. Biol.* 1:43.

Javoy, F., Hamon, M., and Glowinski, J. 1970. *Europ. J. Pharmacol.* 10:178.

Javoy, F., and Glowinski, J. 1971a. *J. Neurochem.* 18:1305.

Javoy, F., and Glowinski, J. 1971b. In J. Domonkos, A. Fonyo, I. Huszak, and J. Szentagothai (Eds.), Third meeting of the Int. Soc. for Neurochem. (Akadémiai Kiado: Budapest), p. 169.

Jequier, E., Robinson, D. S., Lovenberg, W., and Sjoerdsma, A. 1969. *Biochem. Pharmacol.* 18:1071.

Jouvet, M., Bobillier, P., Pujol, J. F., and Renault, J. 1966. *C. R. Soc. Biol.* (Paris) 160:2343.

Jouvet, M. 1969. *Science* 163:32.

Kety, S. S., Javoy, F., Thierry, A. M., Julou, L. and Glowinski, J. 1967. *P.N.A.S.* 58:1249.

Koe, B. K., and Weissman, A. 1966. *J. Pharmacol. Exptl. Therap.* 154:499.

Kordon, C., Javoy, F., Vassent, G., and Glowinski, J. 1968. *Europ. J. Pharmacol.* 4:169.

Kordon, C., and Glowinski, J. 1969. *Endocrinology.* 85:924.

Lin, R. C., Neff, N. H., Ngai, S. H., and Costa, E. 1969. *Life Sci.* 18:1077.

McGeer, P. C., and McGeer, E. 1964. *Biochem. Biophys. Res. Commun.* 17:502.

McGeer, E. G., Peters, D. A. V., and McGeer, P. L. 1968. *Life Sci.* 7:605.

McKenzie, G. M., and Szerb, J. C. 1968. *J. Pharmacol.* 162:302.

McLennan, H. 1964. *J. Physiol.* (London) 174:152.

McLennan, H. 1965. *Experientia* 21:725.

Macon, J., Sokoloff, L., and Glowinski, J. 1971. *J. Neurochem.* 18:323.

Meek, J. L., and Fuxe, K. 1971. *Biochem. Pharmacol.* 20:693.

Milhaud, G., and Glowinski, J. 1962. *C. R. Acad. Sci.* (Paris) 255:203.

Millard, S. A., and Gal, E. M. 1971. *Intern. J. Neuroscience* 1:211.

Mitchell, J. F. 1966. In U. S. von Euler, S. Rovell, and B. Uvnas (Eds.) (Pergamon Press: London) 5:p. 425. Mechanisms of release of biogenic amines.

Montanaro, N., and Graziani, G. 1966. *Dal. Boll. d. Soc. Ital. d. Biol. Sper.* Vol XLIII. 1:42.

Mouret, J., Bobillier, P., and Jouvet, M. 1968. *Europ. J. Pharmacol.* 5:17.

Mouret, J., Pujol, J. F., and Kiyono, S. 1969. *Brain Research* 15:501.

Mueller, R. A., Thoenen, H., and Axelrod, J. 1969. *J. Pharmacol. Exptl. Therap.* 169:74.

Musacchio, J. M., Julou, L., Kety, S. S., and Glowinski, J. 1969. *P.N.A.S.* 63:1117.

Nakamura, K., Gerold, M., and Thoenen, H. 1971. *Naunyn-Schmiedebergs Arch. Pharmak.* 268:125.

Neff, N. H., and Costa, E. 1966. Proceedings of the First International Symposium on antidepressant drugs (Milan), p. 28.

Neff, N. H., Tozer, T. N., and Brodie, B. B. 1967. *J. Pharmacol. Exptl. Therap.* 158:214.

Noble, E., Wurtman, R., and Axelrod, J. 1967. *Life Sci.* 6:281.

Nybäck, H., and Sedvall, G. 1969. *Europ. J. Pharmacol.* 5:245.

Persson, T. 1970. Catecholamine turnover in central nervous system in Reports from the psychiatric research centre, SF. Jörgens Hospital, University of Göteborg. 4.

Persson, T., and Waldeck, B. 1970. *Europ. J. Pharmacol.* 11:315.

Poirier, L. J., and Sourkes, T. L. 1965. *Brain* 88:181.

Portig, P. J., and Vogt, M. 1966. *J. Physiol.* (London) 186:131P.

Portig, P. J., and Vogt, M. 1968. *J. Physiol.* (London) 197:20P.

Pujol, J. F., Mouret, J., Jouvet, M., and Glowinski, J. 1968. *Science* 159:112.

Quay, W. B. 1968. *Am. J. Physiol.* 215(6):1448.

Rech, R. H., Carr, L. A., and Moore, K. E. 1968. *J. Pharmacol. Exptl. Therap.* 160:326.

Reid, W. D., Volicer, L., Smookler, H., Beaven, M. A., and Brodie, B. B. 1968. *Pharmacology* 1:329.

Reivich, M., and Glowinski, J. 1967. *Brain* 90:633.

Riddell, D., and Szerb, J. C. 1971. *J. Neurochem.* 18:989.

Roos, B. E. 1965. *J .Pharm. Pharmacol.* 17:820.

Rosecrans, J. A. 1970. *Europ. J. Pharmacol.* 9:379.

Samanin, R., Gumulka, W., and Valzelli, L. 1970. *Europ. J. Pharmacol.* 10:303.

Sanders-Bush, E., and Sulser, F. 1970. *J. Pharmacol.* 175:419.

Scatton, B., Chéramy, A., Besson, M. J., and Glowinski, J. 1970. *Europ. J. Pharmacol.* 13:131.

Schanberg, S. M., Schildkraut, J. J., and Kopin, I. J. 1967. *Biochem. Pharmacol.* 16:393.

Scheving, L. E., Harrison, W. H., Gordon, P., and Pauly, J. E. 1968. *Am. J. Physiol.* 214:166.

Schildkraut, J. J., Winokur, A., and Applegate, C. W. 1970. *Science* 168:867.

Schubert, J., Nybäck, H., and Sedvall, G. 1970. *J. Pharm. Pharmacol.* 22:136.

Schwartz, A., and Aghajanian, G. K. 1969. *Comm. in Behavioral Biol.* 4:97.

Sedvall, G. C., Weise, U. K., and Kopin, I. J. 1968. *J. Pharmacol. Exptl. Therap.* 159:274.

Simmonds, M. A., and Iversen, L. L. 1969. *Science* 163:473.

Sharman, D. F. 1966. *Brit. J. Pharmacol.* 28:153.

Shaskan, E. G., and Snyder, S. 1970. *J. Pharmacol.* 175:404.

Snyder, S. H. 1970. *Biol. Psychiatry* 2:367.

Spector, S., Sjoerdsma, A., and Udenfriend, S. 1965. *J. Pharmacol. Exptl. Therap.* 147:86.

Spector, S., Gordon, R., Sjoedsma, A., and Udenfriend, S. 1967. *Mol. Pharmacol.* 3:549.

Svensson, T., and Waldeck, B. 1969. *Europ. J. Pharmacol.* 7:278.

Tagliamonte, A., Tagliamonte, P., Perez-Cruet, J., Stern, S., and Gessa, G. L. 1971. *J. Pharmacol.* 177:475.

Taylor, K. M., and Laverty, R. 1969. *J. Neurochem.* 16:1376.

Tenen, S. S. 1968. *Psychopharmacologia* 12:278.

Thierry, A. M. 1968. Thèse de Doctorat 3ème cycle (Paris). Effect du stress sur le métabolisme central des catecholamines et de la sérotonine chez le rat.

Thierry, A. M., Javoy, F., Glowinski, J., and Kety, S. S. 1968a. *J. Pharmacol. Exptl. Therap.* 163:163.

Thierry, A. M., Fekete, M., and Glowinski, J. 1968b. *Europ. J. Pharmacol.* 4:384.

Thierry, A. M., Blanc, G., and Glowinski, J. 1970. *Europ. J. Pharmacol.* 10:139.

Thierry, A. M., Blanc, G., and Glowinski, J. 1971a. *J. Neurochem.* 18:449.

Thierry, A. M., Blanc, G., and Glowinski, J. 1971b. In J. Domonkos, A. Fonyo, I. Huszak, and J. Szentagothai (Eds.), Third meeting of the Int. Soc. for Neurochem. (Akadémiai Kiado: Budapest), p. 168.

Thierry, A. M., Blanc, G., and Glowinski, J. 1971c. *Europ. J. Pharmacol.* 14:303.

Tozer, T. N., Neff, N. H., and Brodie, B. B. 1966. *J. Pharmacol. Exptl. Therap.* 153:177.

Ungerstedt, U. 1971. *Acta. Physiol. Scand.* suppl. 367.

Valzelli, L., and Garattini, S. 1968. *Adv. in Pharmacol.* 6 B:249.

Vogt, M. 1969. *Brit. J. Pharmacol.* 37:325.

Von Voigtlander, P. F., and Moore, K. E. 1971. *Fed. Proc.* 30:677, Abs. 2690.

Weiner, N. 1970. *Annual Rev. Pharmacology* 10:273.
Weissman, A., Kenneth-Koe, B., and Tenen, S. S. 1966. *J. Pharmacol. Exptl. Therap.* 151:339.